CANCER PATIENCE

NIGEL HUGHES

To Ben + Rachel
with my love

Nigel . ♡
22/10/24

ACKNOWLEDGEMENTS

I would like to give my heartfelt gratitude to all the contributors/respondees to my ramblings that have made this book possible.

And big thanks to my editors and incredibly patient proofreaders including (but not excluding) Maria Akinla, Sue Copping, Katie Haselhurst, David Hughan, Laura McClelland, Neil Roberts, Chloe Taylor

Contact: Nigel Hughes
Nigel@outstanding.global
www.outstanding.global

This journey would have been impossible without Ric, my life-long partner and now husband whom I met at Bristol Old Vic Drama School in 1971.

FOREWORD

Before you plunge into reading my candid account of dealing with colorectal cancer 2013-2015, I want to headline that this is a warts and all, very personal, very intimate account of my experience. Written as it happened, I sent it as a weekly update to my friends and family to share my journey and gain support. Unexpurgated, I publish it now to inspire anyone facing their own cancer. It is offered to support everyone experiencing their own journey.

I hope it will be helpful to you personally, to your loved ones, families, supporters - and the medical profession who dedicate so much of their lives to bring us their expertise. Working together and trusting others may help you face one of the toughest challenges of your life.

Read as much as you can bear.

Nigel

SIGNIFICANT DATES:

2013:

March 19 – visit to GP, Dr Hughes, with suspicions.

October 25 – double check visit to Doctor – referral to a specialist. (No letter arrived before departure to India.)

December 17 – Depart for India

2014:

February 10 - Return from India

February 12 - Basel work trip for Roche I call Michael reporting diarrhoea before I board the flight

February 14 - GP appointment to check up on diarrhoea – probable "piles"

February 19-21 - Hamburg work trip for Bertelsmann

February 23-25 - Birmingham work trip for Burtons

February 26-28 - Prague work trip for Deutsche Telekom – need for toilet location awareness.

March 2-7 - New York work trip for Roche

March 19 - Cancelled Maynard Leigh (MLA) work internal meeting – toilet trouble

March 19 GP appointment – locum recommended I see a specialist – date made for 7 April

March 20-2 - EY Impact & Influence (I&I) – toilet trouble (warned Barbara of "piles")

March 23-25 - Birmingham work trip for Burtons (warned team of "piles")

March 28 - David/Hilary funeral - Ric's best boyhood friend (continued nearest toilet awareness)

April 7 - 13.15. Private Specialist appointment at BMI Private Hospital – Mr Keeling diagnoses colorectal cancer recommends immediate biopsy and CT/MRI scans

April 8 - 13.30 MRI scan

April 9 - 08.30 CT scan (Bury St Edmunds), 12.00 Capgemini work meeting in Holborn, London, 16.30 BMI operation in Bury St Edmunds

April 10-11 - Cancelled EY I&I work meeting in London

April 14 - Dentist and hygienist

April 15 - Geneva work trip for PepsiCo – severe toilet awareness and severe discomfort due to biopsy operation

April 16 - 19.00 Mr Keeling calls me at home to confirm squamous carcinoma and makes an appointment for the following evening at 18.00.

April 17 -18.00 Ric and I meet Mr Keeling who explains diagnosis and probable recommended chemo/radio treatment plan

April 18 - Snape Maltings live concert

April 23 - John Godber's (Ric's brother-in-Law) funeral and memorial in Forest Row

May 1-2 - London work trip for EY I&I (alert Ann of my "piles")

May 7-9 -Prague work trip for DT (alert Siobhan of my "piles")

May 12 - Addenbrookes Colorectal Cancer Clinic and a fateful meeting with Dr Jephcott who recommends a treatment plan of 5.5 chemo/radio starting May 26. I ask for a delay and suggest we start June 23rd. She agrees.

May 16-23 - Alan and Tim's wedding in Cornwall followed by a quiet week by the sea – spent researching squamous carcinoma and colorectal cancer and alternative approaches.

May 26 - Raphael Centre Tonbridge with Dr Jenny Josephson to explore mistletoe therapy. She administers intravenous drip and sends me away with a three-month supply of phials and syringes.

May 27 - Addenbrookes CT planning session for chemo/radiotherapy- "Press release" to MLA work team that I will take a 2-month health sabbatical

June 2 - Star Throwers in Wymondham to see Dr Henry Mannings – who supports a complementary approach – no sugar and low fibre diet. AND second opinion appointment at Addenbrookes with Dr Jephcott to confirm that their treatment plan was the correct path. We agreed it was.

June 3 - Trip to London to see Capgemini confirming arrangements for Paris 2-day event

June 4-6 - Bratislava work trip for Deutsche Telekom with Siobhan

June 10 - London MLA internal work breakfast seminar

June 11-13 - Hamburg work trip for Bertelsmann – alert team of my special diet because of my special circumstances.

June 18-20 - Paris work trip for Capgemini Future Leaders programme – ending with me "coming out" with my health sabbatical.

June 23 - Addenbrookes PICC line inserted, chemo bag attached and first daily radiotherapy zap!

June 24 - Roche planning call with Jenny Zhong for tentative ACE team event in September

June 26 - Major reaction to chemotherapy and finally - extraction of automatic pump at 21.00. Followed by a very bad night where my body reacted out of control to chemo.

June 30 - Reported severe reaction to chemo at colorectal clinic after my daily radio zap.

July 12 - Jessica and Judd's wedding

July 13 - Michel & Michel, Simon and Evie visit us in Suffolk

July 19-20 - Carol and Michael visit us in Suffolk

July 23 - Margot from NZ visits us in Suffolk

July 24 - Rob visits us in Suffolk

July 30 - Final radiotherapy treatment

August 2-3 - Jacky and Charlotte visit us in Suffolk

August 5 - First trip to London by car with Ric to see Dr Sosie Kassab at RLHIM (Royal London Hospital for Integrated Medicine)

August 15-18 - Luxury days away at Aldeburgh

August 18 - First Addenbrookes check-up after treatment completed

August 27 - First solo trip to London for Capgemini phase two planning meeting

August 29 - First public appearance at MLA meeting for Gravitas

August 30 – September 9 Back to work – San Francisco and Bonn!

September 13 – Green Light Trust 25th Anniversary

September 29 – The experienced finger at Addenbrookes

October 13 – Dr Sosie Kassab at RLHIM (Royal London Hospital for Integrated Medicine)

THE BEGINNING?

19th March 2013 – Suspicions

Booked a check-up with Dr Ralph Hughes, my GP.

"Good morning, Nigel, how are you?"

I have known Ralph for a few years now and he is also a neighbour. He is tall, at least 6'3", lanky, with a very pointy nose and listens well.

It is hard to be completely relaxed with him because of the nature of the examination that is about to be performed. I also notice it is a bit of a silly question to ask – but how else would he open the conversation?

"Well, I have noticed that there is blood in my stools, and I wondered if you should take a look please." "OK, tell me a little more, how long has this been going on and do you have any stomach pains, cramps, or anything else?"

He puts on "the glove" and finds some lubricating jelly and has a good old look and poke around.

"Mmmm, doesn't look too serious to me at this moment and your stomach feels fine. I suggest you monitor it closely and if it persists we will refer you on."

25th October 2013 - First signs

Visit to GP but this time Ralph is on holiday, so I have to see another doctor.

Decided this blood in my stools and a slight pain when crapping has to be attended to especially as we have now committed to going to India.

Arrive at surgery on time for a mid-morning appointment and am called in by a rather squat and dowdy looking woman in her mid-forties.

"How can I help you?" Is her opening greeting. A bit more efficient than Ralph's.

I tell her about the blood and the slight pain, and she offers to carry out an examination. She, as gently as she can, inserts a finger up my bum and rootles around a bit.

"Well, I think this might be more than haemorrhoids, so I'll refer you to West Suffolk Hospital and let's see what they say. Doesn't look too serious."

I tell her I am off to India with Ric, my husband, in a few weeks for two months.

"Oh well, hopefully, you will be seen before then."

I leave a little reassured that it is not too serious and happy to wait for the specialist to see me, possibly before we go off on our travels.

March 19th 2014 - Trouble Brewing

Having spent December and January in India, with its usual diet and bowel challenges, I became more worried as my stomach hadn't settled. So off I jolly well went to see my GP again. Another locum. He prodded and poked with the usual decorum and concluded it was time for me to see a specialist and we made a date for 7th April.

6th April to 18th April 2014 - Only a week but what a week, except it was 13 days!

Sunday 6th April

A very dear and close friend rings to say he has been diagnosed with motor neuron disease just as we had stepped in the door from another dear friend's funeral where Ric read the eulogy.

Monday 7th April 1.15 pm

BMI Private Appointment with specialist to look at my "piles". Delayed from October 2013 due to administrative confusions and my 2-month sojourn working in India. He pokes around my anus and rectum and unlike possible public perception, this gay man does not enjoy fingers or utensils up my bum! He tells me it is likely to be something more serious - possibly a malignant growth in my colonic canal. I may need chemo and radiotherapy. He is direct, serious and compassionate.

We compare diaries and set a date of Wednesday 9 April for minor op/biopsy under general anaesthetic. At the end of a full and busy day of surgery, he will squeeze me in. He suggests CT and MRI scans too for belt and braces - they are fixed for Tuesday and Wednesday.

Home again to help Ric with the final draft of his new drama "FarmPlay", we want to focus on creativity.

Tuesday 8th April 1.30 pm

MRI scan at West Suffolk Hospital. The nurse notices my Lawshall address and chats away about her daughter who just moved there last week. Home again and review Scene 7.

Wednesday 9th April

I have a coaching session in London as well as an important new client meeting. So, Wednesday is suddenly full. I get to Bury NHS hospital at 08.30, have my CT scan (having drunk the appropriate liquid, not eaten or drunk for 8 hours before) use the "can eat and drink one hour window before surgery rule" as I drive from Bury to Colchester, catch the train to London, complete a one-hour coaching session, scoot to a very successful client meeting, scoot back to Liverpool St station, arrive at Colchester, drive back to Bury St Edmunds BMI (private) hospital in time to be admitted, settled and operated on at 5.30. Made a deal with the anaesthetist that I would be able to walk out and go home around 7.30. Neil my surgeon appears, and proudly shows me my large private room and we discuss the forthcoming procedure. We agree he will not do anything too drastic! I walk to the small operating theatre, lie on the bed, have my anaesthetic injected and s-l-e-e-p descends.

Wake up at 6.35 as promised, back in my room. Eat my pre-ordered sandwich, yoghurt, fruit and tea. Rest for 1 hour. Nurse arrives to check me out and I am walking around the room, having had a pee (one of the 'free to discharge' stipulations.) Agree with the anaesthetist and surgeon that I am fit to leave. Staff Nurse accompanies me up to the exit gate (just in case) where Ric picks me up at 8.20 and home we go by 8.45! Phew!! Sadly, no time to review his latest scene dynamic.

Thursday 10th April

In a moment of wisdom yesterday, I arranged to be replaced by a colleague on my favourite EY I&I job.

Resting at home, the same friend who rang to give motor neuron diagnosis rings again to say his Mum in law whom we are close to "has days to live". A double whammy for them.

Ric and I have plenty of time to review his scene and we are confident he can have an Easter break having reached the interval!

Friday 11th April

I keep my 11 am haircut appointment and struggle to sit in the chair and keep a brave face blaming a "cranky back"! Check with my colleagues in London that the EY course is going well.

Angela, Ric's sister, arrives for the weekend and I keep up the "cranky back" scenario so as not to alarm her.

We have a restful weekend, but I have two things on my mind: the accumulating evidence now being processed in the NHS system that will decide my short-term future course of action. And the stitches up my bum causing acute pain when I crap. I have set myself the target of being fit and well enough on Monday to not only fulfil a telephone coaching commitment to a client who is fighting for his job survival but also conducting a face-to-face coaching session with another client who is going for a big promotion opportunity - PLUS a flight to Geneva on Monday evening, - all without rupturing my stitches or crapping myself by accident en route to and from the office to the underground, DLR, City Airport, flight, cab and finally Geneva Hotel.

Through the weekend Angela enjoys referring to people we know who are either sick or dying and we agree to focus on more positive life aspects!

Monday 14th April

I did it. I made it safely and I kept clean and dignified. I honoured my additional and long-planned hygienist and dental appointments on Monday morning and conducted the phone coaching client call and several client directors' calls. Travelled to London (reached the train toilet just in time) had the 2-hour promotion coaching session, hopped on the tube, DLR, flight, Geneva, cab and reached the hotel without incident! I ordered room service of Chicken salad (following low fibre diet recommendation) ate it gently, and opened all the windows for cooler air so I could sleep.

Tuesday 15th April

Up at 05.30 to give myself time to do what was necessary to ensure my health and safety. Ate the biggest bowl of porridge ever – delicious.

Fantastic full-day follow-up session with CEO and HR Director of new company. I was audacious and warned them I had a tummy upset and may have to leave the room at a moment's notice and HR Director said, "Don't worry we don't want you to shit your pants!"

I was even more audacious and suggested we work in the large banqueting room in the Swiss hotel I had spotted in the morning.
They agreed without flinching, so after lunch we repaired to the conference room.

Both surpassed themselves in their newly unlocked passion and communication and totally impressed and surprised their PAs whom I had invited as audience to the see their final BIG finish presentations. Back in cab, flight, DLR, tube, train to Colchester and 40-minute drive home. YUP I was triumphant!!!

Wednesday 16th April

The big wait. Neil my Surgeon said he would call... No call. After an e-mail prompt to him, he promised to phone me with the results after his lunchtime meeting. No call.

I conduct client director call with a colleague and sell in a whole new experiential event called "Dramatic Shift" (well I am in the zone as it were.)

No e-mail or message from Neil. "When might I hear from you please?" I mail him around 15.30. "As soon as I get home" he replies at 18.15!

7 pm he rings with the news:

"Squamous cell carcinoma, two lesions. We may not need to remove your colon. We will need to do chemo/radio."

I arrange to see him at end of day Thursday at 6 pm. "Wait with a book!" he says.

Thursday 17th April

Ric and I visit the surgeon and get given the lowdown. He says the survival stats are good and we have caught it very early. Make a forward plan for after Easter. At home later I call a cancer survivor good friend, ask for her support in my forward journey, she is just who and what I need and she says all the right things without any panic. I recognise I am in shock and panic and need to work hard to stabilise.

Ric completes his final review of part one and we relax and take stock of everything.

Good Friday 18th April

I compose an important message to send to colleagues who are on holiday in the UK and Argentina. Send texts warning them I have a serious health issue that I need to deal with and likely to take some time off.

Drive a dismal grey route to Snape Maltings for Mozart concert. The weather mirrors my dismal grey thoughts and feelings. We arrive both depleted and desperate and guzzle a cream tea. Walk along a cold and windswept estuary, have supper crammed in at small tables and listen to an appalling concert. The conductor not only managed to suppress three beautiful Mozart pieces but also beat the Britten Pears young orchestra into submission and totally squashed a talented mezzo-soprano.

Arrive home just as the phone rings - Ric's sister "I know you don't like this kind of news, but John unexpectedly died today. His funeral is on Wednesday."

Good heavens!

I recall a poem from 'The Moon Appears When the Water Is Still' – Ian McCrorie

'Life is like bailing a boat with a hole in it.
No matter how fast we work,
No matter how large our pail,
No matter how many friends help us,
Water continues to pour in.

But what if we accept the fact
That our boat has a hole in it
And sooner or later it will sink?

We continue to bail
Without the hope of stemming the water
But because bailing is the stuff of life.
Now freed of the craving to solve
The tragedy of our existence
We can turn our eyes to the heavens above
And bask in the wonder and joy
Of the futility of it all.

Don't worry – things will get worse.'

12th May 2014 - Shock and Awe

I have been sent by Neil Keeling at BMI Hospital to the Excellence Centre at Addenbrookes Hospital in Cambridge. I'm here to see Dr Charles Wilson, the Consultant Clinical Oncologist at the weekly Colorectal Clinic in the Clinical Oncology Department – deep in the bowels (pun intended) of the labyrinth of what I call 'Health City'. Neil explained that for efficiency and excellence, it has been deemed that 'oncology is centralised.'

Ric and I arrive and park in the visitor's car park and trek our way through the endless corridors. My heart and mind are both skipping beats and looping the loop wondering what treatment plan they have in store for me. Neil suggested they may take the Chemo-radiotherapy route to eliminate the possibility of any residual disease lurking around after his surgery where he removed one lesion entirely. I have been given a 60-70% chance of recovery.

We finally enter the full waiting room; it is rather hushed and people in various states of illness are sitting around expectantly. I register and am asked to wait. They will weigh me and take some blood samples before I see Dr Wilson. "We are moving quite fast today, so it shouldn't be long," says the rather over-friendly receptionist. We settle in a quiet corner and begin to observe the activities.

"Nigel Hughes? Hello, how are you today?" But without a pause for me to reply, the sprightly assistant ushers me into the weighing room, and asks me to remove my jacket and shoes, I stand on the scales, and she registers my weight. – About 74 kgs. - I think about 11 and a half stone, which is fairly normal for me. "OK, thank you. Please take this blue slip and go into the bloods room - just turn left and up the corridor, you can't miss it." I obey instructions and wait in a short queue and very swiftly my name is called again and in I go. The male nurse is dressed in his smart blue uniform and sporting a name tag that suggests the possibility of Philippine origin. I comment on his name and indeed he confirms "Yes I am from Manila." He painlessly and efficiently extracts three phials of rich, red blood, presses a piece of cotton wool to the puncture asks me to press hard for a few seconds and tapes it up and off I go back to the waiting room. Ric is looking a little greyer and more alarmed on my return, having had the time to take in the feelings of the waiting patients. I squeeze his hand for mutual comfort as I settle down next to him.

"Nigel Hughes?" A different, blue-uniformed female nurse calls my name and says, "The Doctor will see you now." "OK, thanks, Ric off we go!" and we follow her into another corridor of doors, some open, with people mostly sitting in pairs.

"Please sit in here and the team will be with you shortly. By the way, do you mind if a student joins the meeting?" "Er... ok no problem, thanks."

It is a regular consulting room with a chair at a desk with a computer, two other chairs placed side by side and another two chairs at the back of the room, giving a fairly cramped atmosphere. So, we settle and wait. She leaves the door open and like the other pairs we saw as we walked along the corridor, we too await our fate, nervously. I am wondering what kind of person Dr Wilson is, Neil has told me he is the most experienced that Addenbrookes can offer, so I feel I will be in safe hands.

Suddenly three people arrive. All women. I wonder if this is the advance guard, and whether Charles Wilson will appear shortly.

"Hello. My name is Dr Jephcott. What do you like to be called?" "Er... Nigel and this is my partner Ric." "OK, Nigel. This is Kimberley Bennett the colorectal nurse specialist and this is *** (don't hear the name) who is a student, is it OK if she stays in the room with us?" "Er... yes of course if it helps her training."

"OK good." "Now then we, the MDT." "Um, excuse me, the MDT?" "Oh yes, the Multi-Disciplinary Team. Well, we have looked at your case, studied the histology and scans and have decided that the best way forward with your treatment plan is to do five and a half weeks of localised radiotherapy, five days a week and chemotherapy in weeks one and five.

Our experience tells us that this will provide you with the best way to help cure your condition. May I conduct an internal exam please?" She is factual and pragmatic in her approach.

A modesty curtain is pulled across and she does the business.

"OK. We are satisfied that Mr Keeling removed one lesion, but we are afraid there is evidence that there may be residual disease at the edges. So that is why we are recommending this course of action." She continues in her matter-of-fact tone.

This all sounds a bit more serious to me, and I suspect to Ric, than we had anticipated from our rather gentlemanly conversation a few weeks ago with Neil. So my heart is beating a little faster and many questions come up. But there doesn't appear to be time for me to ask those as Dr Jephcott immediately launches into a long list of risks and side effects that I might experience from the treatment. The list goes on and on. I remember – incontinence, dry ejaculation, shrinking bladder, loss of sphincter control. And much to my surprise, again it feels without pause, I am asked to sign the consent form so that another Doctor can perform a EUA (Examination Under Anaesthetic) tomorrow and I will need to come in next week to be measured up for my radiotherapy treatment.

When I pause for a breath and try to take all this in I notice that due to her manner, I am feeling bullied into submission. In a moment or two I regain my equilibrium and begin to ask some questions. "Is your treatment plan absolutely essential? Is this the only route? Given that I have a fairly clean bill of health up to now and the survival rates you have given me are fairly positive, can we re-shape your suggested treatment plan?"

There is something in her face that signals to me she is not used to receiving these questions. It appears she is used to being the expert in the room and her patients complying with her recommendations. Ric also chips in with some more questions and her face and position harden minute by minute until she finally says, "Well of course you do have a choice." And from out of nowhere she suddenly suggests, "Well perhaps you would like to be seen by a male doctor?"

At that point I reluctantly agree to sign the consent forms, knowing that at least we can get the process started. I sign. She leaves and we are left with Kim, the support nurse who sympathetically tries to explain the situation again, with more compassion, allowing me to hear more.

Ric and I get up to leave. We walk down the corridor towards the main exit, and I stop and say to Ric, "I need to have a cup of tea and think this through for a moment, OK?" We head towards the food court, order tea and sit in silence for a few moments.

"OK, I need to buy some time. We need to find the support nurse and see if we can delay the start of the treatment. It feels we are being pushed by NHS protocols and targets and they seem to have forgotten there is a human being inside here."

We retrace our steps, catch Kim, the nurse, and ask her if I can buy at least three weeks. I need to get a second opinion, but more importantly, I need time to digest this important information and allow myself to catch up. We wait.

"Yes, Dr Jephcott has agreed you can delay by 21 days, but no more."

Phew!

16th May 2014 – Letter from Neil my surgeon

'Hello Nigel,

I think Prof Tekkis is a nice enough chap, his rep is based on lots of number crunching and data analysis rather than surgical ability, maybe this has come on since he was a trainee?

The treatment for this condition is quite aggressive, but for a reason, the condition is curable and once completed the side effects are pretty minimal. David Cunningham has a main interest in UGI cancer, but his treatment would be no less aggressive. I did try to prime you for the treatment.

Not sure why Nicola is doing repeat EUAs on all of the patients we send - it was for a research project maybe that continues?

Hope all went as planned, but personally I would be itching to get on with treatment.

Best wishes, Neil.'

26th May 2014 - Dr Jenny Raphael Medical Centre

After my research in looking for complementary approaches, I have been recommended that I consult with Dr Jenny. She is a highly respected medical doctor following anthroposophical methodology.

Her first question when looking at my sheet – "Did they close up or give you a bag?" – Slightly threw me.

"Wonder why they didn't go in and get it all out? One polyp gone but didn't get the other? Better to get it all out.

Can you ask them this question - What is the reason they are not considering another operation to remove what's left of your rectal tumour? "

She agrees the radio/chemo route presents many risks to other organs and another operation, although uncomfortable and possibly inconvenient for three months (with possible temporary colostomy bag) may not endanger other organs short/medium and long term.

She suggested St Marks London did innovative colorectal work back in the 70s. Dr Kiko Rutter – but suspect he is no longer a practising surgeon.

"Need to get you to Paracelsus for a whole checkover. - Germany may be a viable alternative at Paracelsus, Kranken Haus, Baad Liebenzell – near Stuttgart."

Jenny gave me her Holistic view:

Low grade heartburn – possible stomach ulcer.

Food groups:

- C1 = Chili, Curry, Citrus – impacts on stomach

- C2 = Coffee, Chocolate, Cheese – impacts on liver

- C3 = Cucumber – impacts on gall bladder

Tingling feet – lack of B12/folic acid

My Actions:

1. Explore St Marks London lower rectal specialist
2. Ask Dr Jephcott/Fernhead for Oxford specialist
3. Explore Paracelsus

Conclusion:

All hope is not lost – I can participate in my own healing and if I find the right approach I may not have to go through the nightmare scenario described by Addenbrookes.

Came away with a reality check – I do of course have cancer that needs treatment! And I have lifted spirits with a view to working with this rather than surrendering to mainstream "abusive" attack.

28th May 2014 - Project Nigel

The other perfect storm. The rain is lashing down in glorious celebration, crying for me and people like me who are struggling and confused.

"Farm Play" Ric's latest drama project is in the birth canal – just one more gentle push and it will be born, kicking screaming, howling and yelling into the world. The upturned back garden where Nigel our builder neighbour is preparing to install a long-awaited shower in the guest suite - is a sign of the holes and tunnels in my confusion. The rain is pouring in and filling up the tunnels, thunder and lightning rumble and flash and the mound of Suffolk clay is saturated and waiting to fill the tunnels. My office is also upturned and inside out. I have to clamber over builders stuff in order to work.

Matthew Manning says, "Cancer is chaos". Well, it certainly has manifested here! I feel upturned, inside out, spilling over, mess and rubble. Shereen and Alesha are about to arrive for a summer holiday – unprecedented but adds to the chaos. AND "The gang" is expected at noon on Saturday for a 24-hour blast. More chaos, more thunder and lightning.

Every cloud has a silver lining. Does it? I wonder if Mr Keeling had taken it all out if we would not be needing the aggressive chemo/radio treatment that is almost inevitable. Try as I might avoid the terrible action that has been recommended it seems at this moment anyway that the Centre of Excellence route at Addenbrookes is the option. "But don't make decisions in the darkest hours" says Mathew Manning.

I have been marked up, tattooed permanently, measured and I have practised the tunnel. The radiography staff are kind and gentle, compassionate and caring. Even Lindsay sounds convinced that the mistletoe therapy is complementary to chemo/radio.

Fess up Nigel, the time has come to face the fact that this is the big one for you. I was saying "OK it feels like there is another big project in me" little knowing that "the big project" is – ME.

The compassion, patience, understanding, unconditional love and support I give to others all needs to be directed at me for the moment. Humility, vulnerability, understanding and surrender seem to be words that are "My gift in the wrapping". I like to say wisdom is the gift when I hear Mathew Manning's visualisation but maybe that is the wisdom; to recognise humility, vulnerability, understanding and surrender - my gift to myself.

These next few days will be a challenge of everything and trying to stay present and gentle.

The rain is raining, the puddles are filling, the ground is saturated, and the skies are heavy. "Farm Play" needs to be off. Ric and I need to have confidence that we have made the right decisions, and his play is born. Rob will be Rob and his reaction will be what it is. The rain will stop. Maggie, Rich, Clive and Sue – THE GANG - our next summer weekend guests will herald some sunnier days.

My mind will be more peaceful once I have made my decision. NOT deciding is not an option. It is the constant questioning that is the storm. I am looking into the eye of the storm now. If I face up to the fear, the uncertainty, the doubt and find a way to come to terms with a decision that I can stand behind, then I will gather the right support around me to weather the storm. There may still be grey skies, more rain clouds, more thunder and lightning, but at least it is energy. And as I have always said *emotion is energy in motion.*

'See the possibilities in everything and anything is possible' – even this, PROJECT NIGEL.

THE BEGINNING? - THE RESPONSES

Hello Nigel,

Just returned from a week in the Dordogne at Deidre's house. Deidre's woods and meadow were great, and the latter was simply roaring with butterflies. Lots of jays and we heard the sound of the hoopoe but never actually saw one. Also, attached some photos of orchids (v common) and just-gone-over lizard orchids. Lots of broomrape(s), reminding us of that beautiful evening when we were with you last.

We are thinking of you and sending love and strength. Sue and Clive

*

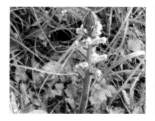 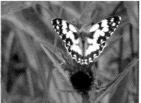 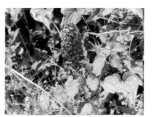

28th June

Hi Nigel

I can't help but feel completely inadequate in providing even the minutest kind of support to you in this leg of your journey. I try to say the right things, but really wonder what good it does. Especially when you do so much for me, for others, even at this time.
Miss you, love you, thank you for being my mentor.

Steeve

*

Dear Nigel,

We, along with many others we are sure, have had you very much in the front of our minds this week. We do hope your treatment has begun well and that it has been manageable for you.

I dreamt of you and Ricky this week and in the dream was aware of how hard this must be for Ricky too - to stand by while you go through these big hospital procedures.

No need to get back to us - but we are here! Look after yourself dear N.

With love C and M

WEEK ONE - THE TREATMENT

Monday 23rd June - Saturday 28th June

"Climb every mountain"
Climb every mountain
Search high and low
Follow every highway
Every path you know.

Climb every mountain. Ford every stream
Follow every rainbow, 'Till you find your dream.

A dream that will need
All the love you can give
Every day of your life
For as long as you live.

Climb every mountain, Ford every stream,
Follow every rainbow, Till you find your dream

Climb every mountain,
Ford every stream,
Follow every rainbow,
Till you find your dream"

Well Saturday 28th June is the anniversary of World War One beginning –
and I feel that this Thursday and Friday I was in my own internal world
war. My dream is not for my war to continue for four years, not even for
four months!

Day one

Having started on Monday 23rd June with optimism and hope with all the preparation and good wishes of all my friends, family and colleagues I felt I was ready for anything and everything. I had taken second, third and fourth opinions. I had done my own risk assessment and made some strong choices about the way I wanted to do this – without being overly controlling - but certainly putting my own personal values, ethos and philosophies into practice. And of course, including Ric in all discussions and decisions. My goodness, the value of a long-term relationship built on trust, mutual respect, and fathomless love. My heart is overwhelmingly grateful.

Patience is and never has been one of my greatest qualities, and this week it has been necessary to add it to my repertoire. Patience, acceptance and flexibility are all being tested along with vulnerability and openness. I have met incredibly caring and genuinely helpful staff at 'Addenbrookes Health City' in Cambridge.

On approach, it looks like an industrial unit. Blocks and blocks of concrete and glass with tall chimney towers, multi-story car parks and miles and miles of long and crowded corridors with confusing signage. The health factory has over 6,000 people working in it, all concentrating on doing their best with years and years of investment poured into their specialism.

The corridors can be airless, and I wonder as I patrol and search for my department how many germs are circulating, unable to escape. Hand cleansing dispensers litter the avenues and go mostly ignored. Continuing my patrol and search I get the occasional glimpse of a person on a bed with various machines, drips, bandages, eye patches attached. Wheelchairs of various kinds are pushed by caring volunteers of all shapes and forms, sometimes the pusher looking no healthier than the pushed!

We arrive at 08.45 on time at Level 4 vascular access. A functional name for a functional unit. Two receptionists greet us and send us along to find Level 2 lift – where we will find another reception desk. There is confusion as the warm and friendly receptionist has my name on the list but cannot find my medical notes. She makes several calls but no joy. The notice on the wall invites me to drink plenty of water while waiting. The water holder is empty and there are no cups, and some strange TV channel blasts out a home and garden programme, presumably to keep our minds occupied while we patiently wait. After some searching no notes are found until I suggest that they may be with oncology as I am about to have a chemo bag attached to my PICC (Peripherally Inserted Central Catheter) line then go to radiotherapy for my first treatment. "Don't worry Nigel you go ahead and get your PICC line inserted, and we will find the notes."

I enter an open space with several sets of green plastic curtains displaying a no-entry sign and 'Please knock before entering' posted on them!

A man who tells us he is from the Philippines called Aldwyn approaches us, and invites us to sit down, but no chairs. After a confusing moment of looking at a crumpled bed in the far corner and two females lying on beds in the other two corners, he emits a very high giggle and finds three chairs. He looks at us and in another confusing moment asks, "Which of you is Mr Hughes?"

I respond, "I am - and this is the other Mr Hughes, of 43 years."

Another piercing giggle and we have efficiently established our relationship and whose arm he needs to insert the PICC line. He explains the procedure and possible side effects at high-speed punctuating each paragraph with what is now becoming an infectious giggle.

Basically, he inserted a fine tube into my upper left arm and wiggled it along one of my central veins (using ultrasound) until one end is placed into the muscle wall of my heart. This will enable the Chemo to have a direct hit on my blood supply automatically for 96 hours! At the end of the five-minute explanation, the three of us are delightfully bonded. I sign the relevant paperwork. This hospital, I have come to learn, like you to take in multi-faceted information and instructions and expect you to sign permission forms immediately. I comply, trusting that Ric and I between us will remember the vital information.

He takes me into an almost separate room where he begins to chatter about *his* new husband, also from the Philippines, and his recent trip to Berlin where he stayed up until 7 am most mornings before attending his three-day training conference. I am slightly alarmed as he shares this story with me and another nurse who has appeared, who is eager to hear his stories. But this is a man of great skill and well-practised techniques as he painlessly inserts my PICC line which will carry my fatal cocktail to the muscles surrounding my heart. "You may feel some side effects as the local anaesthetic wears off in a few hours but don't be alarmed, take a couple of paracetamol. Your dressing will be changed in 24 hours and then weekly. - Off you go to X-ray to see that I have put the line in correctly. Goodbye, see you shortly."

And that's it. I leave the bay and deduce, by the sneaky glances of the two female bedridden corner patients, that our conversation has been totally public. Back to reception, down to the ground floor, along the corridor where to my surprise there is only a four-minute wait. Quick x-ray snap and back we go to Aldwyn who gives it the all-clear. And with a giggle and wink - off we go to Radiotherapy.

The process begins again: check-in, name, and date of birth, first line of my address. "Please take a seat and the Doctor will be with you shortly."

Relatively quickly we are ushered into a private consultation room by Rachel who has difficulty in writing up my notes and answers to her questions due to a huge bandage on her right arm inhibiting her mobility. "Careless DIY accident" she says before launching into the explanation of the Radiotherapy process and accompanying possible side effects, ending with a flourish and hands me the consent form. I pause and ask a few points of clarification, Ric double checks some hinted at implications, and we are gently escorted back to the waiting room. Rachel has a pleasant, warm and human manner and the 10–15-minute consultation process does not feel rushed. She wishes me well, gives me her numbers to call if I need.

Waiting for the first Radiotherapy treatment was a strange mixture of excitement and relief. I had met 'Timo' my radio machine and insisted that I have a trial ride two weeks ago. I had asked numerous questions, been measured, and tattooed on both hips and on my pubic bone – marks that will now never disappear. In each treatment I will have a CT scan to assess my current state and check I am in the correct position thereby minimising any accidental impact on any other internal organs (!). Nicola the tall and lanky chief radiologist calls my name and with a nod to Ric, off I go into LA4 to be zapped. 'Timo' awaits. A big bubble machine with a hard black plastic-coated bed at the end of a cold and dimly lit room. Nicola and Poppy, the assistant radiographers, ask me to remove my shoes and trousers, request my name, date of birth and first line of my address. Apparently, I answer correctly, and they are happy.

I am invited to lie down and line myself up with the correctly positioned head, knee and ankle rests. I need to slide down my underwear and they deftly place a piece of kitchen towel over "my privates". Their efficient record-keeping proves successful. I am in the right position, relatively comfortable and can take a deep breath to settle in for the sequence.

They reiterate what I have been told before and it tallies with my memory. First, the bed will retract into 'Timo', he will take a quick CT scan, and there will be a pause while the computer checks everything. I will then hear some strange growling noises and some bleeps as everything is double checked and with a whir and a whoosh I will be propelled slowly back again into the tunnel. More bleeps, more whirring and more growls, then the 318 second treatment will begin. It will be painless. They disappear out of harm's way into the control console with a cheery "See you later!"

As I enter the tunnel I breathe deeply, sending soothing messages to my unconscious and conscious, a routine I have practiced daily since my introduction to 'Timo'. I focus in my mind's eye on my sentinel – the bee orchid – I silently mutter my thanks to the phenomenal advance in technology and masses of investment of time, money and people's dedication that is making all of this possible. I truly feel the impact of the 21st century. My traditional and natural values are truly being tested and yes, I surrender.

All goes according to plan and within five minutes I am out of the tunnel, being invited to sit up, get dressed and am free to go. I thank them and depart with a "See you tomorrow Timo". I am shaking and stirred up. I sit for a moment's silence next to Ric, we breathe together aware of each other's stress and distress, I take some more Rescue Remedy and off we go to the Chemo Day Centre down the corridor and around the corner.

I think it is 12.45. To eat lunch or not to eat lunch? I decide to check in at yet another reception desk – name, date of birth, first line of your address. "Hello Nigel, please take a seat, we won't keep you waiting too long." We sit in a small alcove, and I take a moment to recover and catch up with this morning's proceedings, reeling a little and my insides trembling.

I also notice that I need a pee and am hungry and thirsty. I go to pee, Ric goes to the WRVS kiosk to buy water and apple juice and when we both return, we take another deep breath, look at each other and I open my lunchbox. He has made me delicious sandwiches with homemade bread and veggies from our garden, accompanied by home grown fruit. Yummy.

"What a great satchel". "Thank you" I say, "It was given to me by my Indian friends." "Oh, have you been there?" she asks. We have a conversation with Christine who is with her mother and sister-in-law. Christine's mother is being treated. Christine is on her annual two week visit from Canada. We ask her about her place and have a very interesting mutually inquisitive dialogue. Just as Mother and sister-in law exit from the treatment room my name is called. We part almost reluctantly.

"Please follow me and sit in the far corner chair over there." Another world opens up before us.

WOW! - I instantly label it the Chemo Laboratory. This is yet another new situation and another new set of circumstances to take in, understand and digest.

As we enter there are a series of beds and easy chairs around the long room filled with harsh fluorescent lighting – maybe 20 altogether. Various people are attached to various lines, some alert, reading books, doing crosswords, some comatose, their monitors bleeping.
There is a respectable and quiet hush, and conversations are conducted in low intimate tones, apart from one conversation, due, I imagine, to the hearing ability of the patient. All ages, all shapes, all sizes.

Some have accompanying adults, some are alone. One woman we are told who has a particular and apparent skin condition is 100 years old today. "She received her telegram from the Queen when she wasn't wearing any knickers!" It feels like a laboratory, with humans as the experiment. I gulp. We settle in the corner. Sanjay a round Indian man approaches us, and the usual routine ensues: ID, information, side effects warnings, and of course the consent form to sign. My heart by now is beginning to race a little and my mind is in disarray with too much information, my senses are overloaded with incomputable sensations, and I am beginning to spin. I have to hold Ric's hand to steady myself and involuntarily, my first tear drops and dribbles down my left cheek. He is looking a little wild eyed and ashen and the shock and enormity of the power of cancer hits us both.

The surprise being offered by Sanjay was not pre-warned. I have to take 4 pills now – 2 to ensure the chemo will be assisted to settle in my body and 2 anti-nausea pills. I will also need to take these four times a day for the first five or six days AND one antibiotic pill twice a day for 35 days. He hands me a package containing the mountain of medication (plus something to counteract diarrhoea!) I protest and challenge if all this is absolutely necessary. "Will I not be overloaded with drugs and chemicals?" "How will my natural system know what to do?" He assures me this is best practice and gently advises me to stick to the rules. "Your chemo has not arrived yet, so relax. We will be back shortly." "What time did your PICC line get inserted?" Apparently there has to be a gap of at least an hour before chemo can begin. About fifteen minutes passes and Claire arrives, just as Ric has gone to find some water. I ask her to wait because my information absorption rate is full. I tell her I cannot guarantee to remember anything she might tell me – knowing there will be another extensive briefing, side effects warning and consent form to sign.

We wait and she makes polite conversation sharing that she is being promoted to a new unit in three weeks' time and is off on holiday on Friday "but not packed a thing". Luckily Ric arrives. I am to have two treatments, one now - Mitomycin that is bright purple in colour, she will insert manually, and it will take about 3 minutes, followed by a dose of Fluorouracil (5FU) that will come in by a drip first now for about 20 minutes, then they will attach the remainder to my PICC line and will give me my portable pump and a bumbag to strap around my waist. 5FU will administer itself automatically for the next 96 hours.

I gulp again and try to take in this new information, make friends with the new drip that has appeared, ask to hold the Mitomycin for a few minutes to be acquainted before we start. She accepts all my conditions and is warm, open and empathetic. She rattles through the possible side effects as she personally injects. We are off. I breathe as much as I can surrendering to this alien environment and alien intrusive medication. Ric holds my hand breathing with me. I can only imagine what is going through his heart and soul. We have talked over everything, and he has respected my decisions

BUT THIS IS HARD, HARD, HARD.

Cancer is the 21st century disease and we have both succumbed – he 10 years ago – me now. HECK! Who would have thought that with all our "good life" we would both suffer? AND this is life as it is not how we would like it to be. Acceptance, grace, humility.

At least now, with my chemotherapy Joey bag strapped around my waist that will drip lethal chemicals into my system automatically over the next 96 hours and with my radiotherapy five times a week for 5.5 weeks we have begun my journey to full recovery.

I want to get home to peace, nature and tranquillity as soon as possible and give my spirit the chance to catch up on the day world war one began in my body.

Day two and three

Tuesday and Wednesday in retrospect were relatively easy compared to what subsequently transpired. In and out of the radiotherapy room and the usual sequence with 'Timo'.

Day four

Thursday was another matter. I had an appointment at West Suffolk Hospital Dermatology clinic that we had tried to move unsuccessfully to Addenbrookes, so that all my treatment could be under one roof at 'Health City'. A suspicious spot on my ear had been troubling me for a few months and a small skin horn had appeared on my right shin. As it happened under examination by a young male registrar who coincidentally, works at Addenbrookes, they were declared benign. Future surveillance will be kept. On exiting that appointment there was a message from the tall and lanky Nicola at Radiotherapy that 'Timo' had broken down and my appointment would be delayed until 4.45. I confirmed my attendance and we drove home. But my chest had begun to feel a little tight and uncomfortable. I kept breathing and tried to integrate this new experience. At home I took my temperature, and all was below normal as usual for me. I poodled around taking it easy and doing some desk work and a little weeding in the garden. We left for Addenbrookes around 3.30 in time to reach there for my 4.45 'Timo' session. As I was driving my chest became more constricted and more painful and as advised we telephoned the emergency line who suggested as we were nearer West Suffolk Hospital that we should go to A&E there.

Although doubtful that this was the right action I checked in to A&E, told them my case history at reception and alerted them to my chest pains. Ric parked. Within five minutes and just as Ric arrived, I was called in to Triage. I explained my circumstances and the nurse took blood pressure, temperature and an ECG. All proved normal but having reported in I had to be seen by a doctor. He came shortly and I had to start at the beginning but knowing in my mind that the best and right course of action for me to take right now would be to get to Addenbrookes Day Care ASAP. Patiently and gently I said I would like to be discharged and make my way there. Of course, he was a little alarmed at this suggestion wanting me to stay with him, get blood tests and stay under observation for six hours. This would throw my schedule out the window and I did not want to interrupt the flow.

With gentle persuasion from me and a few words separately from Ric outside (unknown to me at the time) - we escaped and set off for Addenbrookes.

Against advice I went straight to the Chemo Day Centre and was met with a cheery "Hello Nigel" from the receptionist. "Sorry for sending you to West Suffolk but glad you are here now. How are you?" I said I had stabilised and that tests were OK and handed her the report from West Suffolk. "Great. Why don't you pop along to Radio, have your treatment and we will see you after." I proceeded to the Radio department, checked in where they said it would be about six before 'Timo' was up and running but as soon as he was, I would be seen. I had an hour to wait.

Around 6.15 "Nigel, come into LA3 and we can do your treatment". "Sorry to hear about your day so far. How are you now?" Poppy showed me in to an almost identical set up and I was met with an identical 'Timo'.

The usual procedure and when completed Poppy said that Day Centre were waiting to see me now. I returned there and was welcomed into the empty Chemo Laboratory and asked to lie down on one of the empty beds. A young American/English trainee nurse took blood pressure – which by now was climbing - my temperature, which was normal and attempted to set up the ECG monitor with considerable difficulties. Another nurse appeared and eventually they sorted the octopus-armed leads out. "Can't really tell my right from my left" she said sweetly.

Once the report had been printed there was a little huddle around it by two female and one male nurse and a registrar Anna. Anna approached me, introduced herself and asked a few vital questions. I was waiting for bad news. Fortunately, she said the ECG looked clear and normal and though my blood pressure was rising it was not alarming. But she said under consideration we think it would be wise to disconnect Joey – my Chemo bag and line. They would also take bloods and have them sent urgently to the lab and would let me know ASAP if anything unusual was found. I felt relieved in that moment, not knowing what was yet to come. After about 15 minutes Receptionist/Triage Nurse came and detached my line and took bloods. "Phew" I said, "I'm glad that has been done it feels like my body has had enough chemo." They checked they had my number and knew that I was staying on site at Kingston House. Ric in the meantime had moved us into our self-contained one bed apartment and was cooking supper. It was ready almost 2 hours ago – when I looked at my watch it was almost 9pm! With a few words of assurance and consultation Matt the male nurse who was involved in the earlier huddle around my ECG results said "I'm sure we have made the right decision. This can happen with PICC line chemo. The symptoms may last for 24 to 36 hours. And we will see you tomorrow."

With some relief, I staggered through the long corridors getting lost on the way, crossed the small park and called Ric to say I was almost there. As I rounded the corner there he was hanging over the balcony with my shared relief showing on his face. I fell into his arms on the doorstep and burst into tears, climbed the stairs, found the bathroom just in time and threw up!

He had made the apartment look as much like home as possible. He had spread two colourful Indian bedspreads, placed flowers, laid out our fruit and vegetables in the kitchen and hidden the TV behind a rather dubious romantic picture of what reminded me of Iceland. Our freshly picked herbs were struggling to revive in the plastic container he had found to put them in. A metaphor of how I was feeling. Rather droopy and surrounded by plastic! I began to settle and told him the story of the last 4 hours. I ate some delicious spaghetti he had made and some fruit and began to perk up. My chest was still tight and felt very restricted, but I was sure that these symptoms would decrease gradually through the night....

They didn't.

11 pm was bedtime and we snuggled down in our two single beds for a well-deserved good night, hoping against hope that we could catch up on some recent broken nights. My chest was still aching, and I was a little concerned. I checked that my mobile was on and that there was sufficient signal in case the labs called to say they had found something in my bloods. The chest pains increased, the tightness became a bit like a clamp – a severe dose of heartburn or indigestion.
There was no extraneous pain elsewhere, nothing in my back or head or neck and I firmly believed it was my body reacting to the toxins and not able to deal with them effectively.

Miraculously I heard from Ric's breathing that he had fallen asleep – unusual for him as it normally takes him ages and ages. He must have been whacked and wracked and fortunately, his mind and body escaped into slumberland. For about two hours I did everything I could to manage the discomfort. I breathed deeply. I visualised my bee orchids. I walked around our five-acre meadow in my mind. I strolled through Crooked Wood, Golden Wood and Frithy Wood. I called upon the spirit of the mistletoe therapy to help boost my immune system. I pictured all my friends and family in a BIG circle around me and I called them one by one. There are many! I created an outer circle of the practitioners who are now involved in my healing process, I saw 'Timo'. And I saw the remnants of Joey being gorged by the hospital incinerator and I thanked him for the work he had done so far and insisted it was my turn now to re-claim my body and help the toxicity pass through effectively and efficiently but as quickly as dammed possible. The tightness came and went in waves, some big, some not so big. I even thought of millions of women around the world who go through contractions and although unsure of exactly what kind of experience they might have in their labour, I empathised hugely.

At some point I found myself saying out loud "I don't know what to do, I don't know what to do, I don't know what to do." I was reminded of my desperate time up the Mahakam River in Borneo when I had some strange tropical disease that wracked my body and sent sharp laser pins into my eyes and head and how we were tenderly rescued by a non-English-speaking Kalimantan paramedic who gave us home and help for three long days. But this was different, very different. Somehow in Borneo in that environment to get a tropical disease was explicable, unbearable, but explainable and I had some points of reference.

There was enough difference in the sounds, the heat, the air to let my body know I was in unfamiliar circumstances – I was way upriver and out of reach of a hospital with no means to get to one if I knew where to go - and it had to cope in a new way with new bacteria that it hadn't before encountered. But this time I was in Cambridge, England, albeit in a strange and comfortable flat on the edge of Health City. Here I was in a comfortable bed in a comfortable room with my best friend by my side and resources within easy reach. Even though I knew that to go back to the Day Unit would be futile – what would they do? Administer more drugs, take more bloods, and attach me to another machine to assess another whatever? So I lay and breathed and breathed and tossed and turned until I could not do it on my own anymore. My cries of "I don't know what to do" must have got louder. I was half conscious that if I said it loud enough, then I might possibly wake Ric, something I am always reluctant to do when he is sleeping, because we both know once he wakes it takes him at least another three hours to go back to sleep.

BUT.

"Ric. I don't know what to do. Ric. I don't know what to do. Ric I don't know what to do. Ric I don't know what to do. Ric I don't know what to do. Ric" – he woke up. From that moment on he was brilliant. He took charge of me, listened to my situation and talked me through an excellent reality check of what he understood my body was going through. Step by step we walked a new path of assimilation. For two hours. Until I was able to settle, and we both fell asleep and woke at 9 am.

PHEW!

Day five

Friday 27 June. My Rad review with Rachel was set for midday and I was asked the night before I had the chemo disengaged to report early so they could take more blood. But my bloods had been done, the hospital had not rung in the night with bad news, so I could assume everything was OK. We confirmed our respective reflexology with Kelvin at Maggie's Wallace. Ric at noon, me at 1.45. Had some breakfast and a few quiet moments before I went off. Ric was to return from his session and make lunch. I would return from my various appointments eat lunch, have my reflexology and then we would get home as fast as we could before getting caught in the Friday afternoon Cambridge exodus. Not quite what happened? Of course not.

I checked in at Radiotherapy unit – they immediately sent me to get more bloods done. Then there was a slight delay as Rachel was not quite ready for my review and I saw her patrolling the corridors with paperwork. She passed me "Hello Nigel. Dr Noble – one of the other oncology team - would like to see you before you go today, just to check you over after yesterday. I'll come back and find you in a minute."

Sometime later after patiently waiting for my 12.45 'Timo' spot I was unsure which card would be pulled first, Rachel for Rad review, Dr Noble or 'Timo', so I had to prepare for all eventualities. I took my pre – 'Timo' rescue remedy, went for a pee, didn't eat and didn't drink too much water. Rachel called, walked me down to another unfamiliar corridor, invited me to take a seat and off she went. She went to and fro three times before stopping and saying, "We thought Dr Noble was going to see you now, but something has come up." "Not a disciplinary I hope."

"Oh no. Come with me we will do your review, get you into your treatment and by then we hope Dr Noble will be free."

She asked me the usual questions about various side effects and the only one I could confirm, apart from my chest/heart condition was throwing up once at 9 pm last night. She seemed pleased that at least she could tick one box for me! We discussed the fact that neither Ric nor I had heard of the possibility of the Chemo creating chest tightness, but she confirmed that it was one of the lesser side effects. I wondered how we had missed this. We agreed that I had imbibed the majority of the dosage and that the rest that was thrown away should not affect my treatment in the long run. "There may be other things that we can do." We clarified her role as opposed to another nurse and she confirmed that she was the Radiotherapy support nurse and as most of my sessions were radiotherapy, I would have my reviews with her. Her bandage had decreased in size, and she showed me her healing right hand wound. She was still pleasant, still warm, and still compassionate and still giving the impression that she had all the time I needed.

When we finished, she strode me off back to 'Timo' where Nicola and Poppy were waiting to greet me, concerned about yesterday's events. Poppy was particularly surprised to see me wandering the corridors at 9 pm last night. I assured them I was feeling much better and ready for my 318 seconds. All went according to plan, and they said that Dr Noble would see me now. Poppy escorted me back to one of the new but now familiar corridors where once again I was asked to wait. Waiting allowed me and my system time to reflect, catch up and re-assess. My chest pains had eased considerably, and I could feel less toxicity attacking me. Relieved, I even dropped my shoulders for a few minutes.

I looked at my watch and realised I would neither make lunch on time nor my reflexology session. I called Maggie's Wallace and alerted them, "No problem just get here as soon as you can." They are used to this no doubt. Rang Ric but realised his mobile was out of battery because neither of us had brought our chargers, so had one second to say. "I'm OK will be late" before the line cut.

"Nigel Hughes" a male voice called from the end of the corridor. A 5' 10 tall, lean, dark-haired man with blue/grey sensitive looking eyes in his early forties greeted me with a very warm handshake. "I'm so sorry to have kept you waiting for so long, but I have been with you reading all your notes and pondering your situation." Sounded like a good start to me.

"Please come in, take a seat and we will assess the current situation to ensure that everything is going in the right direction. So sorry to hear about your day yesterday, sounds like a full one. I'm sure you have told the story many times already, but it would be useful to let me know, I would like to hear it from... you."

I told him. He was taking notes and looking at results and when I stopped for a moment, he assured me that he was listening. He asked me, "If you were to describe your symptoms yesterday as if somebody had done something to you, how would you describe it?" Good question. But I couldn't answer it directly. "Well, my sense is that I had a surfeit of chemicals pouring into my body." "I am not a drug taker and I notice that if I ever have to take any drugs, I usually take less than the prescribed dosage. I believe my system is relatively vital and clear. So, I think it was my body saying – enough now thank you, I can take over." He listened intently and absorbed. "Matt made the right decision yesterday to remove the Chemo. You will not have lost anything from not having the little that was left, it was due to be taken off today anyway, so you only lost a few hours and a few milligrams.

Yours is an unusual case and we have the perfect window of opportunity to take stock and re-assess before the next chemo round. We will talk about it when Dr Jephcott returns – she is away for two weeks and in discussion with you we will make a proposal." He said the magic words that I have heard several times "Yours is an unusual case" … I challenged him and said that in my initial discussions with Dr Jephcott, I'd suggested that maybe the standard approach was not the way forward. He reassured me that he agreed with the initial and standard approach and that now there may be room for some flexibility. I suddenly felt I had a man with half an open ear to some flexibility, a move away from Dr Jephcott's rigidity. I certainly would not want to endanger my heart again. I thanked him for his time and care and his listening and said I felt I had reached another stage on this journey due to this conversation.

NOW. What to do next? It's 2.15. I'm hungry, thirsty, and late and decide that I will go to reflexology to see if there is still time and space for me. I need some TLC and even if Kelvin is useless, it will be an opportunity for me to land. I send Ric a text just in case his phone has a tiny bit of juice saying, "see you at 3.15." A gentle and caring man gives me a very sensitive reflexology session and it does the trick. I arrive back at the room and tomato soup with veggies is waiting on the table. Ric is packed up and ready to take us home ASAP. I eat my soup. Lie down and we leave by 4pm. Yes, yes, yes. Already the chest pressure is easing, the chemical flow that is doing its extraordinary work is lessening and as we leave Health City behind us and join the Cambridge exodus, I don't mind sitting in a traffic jam for a few minutes. We arrive home within an hour, and I relish the clean, clear air and go to say thanks to my bee orchids in the wildflower meadow. They are beginning to fade. But one Pyramidal Orchid is now shining brightly.

Home sweet, sweet home. We have created our own haven. It truly welcomes us even though the weather is cold and miserable. I have climbed at least one mountain and with fabulous assistance have forded several streams and followed many rainbows.

I am on my way to find my dream...

WEEK ONE - RESPONSES

Dearest Nod.

And dearest both of course because there are two of you on this journey! (And many more of us walking by your side!) What lovely ramblings from a lovely man.

It is so powerful to witness how a threshold such as a challenge to our very mortality draws us so far into the Outer world of Knowledge and Learning so that we can do our best for ourselves; and yet so far into our Inner world where the need to find a meaning for what is happening becomes very profound. Nature is a wonderful support and the bee orchid a massively appropriate symbol for you Nod.

It seems both so flamboyant a flower with a real statement to make, standing erect in all its glory and yet so delicate and fragile hanging on to its little triangular umbrella.

I found out it means 'Industry' in the language of flowers and that is such an apt description of you! Like the bee itself. By its very mimicry the bee orchid demands to be noticed, looked twice at until the observer really sees what it is. It's not pretending, it's real. Like you in your ever adapting and evolving journey, bringing the skills you have to the people you have, with such love and dedication.

May all go well for you on Monday and the ensuing weeks. May you still be able to notice the daily miracles even at the bleakest moments.

Best love, strength and good thoughts to you and Ric. Lindle

PS: let me know if there is any way I can be of use, and I'll see what I can do.

*

25th June

Dear Nigel

When you told me that you had received some 'challenging news' you mentioned 23rd June, and this date has lodged in my mind. I do hope that you and the doctors have arrived at a way forward which feels right and bearable. Jess and Judd loved their visit to Lawshall over the weekend, and Jess was entranced by your garden.

I hope that despite the Orchid Project you are enjoying our beautiful county at the most beautiful time of year. We walked along the meadow beside Lineage Wood yesterday; it is filled with pyramidal orchids – mostly deep purple/pink, but some white too. The most amazing show of orchids I have seen and well worth a visit (and tea at Bright's afterwards?).

Much love to you both, Amanda

*

30th June

Oh goodness, Nigel! I had no idea this was going on for you. I scarcely know what to say, so I will sing very loudly and shed a wee tear. Such a brave journey you and Ric are taking. And you write so beautifully. It must be a good way to process what you are going through.

Please keep us in the picture. Good luck, keep being brave. I hope the chemo works and you are only going through this for the shortest amount of time. Big love to you and Ric. You are both in our thoughts, hopes and hearts.

Josie & Steve

*

1st July

Hi Ric, hi Nigel,

I was really sorry to hear your news yesterday and am imagining you now resting at home in Lawshall, so I hope that's the case.

Josie and I were both really stunned and are hoping (and praying) although I'm not normally the praying sort, that you make a full, fast and absolute recovery.

On top of everything else I know it must be really stressful. Josie and I had a similar situation a couple of years ago and Ric, I know that for the partner, the stresses can be very acute. So I really want to stress that we're thinking of both of you and sending you our love.

It goes without saying too of course that we'll do absolutely anything we can to help. In any way at all. I'm not sure what that would be or what form our help would take, especially as we're so far away, but if there's anything we can do, please do let us know.

Lastly, I'm not sure you'll remember this, but one time when we were in Lawshall we went for a walk early in the morning through I'm guessing what the larger estate was. We walked through forest and gullies and meadows and paddocks for a couple of hours. I remember your boots were muddy and well-worn from doing these long walks and we bumped into various people along the way. I really enjoyed it.

But what I really wanted to say is that when we're back in the UK we can do it all again and I'll be looking forward to that. More walks and cold lunchtime beverages. More great conversations and more of Ric's amazing garden fare.

Like you say, climb every mountain and keep in mind that we're right there with you, every step of the way.

Our love to you both,
Steve and Josie

*

2nd July

Yep. I read it this evening at the office. To tell the truth I thought I would speed-read it, nine pages would be a challenge. But I read every word.

It felt like a slow dawning of reality, a darkening despite your resolve. And Rick always supporting by your side, or in the background creating a loving nest.

It seems like it could be a lonely path you are walking, but it is populated by loving people. That cannot alleviate all the challenges, but I hope it gives meaning and solace.

With love
Stu~

*

Dear Nigel,

I hope that you will feel better soon and become well again. Although we speak of cancer every day in this workplace it is always disappointing to hear of someone close coming under its grip. You are very courageous, so stay strong! I enjoyed reading your story of week 1 (really, that was only the first week?!) and getting some perspective on what it is really like for patients. You are lucky to have Ric and family and friends to support you. Try to enjoy life as it is as best as possible. I am sending you a picture of the mountain you will conquer. Enjoy!

Take care, Carmen

*

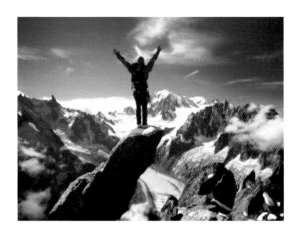

Hello darling. Read your pages and my goodness I can feel the vulnerability that Thursday and Friday brought you.

Golly gosh babe. I hope that this week is easier. Why is your case unusual? I mean given that it's you it would be of course, but what exactly is unusual about it?

I must say your account brought my experience into focus again quite vividly. You meet so many people, some of them just wonderful, it's a big cast of characters. I remember the bewildering newness of every next procedure, how exhausting it is, how one's resilience is tested over and over. After a while, you feel like an old hand. A very old hand.

Finding a way to be at peace with the mixture of allopathic and homoeopathic is a journey in itself. The amazing progress that has been made in treatments, and understanding the complexity of it all is demanding and astonishing.

I remember making a decision that, although I would stay alert and awake and continue to ask a million questions and push against some things, overall I would surrender and accept healing in this challenging and unfamiliar form.

45.

I feel for you - dancing with Patience, Vulnerability, Surrender, and Acceptance. And you are a dancer Nigel. You have grace and dexterity of spirit.

Not a time to lead or follow - just dance.

Your doctor sounds like he really heard you and the relief will go a long way to working with the next phase.

Sending you huge love and holding you in my heart.

Blessings from Cricklewood Veronica Xxxx

*

9th July

Hi Nigel,

I read through both of them together. An incredible read: you express the challenges and your optimism so well. I like the humour too ("Not a disciplinary")!

One thing you mention is the 'surprise' at you (and Ric) having this when you are fit and healthy but from at least a dozen people I know who are going/have gone through this it really is a lightning that strikes randomly (even if they do theorise some 'proneness'). What has mattered as far as I can see - and certainly in Anne's case - is that the treatments themselves are such a challenge that being fit and healthy is a key perhaps not in avoiding cancer but in being able to deal with the cure. I have a friend going through it now who was an athlete (who even managed to train for and run the Great North Run during his treatment while skin was peeling off his feet!) and he's had it rough and is getting through because of that healthiness where he might not otherwise have done.

Really inspiring read Nigel - thank you for the privilege. Keep them coming. And yes I did sing, but I found Carol King easier to relate to than the Von Trapps!

Love John x

*

Dear one -

You really expressed everything so clearly and viscerally. I hate to sound like former President Clinton, but I could "feel your pain." I could also feel your deep love and respect for the amazing Ric. Your relationship sent me into tears of joy for you. I shed a few other tears for the process you've navigated so beautifully. It seems that the way you embraced the vulnerability of the situation was completely self-empowering, as was your surrenders to various realities.

I can't tell you how moved I am and how grateful to have been able to read your two weeks. I look forward to hearing more about your process & healing. San Francisco in September? Did I mention to you that I have a dear friend there who is connected to all of the hospitals & Doctors in town, should you want to explore any part of your treatment? She's also well connected to alternative practitioners, I'd love for you to meet her. She's wonderful.

Again, thanks for Week One & Week Two. Love to Rick!

Love,
Sal

WEEK TWO

As different as chalk from cheese but with a sting in the tail!

Having been through the mill, dragged through a hedge backwards and climbed a very steep mountain in week one, week two felt like sitting on a plateau observing the view. Except the view was inside and I needed to get to it. I have spent many hours being, not doing.
As it stretched ahead of me it looked like a simpler journey, literally travelling daily for 50 minutes each way along the A14 to Cambridge, check in at Radiotherapy, have my bloods taken on Monday to ensure no unintended consequences were accumulating from last week, change my PICC dressing on Tuesday and look forward to a Rad Review on Friday. And it almost worked out like that, until Saturday evening.

On Monday I woke up feeling vital, alive, clear-headed and bounding with energy. It was a glorious sunshine morning, and we needed some eggs. I set off on my egg hunt. Here in Suffolk, we have a tradition of local people selling their homegrown produce on their doorsteps, or in home-made cabinets placed at the side of the road with honesty boxes. I had three chances to find eggs for sale at 7.30. My bike had been recently overhauled, so it was in perfect condition and even my tyres were inflated to their correct psi. I donned my spanking new Cambridge blue peaked cap, didn't risk wearing my shorts, just in case my skin was still sensitive from chemo, and off I rode. Our resident song thrush gave me an operatic send-off. Having been disappointed that the two nearest eggs for sale opportunities were not open for business it would be the furthest point of sale 2.5 miles away at the other end of the village that just might have theirs out.

I felt encouraged, slightly anxious that my heart may develop a flutter or an ache, but I took it gently up the hills (whoever said that Suffolk is flat obviously didn't do it by bike!). And yes, in Brands Lane I caught the back of the egg lady disappearing into her blue-door bungalow; she had just placed a dozen eggs in her roadside cabinet. "Hooray, hooray" I puffed out loud, stopping her in her tracks. "These are definitely the best eggs in town" "Oh my goodness" she responded extremely shyly. "Shall I give you the £1.50 or put it in the pot?" "Oh, thank you I'll take it." And she scurried into her kitchen. Both of us very happy.

Cycling home, I felt I had achieved a major expedition and was not only glowing with sweat, but also pride. My first independent activity for over 10 days. At 08.30 I made two boiled eggs for myself; Ric was having a well-earned lie in and his sister Angela who had been visiting for the weekend had not yet appeared. Bliss. A very good start to a very different week. Eventually both appeared, had their boiled eggs, Angela packed and left. Ric and I sat down to make our week two plan.

The idea was for me to travel alone in and out to Cambridge, have my daily treatment and any additional explorations that may come up. Ric was to start work on draft 5 of "FarmPlay". He had received comments and instructions from the dramaturge he has been working with to make some additional trimmings and changes. We both agreed it is essential he gets back to work. I was out of Ric's hair for about four hours and when I returned, we swapped stories and reviewed his progress. Ric has a sharp mind. After initially being slightly resistant to this new task, he managed to achieve some excellent cuts in the early scenes and even surprised himself that there was an improvement. In the meantime, I accepted some discomfort, rested when I needed and found myself entering a new rhythm and phase of my treatment. The rotating radiotherapy team continued to be attentive, caring and as personal as they can be in these circumstances. But something was stirring. I needed to be mindful of where a toilet was in every location and needed to time my journey exactly.

In the meantime, Orchid Project Nigel hatched a new idea. On Tuesday morning, another stunning bright clear and sunny start to the day I took my iPhone and snapped a series of pictures of my morning walk. I sent these to my filmmaker mate Duncan, accompanied by a list of the birdsong that I hear as I walk. He made it into a video with soundtrack lasting exactly 318 seconds. Something I can now use in my daily Rad treatment and as added value I sent it to the MLA work team to offer as a morning start to Company Day, making an impact with my virtual presence.

Friday is Rad Review Day with Rachel. As planned Ric accompanied me so we could have four ears on the case. We checked in and I was sent to bloods, Ric went off to Kingston House to check it out and refresh supplies so we could have lunch there after Rad Review and my zap. As we were waiting in the corridor queue outside bloods, Rachel walked towards us cradling her right arm. "Hello Rachel, shall we see you after bloods and before treatment? Or what is the sequence today?" "Oh, I'm so sorry I have to go to the clinic to get my hand seen to, it is ****" and she used a word that I didn't understand but obviously she was in pain and concerned. She showed us her right hand and indeed it was not looking too great around her stitches. "I may be back in time to see you but if not, Dr Wilson will see you." "Ok, good luck" I said and off she went. WELL. Unfortunately for Rachel, her hand was causing her pain, but a happy accident for us. It meant we would be seeing the head honcho Dr Charles Wilson; under whose care I was promised to be at the beginning of this whole process. The list of questions that we had put together would now have added relevance.

Bloods were done, 318 seconds of Radio were uneventfully completed apart from the fact that I was introduced to a new male team member, Paul.

He had the warmest hands so far of all the team which I commented on, and Poppy retorted with "Well as we know cold hands, warm heart in my case." "Oh" I said "Does that make you are cold-hearted Paul? "They were up for the banter and a few kind jokes later 'Timo' was set to work.

Just as I was tucking into my delicious lunch box: "Nigel Hughes?" The call from along the corridor "Dr Wilson will see you now." I enter the office, the same consulting room that I saw Dr Noble in a week before after my heart incident. "Hello, we met in the corridor a few weeks ago and this is my partner Ric." Dr Wilson is a man in his late -forties, medium height, fairly chubby face and body and with intense, yet gentle eyes. "Please take a seat and let's see what we can do today." His attention is mostly on my file, but he does take me in and acknowledges Ric's presence. "Let me see. How are you today?" I say I am recovered from last week and feeling almost like myself. "Tell me more about last week." I describe the recovery process I went through since the removal of the bumbag. He is very interested and listens with great concentration, and I feel he is taking in more than what I am saying.

"Can you give me an exact picture of the existing lesion we are treating as I want to visualise to help my recovery?" He pulls out a pencil sketch that Miss Nicola Fernhead drew after her EUA – "Perfect. That really helps" I say as the three of us examine the picture and have a detailed discussion about it. We almost get to the bottom of the 'unusual case' story and later realise there is another level of detail we need to ascertain to get a full and even clearer picture. But for now, I am satisfied.

We discuss the heart incident at length and again he confirms that this can be one of the expected side effects and re-iterates that we took the right course of action by removing Joey before any further damage.

When I raise the question of week 5 repeat of 5FU chemotherapy and I would be very nervous if that was still the recommended course of action, he responds with "Well we are thinking that it may not be necessary." "The Mytomicin and 5 FU have more than likely done their work by now. "But let me discuss with Dr Jephcott when she returns next week. You are officially under her care and politically it would be better for us to include her in that discussion."

My heart, soul and spirit lighten considerably. This feels like another very important turning point. A man, like Dr Noble last week, who is prepared to listen, respond and be flexible. There is a list of four other points that we have prepared and as I announce we have more questions he genuinely stops for a moment and is engaged in our need for clarification and is enthusiastic in our curiosity. At one point over a discussion about acidophilus he at first recommends I don't take it, then checks himself and admits that his opinion is not based on any fact. He re-considers and we have a full discussion – his comment is 'that it may just compromise the good work of the radiotherapy and he would be very willing for me to take it as an antibody booster - but could I continue after radio is completed?' We make a deal. We also discuss other dietary concerns and create a balanced approach to the recommended low-fibre diet.

Killer final question: "My diary is calling, and I have an offer of work in San Francisco with the Global Oncology Team 1-3 September. Can I accept?" "Well... yes, I see no reason for you not to. You may not be bouncing around, but I think you will be OK."

YIPPEE!

All being well and still with some big warning signs that the next few weeks may not be plain sailing we leave the meeting with renewed hope and vision.

We celebrate with a lunch of Heinz tinned tomato soup, carrots and asparagus in our Kingston House apartment, have a short rest and wend our way home.

Saturday, I felt a sense of liberation with the hope that chemo 2 would not now happen, I also felt more in tune with the exact location of the possible residual disease that we were treating so I could focus on it and assist my recovery. We enjoyed a day, and I went market shopping alone, having a toilet break halfway through. We even watched Dolly at Glastonbury on BBC iPlayer – what an extraordinary woman and brilliant performer she is. She doesn't need any of the flashing lights, video, multimedia background that other performers seem to employ to enhance their performance. Just Dolly and her excellent band and backing singers. Around 9 pm there was a brilliantly multi-coloured sunset over our meadow and the song thrush was in full sweet throttle. So off we went on a gentle evening stroll around the meadow to breathe in the dramatically changing sky of blue, grey, black-lined clouds with shafts of golden sun piercing through and hitting the meadow swaying grasses. Awesome.

In a flash, I said to Ric "You just carry on. I won't be a minute." I had the sudden urge to have a crap and no time to dash to the nearest toilet. I crouched in the grass and let rip! This has become a bit of a pattern now, about an hour or so after eating I need to go. But poor Ric was unaware of my predicament and wondered what I was up to. There had been talk of incontinence being a possibility and now I understood. So, from now on I will need to be even more aware of my surroundings and any evening plans will have to be within easy reach of "the facilities"!

The sting in the tail!

I followed him down the path apparently looking rather ashen due to a sharply stinging bum and hand in hand we wended our way home.

When you're down and troubled
and you need a helping hand
and nothing, whoa nothing is going right.
Close your eyes and think of me
and soon I will be there
to brighten up even your darkest nights.
You just call out my name,
and you know wherever I am
I'll come running, oh yeah baby
to see you again.
Winter, spring, summer, or fall,
all you have to do is call
and I'll be there, yeah, yeah, yeah.
You've got a friend.
If the sky above you
should turn dark and full of clouds
and that old north wind should begin to blow
Keep your head together and call my name out loud
and soon I will be knocking upon your door.
You just call out my name and you know wherever I am
I'll come running to see you again.
Winter, spring, summer or fall
all you got to do is call
and I'll be there, yeah, yeah, yeah.

You've got a friend

WEEK TWO - RESPONSES

8th July

Sounds like a completely different and better week which is great news.

I completed a race for life at the weekend, one of the ladies that ran in my team I had only met for the first time that day. After getting to know her it turns out she is a nurse at the local hospital, in fact, she is the manager of the cancer unit. Had an interesting chat with her she is extremely knowledgeable. Any question I'm sure she would be happy to answer.

Sandra Xxx ●●

*

9th July

Dear Nigel

What a difference a week makes'

So glad things are easier. So lovely that the two loves of your life, your Ric and your beautiful garden, paths and fields, are such a comfort and source of joy in your hour of need

And on the horizon, the possibility of not having to have chemo (yeah!) and a possibility of work, which you are so brilliant at, in a glorious place. Double yeah!

Linky and I send you both all love, Bridge xx

*

14th July

Hi Nigel

Well, that was an epic read and I hope you are considering turning it into a book later. It did bring back many memories, but in a strange way I found it comforting to re-live the cancer path I trod with David. It is also interesting to hear your feelings as David found it difficult to talk about how he felt and just wanted it all to go away. Like you, he hated the thought of anything unnatural invading his body, but there are times when you just have to compromise.

I look forward to the next instalment and hope that your treatment is progressing without too many unexpected side effects. It's devastating how cancer can suddenly and unexpectedly take over one's life, but you sound as though you have a very positive attitude and with Ric by your side you will conquer this. Just hang in there with the chemicals for a while as the doctors recommend!

Love to you both
Jacky xx

WEEK THREE - HUMAN FRAILTY

7th July – 13th July

Imagine you are sitting in the Radiotherapy waiting room, about 30 comfortably padded blue chairs set in two banks facing each other with a coffee table in between scattered with daily newspapers and magazines. No TV, thankfully, blasting anything. There is a silent screen in the corner flashing various messages about nutrition, diet and bulletins on specific and general oncology-related topics.

Humankind at large. What I notice and have been noticing in the hours and minutes that I pass here awaiting my name to be called for my 318 seconds, is each individual's coping mechanisms. Some, like me, stay relatively private and contained, with an occasional nod to their companions on arrival and departure, others love to talk their story out to anyone who is willing to listen and share their journey. I hear intimate details of treatment approaches, resultant side effects and how each individual is dealing with it. It is apparent who's there with loving companions and partners and who is being supported by a compassionate hospital service driver. Cancer is a great leveller. There is an unspoken sense of togetherness and a feeling of mutual understanding for each other. All sorts of people are here to face the challenge of all sorts of cancers and a variety of obvious and hidden symptoms.

This Friday morning almost at the end of my third week I am waiting for my slot. In the corner, I notice someone I have not seen before. She is small and fragile, almost sparrow like in build, white tousled hair dressed in a pink cardigan. I guess she may be around 80 years old. She is sitting alone in the corner and breathing rather shallowly.

She is one who does not meet the gaze of others and stays quiet and contained. Her name "Joan" is called and with supreme effort she rises from her chair, pulls out her walking stick and begins her slow walk to LA3. "Thank you kindly. I can manage". She gently refuses the arm of the radiotherapy technician. As she passes, I notice the tell-tale signs of her condition, red marks on the left side of her neck.

She disappears into the treatment room and my attention is taken by the man on my left describing in minute detail his story to a sympathetic listener. I try to shift my focus back on myself to prepare for my turn. But he is a natural story-teller and keeps me (and others I suspect) gripped with the ups and downs, not only of his condition and the vicissitudes of his travel experiences, but also his fears for Saturday, tomorrow, when the main entrance will be closed for maintenance and how he will get to this department etc. I am rapt and am a little surprised when my name is called out – he has compelled me to surreptitiously listen to him for nearly 25 minutes!

Poppy asks me to take my seat in the waiting area just outside LA3 to remove my shoes and she will be with me in a moment. The moment takes a while longer than usual and I notice that due to the distraction of the storyteller I have omitted to have my usual pee before treatment and my bladder is slightly calling. However, Rachel appears, and we begin to make conversation and arrangements for my regular Friday Rad Review which she will conduct this week before she goes off to have her occluded (aha that was the word she used last week) hand.

Just as she is showing it to me, Joan, this time fully supported not only by her walking stick but also on the firm arm of Poppy, shuffles past. She is in severe distress. Her neck is now scorching red and raw, and her eyes are not only determined, but also full of perplexity.

I take a huge deep breath and hold it firmly as she passes, and I inadvertently clutch Rachel's bad hand. She lets out a strangulated squeal and pulls her hand from mine. When Joan has passed, I release my breath, apologise to Rachel for hurting her and a waterfall of tears pour from my face, and I let out an almost silent howl. "Oh, my goodness, oh my goodness, what courage and dignity she has. This puts everything into perspective." Rachel places her good hand on my left shoulder and says "Yes, we see and endure all sorts here. Yes, it is shocking. But tomorrow is Joan's last treatment, and she will be all right, she will be all right." As she says it, I am not convinced whom she is reassuring.

I take a few more deep breaths and she ensures me that I am relatively stable and fit to have my treatment. I have forgotten my tight bladder and go for my zap. After my zap, I have my Friday Rad Review and we look at my situation and she gives me enormous acknowledgement for my progress. She assures me I am doing really well. We talked about the recovery period after 30th July, and she advises that my bowels and bladder may well need a bit of re-training in the first few weeks of August. She also wishes me well for the next two weeks as she will be on holiday next week and as she bids me farewell says, "Charles will see you."

Meanwhile, the beautiful song thrush has finally diverted its attention away from full operatic aria to snail hunting. So rather than hearing its song we hear the tap, tap, tap on the path as it finds and excavates a snail shell for a succulent snack. But we have a glorious replacement. A garden warbler and a white throat are now competing in the operatic competition. Almost the same but subtly different they trill their rippling songs in the oak tree. They have been joined occasionally by a charm of goldfinches and a small family of long-tailed tits. Up the lane on my morning walk we have the chiff-chaff with its staccato calls complementing another melodious white throat.

Tuesday was the main medical event for me apart from having to be extremely vigilant about managing my growing incontinence. After the lengthy consultation with Dr Wilson (Charles) last week I had a dressing change appointment for my PICC line. I sent a note to Kimberly, the chemo support nurse, on Monday as we were all prevented from travelling to Addenbrookes and Cambridge due to the Tour de France passing through. I asked her if instead of changing the dressing on my PICC line if they would consider removing it entirely. I received a positive response almost immediately. "Yes, Dr Wilson says PICC line can be removed on Tuesday."

I checked in at Radiotherapy reception who then passed me to the Day Care Centre and within ten minutes, just as I was tucking into my sandwich (is this a pattern emerging?) "Nigel Hughes?" "Hello, I'm Bernadette. I have been asked to change your dressing today." "Oh" I said, "I believe we have clearance to remove the PICC line." "Oh, OK just give me a minute and I will check for you. You can finish your sandwich if you like, I'll be back." Three minutes later and one sandwich gulped. "Yes, you are right, follow me." And off we went into a private room set up for PICC line removal. "This will be quite simple and should be painless. All I need to do is detach the catheter and gently pull out the 48 centimetres of plastic tubing. It will only take a few moments." Unusually she does not ask me to sign a consent form! As she set to work, I asked her where she came from – "Philippines, one of the larger islands." And we talked about the challenges of living in a hurricane and earthquake zone. And I regaled her with my story of when I was staying on the 21st storey of a Manila Hotel, I suddenly found myself in the middle of the night being turfed out of bed and landing on the floor. A 6.8 Richter scale earthquake had struck. She responded with her experience of being caught up in a 9.8 earthquake followed by hurricanes. And within a few minutes sure enough the PICC line had been carefully and painlessly removed.

"Hang on a second before you throw it away. I need to look at it and thank it for its work before you bin it." "Goodbye PICC line – I hope not to see another like you again but thank you for your work." Bernadette giggled and found herself also saying goodbye to it and ceremoniously binned it. Phew! I felt a strong sense of freedom and relief and looking forward to immersing myself in a warm bath in 48 hours once the hole in my arm has closed up. Another milestone, another turning point and another step on the way to my full recovery. We will see what the MDT come up with once Dr Jephcott returns next week.

I was also looking forward to attending the wedding on Saturday of our relatively new farmer friend's daughter. She, an English rose, was marrying into a Jewish South African family. I had been asked and agreed to be MC for the wedding but had sadly had to withdraw due to the uncertainty of my state. And I made the right decision as it would be embarrassing to say the least to be in mid flow when a sudden call of nature bellowed at me. It was a glorious and quirky celebration. A ceremony marquee had been constructed in and around the apple orchard. Straw bales had been covered with clean sacking and tied at the end of each row with a full sprig of oak leaves. They were using the symbol of the oak tree as a metaphor for their love and commitment. They had also created a fusion of cultures, some Jewish traditions including the reading and signing of the Ketubah (the marriage contract), the 'stamping of the glass' followed by a hearty Mazel tov and a gallop down the aisle by bride and groom accompanied by a traditional Hebrew song played on the fiddle with much cheering and clapping from the assembled crowd.

Later we were all invited into another larger marquee for the wedding breakfast. Each table was named after either a South African tree or an English tree and members of the South African guests were equally distributed at each table with English guests, just like the English roses mixed with South African flowers at the centrepiece of each table.

Even here three miles from home, the spirit of cultural exchange for mutual understanding was taking place. Unfortunately, I had to leave the celebrations early to avoid an accident.

To follow that, on Sunday we had invited four friends to join us for lunch where to our great joy and delight we had a world-renowned flautist give us our own private concert in the luxury of our sitting room. Schumann and Vivaldi filled our spirits. For a moment I thought of Joan, how was she spending her first day after the completion of her treatment. How was her spirit being replenished?

"Hello in there."

We had an apartment in the city.
Me and my husband liked living there.
It's been years since the kids have grown,
a life of their own, left us alone.

John and Linda live in Omaha.
Joe is somewhere on the road.
We lost Davy in the Korean war,
I still don't know what for, don't matter anymore.

You know that old trees just grow stronger,
and old rivers grow wilder every day,
but old people, they just grow lonesome
waiting for someone to say,
"Hello in there. Hello"

Me and my husband, we don't talk much anymore.
He sits and stares through the backdoor screen.
And all the news just repeats itself. Like some forgotten dream.
That we've both seen

Someday I'll go and call up Judy.
We worked together at the factory.
Ah, but what would I say when she asks what's new?
Say, "Nothing, what's with you?
Nothing much to do."

You know that old trees just grow stronger,
and old rivers grow wilder every day,
ah, but, but old people, they just grow lonesome
waiting for someone to say,
"Hello in There. Hello."

So if you're walking down the street sometime
and you should spot some hollow ancient eyes,
don't you pass them by and stare
As if you didn't care.
Say, Hello in there. Hello.”

WEEK THREE - RESPONSES

You're an inspiration dear friend

Martin C

*

Dear one ~ thanks for this account of week three. As I've mentioned before the way you tell your story makes it all so clear that I can see you sitting & waiting, and having your pic line removed. I am so glad for your wonderful progress & will pray you will easily avoid future accidents...

Did I mention to you that I had a wonderful lunch with Ronnie. It was so delightful to see her. We took our time ~ it seemed like old times.
Sending you love ~ hope you have a lovely weekend,

Sal

*

Thank you so much for sharing your experience in such a meaningful way. I am humbled. Your words make me more aware that our life experience is so much governed by our bodies, and it's amazing that bodies are living organisms that can change and heal themselves, and that there was a hole for the PCC line that will just heal, and new body tissue will grow and fill up the hole, and that process can be seen, it's on the surface but a whole lot more is going on inside, I imagine all your body processes must be in hyperactive mode (no wonder your bladder is affected) as they are now being programmed to combat the cancer ... amazing

Big hugs to you and Ric from Taymour and I

*

Hello, you - How strange to say that I love reading your words when they come from a place of you being ill. Yet they carry with them such hope, such courage, such humanity...and such a feel for the countryside and birdsong around you.

I want to ask you something: For the past month or two, there has been a blackbird up on a chimney singing the most beautiful 2 hr song in the quiet when the squawking seagulls have gone to feed- late afternoon- and he has been lifting my spirit every evening. Suddenly he has gone, and I miss that song so much. Someone said that the male blackbird sings to court his lady and he stops mid-July because the job is done! She's his!

Any thoughts?! He's certainly won me over but I long to hear him again.

I send love - Linky too. Bridge xxx

*

Dear Ric and Nod (have I got this right?)

Thank you so much for your very kind email.

We learnt from the "girls" speeches that as a couple Jess and Judd are known as 'Juddica'; as in "are Juddica coming too?"!

The thunderstorm was extraordinary, and the rain fell as the band began to play, so everyone joined in. Traditional Jewish wedding dances mingled with our traditional country dances, and we finished with the wonderful circular Jewish dance where the bride and groom are honoured with clicking fingers and backwards stepping bowing. Truly amazing.

And then Judd set up the electro-swing stuff!

And then we went to bed. But happily no power cuts at Bright's (though we did have a generator). Sunday bought a touch of Glastonbury to the garden, but all was well in the marquee where Robert and I celebrated our 30th wedding anniversary with Gaddies, campers and many old chums. And now I am sitting in the office as if it was all a dream!

Nigel - I hope this week is, shall we say, tolerable, and I am honoured to be included on your list of caring chums.

Much love to you both, Amanda

*

Hi Nigel, Hello OVER THERE!!!!

What an inspiring, gripping and tender piece of writing. So amazing to be able to see inside your world and walk around in it. Flipping hell .... what a tough old couple of weeks. Wishing you more relief in this week coming up. Ahh....made me laugh you had your own flautist performing for you.... I'd expect nothing less!!!

Love to ya Mr. H.

Ann xxx

*

Nigel my darling. Thanks for another huge dose of humanity which I have just read before going off to work here in beautiful Hanoi. It's hot and sticky and in the evening the streets throng with the chatter of large groups of young people sitting on low stools eating drinking and laughing. Lots of laughing.

My thoughts are with you as I take my morning run around the Hoan Kiem Lake and watch the old ladies dance with fans and the couples rumba at 6.30 am and the boys play badminton on street corners.

Loads of love and healing to you - you big old softy!

Xxx Rob

*

Thank you Nigel. I've just read this, sitting on my balcony listening to a mower, not (sadly) a whitethroat or thrush. It brought tears to my eyes - thinking of Joan, and the wonderful wedding, and you travelling so vibrantly through this ordeal.

Thank you. Much love ...

Oh look - A dragonfly has just visited me, and the goldfinches are twittering nearby - so that's good! Here's hoping the Capgemini gig comes off – thank you for asking me. You see nature can do it!!!

Siobhan Xx

*

When I read your stuff it made me go to this quote:

'As it is, we are merely bolting our lives—gulping down undigested experiences as fast as we can stuff them in—because awareness of our own existence is so superficial and so narrow that nothing seems to us more boring than simple being. If I ask you what you did, saw, heard, smelled, touched and tasted yesterday, I am likely to get nothing more than the thin, sketchy outline of the few things that you noticed, and of those only what you thought worth remembering.

Is it surprising that an existence so experienced seems so empty and bare that its hunger for an infinite future is insatiable? But suppose you could answer, "It would take me forever to tell you, and I am much too interested in what's happening now." How is it possible that a being with such sensitive jewels as the eyes, such enchanted musical instruments as the ears, and such a fabulous arabesque of nerves as the brain can experience itself as anything less than a god? And, when you consider that this incalculably subtle organism is inseparable from the still more marvellous patterns of its environment—from the minutest electrical designs to the whole company of the galaxies—how is it conceivable that this incarnation of all eternity can be bored with being?'

~ Alan Watts, "The Book: On the Taboo Against Knowing Who You Are"

Lots of love, Margot

WEEK FOUR - THE SCREWS TIGHTEN

13th July to 20th July 2014

"When the going gets tough the tough get going" – Do they? I'm writing this on the morning of Monday 21 July, looking back on week four and entering week five with a huge amount of trepidation and some reluctance. Only eight more zaps to go, but we need to heed the warning signs that things may be more difficult.

Having got through last week without too much of a hitch and a restful, nourishing weekend where our dear friends Michael and Carol visited, I need to give huge acknowledgement to Ric who terms himself "The Reluctant Carer" but is doing an absolutely brilliant job of being respectful, sensitive, loving, patient and full of humanity. This is probably more difficult for him to witness my pain and discomfort than for me to experience it. Well, it's different, I guess. He sees the aftershock of me having had a painful bowel movement (like shitting shards of hot glass) as I cower in the corner fireside chair in our kitchen breathing deeply to regain my equilibrium. And sometimes he has to literally clear up the mess. Again, our relationship is being tested to its limits.

This is very gory. Because of the impact of radiotherapy and its positioning, I was warned that I might experience sunburn, tenderness and breakdown of the skin in and around my anus. All are happening now to some degree. "The radiotherapy has to escape somewhere, and it will escape through your bottom." They are right.

I have been given three creams E45 for the tender and unbroken skin, another for the broken and reddening skin and a third for the anal aperture to act as a numbing agent for when I pass a motion – have a crap! Because of the location, even fairly flexible me, cannot exactly see where these three options can be applied, so Ric tenderly makes the applications. I said to him "You either have to know someone extremely well – or not at all to do this." We have found a position on the bed where I can lie carefully on one side, gently pull my cheeks apart so he can use cotton buds and apply the creams to the various parts. It tickles and it stings in various degrees, so I have to wiggle my toes to counterbalance the extraordinary sensations and try not to pass wind directly into his face! Then I lie still for ten minutes or so before I can get up and start my "John Wayne walk" as promised by Dr Wilson.

The other huge challenge is, as I have described before, the sudden and unavoidable need to rush to the loo and crap again – maybe up to four or even five times in the morning in the space of 90 minutes. This morning, I was on a client call in my office and the overpowering urge
overtook me and I could neither ring off nor get to the loo in time so I stepped out of my office door into the garden and did my business – without (I hope) alarming my caller. I had just finished my crap and the call when suddenly our good friend Kate appeared round the corner and discovered me! "Oh my god, go away" I shouted at her with some force. She instantly recoiled and dashed off. I had been calling for Ric to come and rescue me and she thought I was calling her name so came to investigate. I recovered, Ric came running I told him what had happened – he scampered off to apologise to Kate and then came back and helped me clean up. I recovered my self-composure just in time to receive another client call which went off without a hitch!

On a better note. After all that I prepared to gather myself together again to face the 50-minute journey to Addenbrookes to receive my 318 seconds worth.

I was shaky but determined to continue with my independence (and control) and convinced Ric I was in a good enough state to drive. I left him to concentrate on revising Scene 11 – only two more to go.

The journey to Cambridge is carefully planned and timed as is my walk from the car park to the Radiotherapy reception. I know if there is the slightest hiccup or traffic jam that I may be in trouble. It feels a little like a relay race – with me passing the baton to myself at different staging posts. There are points of no return. I check at each stage how my internal organs are doing and make the decision to find a stopping place or move on to the next stage. One obstacle that does present itself is the intermittent appearance of speed check cameras.

If I drive sensibly along the A14 at 75 mph I know I can not only stay within the law, but also reach my timings. But occasionally I notice I have strayed over 75 mph as I am lagging a little behind time and increase to 80 mph. The sneaky Cambridge speed camera van decided to place itself in a new layby this morning and just as I caught it in my sights, I also noticed I was doing 79 mph! Bugger. Well, we will see. Fortunately, I arrived at the 'Health City' car park just within my bowel and bladder limits and luckily enough found the perfect parking place so I could make my calculated journey to the first available loo – just in time. Breathing a sigh of relief, I navigated the endless corridors and even assisted a (rather attractive) first timer on his nervous journey to Oncology – yes even in this state I am aware of my libido!

A small confusion with Radiotherapy – Nicky sidles next to me in the blue chaired thirty-seater waiting room. "Hi Nigel, have you had your PICC line changed?" "Had that removed over two weeks ago!" "Oh good." And off she scuttled. Then Charlie came and sidled up. "Now then Nigel we are just checking about the final chemotherapy you're supposed to have today." My heart skipped a beat, turned a somersault, leaped into my mouth, rebounded around the waiting room and landed with a thud in the pit of my stomach.

I took a deep breath. "Well, we discussed that with Dr Noble at my Friday Rad Review, as Dr Wilson had been called away for IT training (!). I reported suffering from a degree of neuropathy particularly in my left leg and toes. He did a careful and thorough examination and found that everything was in good order. But the fact that I had reported it rang more alarm bells and he could almost guarantee that I would not undergo more 5FU – the chemo drug that caused my severe heart reaction. Please check. Immediately."

I could sense at least 15 pairs of ears eavesdropping this conversation as I tried to stay calm. "Ok I will just have to double check because we cannot proceed with Radio today until we have clearance. I'll be back in moment." I let out a silent scream of anxiety and confusion and my mind went from panic to surety, back to panic and into deep fear. I broke into an instant sweat. I rehearsed several conversations. I noticed one or two glances coming my way and avoided their gaze – trying to maintain equanimity. This would blow all my plans, preparations and hopes of a smooth and early recovery. About three minutes of deep turmoil ensued. – Perhaps I was NOT one of the tough after all! I had already written the litigation application, imagined my conversation with an eminent barrister friend of mine in Canada and got her on side to do battle for me by the time I heard "Nigel Hughes" from LA3.

"It's OK Nigel, no more chemo has been confirmed by the MDT. We can proceed." Much to her surprise, and I suspect to one or two of the patients following this action behind me, I gave her a BIG hug as I let out a shriek of joy!

My 318 seconds were administered and lo and behold Rachel appeared. No bandage, no sling and a big smile on her face. "Well Nigel, it seems you are doing really well." We talked over the remaining sessions and the application of the various creams and created a plan of action.

"When the going gets tough"

When the going gets tough
The tough get going, tough, tough, huh, huh, huh
When the going gets tough, the tough get ready
Yeah, ooh, du da do da

I got something to tell you
I got something to say
I'm gonna put this dream in motion
Never let nothing stand in my way
When the going gets tough
The tough get going

I'm gonna get myself 'cross the river
That's the price I'm willing to pay
I'm gonna make you stand and deliver
And give me love in the old-fashion way
Woooh
Darlin', I'll climb any mountain
Darlin', I'll do anything

Ooh, can I touch you (can I touch you?)
And do the things that lovers do
Ooh, wanna hold you (wanna hold you)
I gotta get it through to you, ooooh
I'm gonna buy me a one-way ticket
Nothin's gonna hold me back

Your love's like a slow train coming (slow train coming)
And I feel it coming down the track (whoa)
Darlin', I'll climb any mountain
Darlin', I'll do anything
Ooh (ooh) can I touch you (can I touch you)

And do the things that lovers do
Ooh, (ooh) wanna hold you (wanna hold you)
I gotta get it through to you (ooh)
'Cause when the going gets tough
The tough get going
When the going gets rough
The tough get rough

Darlin', I'll climb any mountain
Darlin', I'll swim any sea
Darlin', I'll reach for the heaven
Darlin', with you lovin' me
Oooh (ooh)
Oooh, can I touch you (can I touch you)
And do the things that lovers do (can I touch you)
Oooh, wanna hold you (wanna hold you)
I gotta get it through to you

When the going gets tough
Going gets tough
Going gets rough
Going gets rough

WEEK FOUR - RESPONSES

21st July

"When the going gets tough
The tough go shopping?

Oh yes! - Trouble is there is a sale at my favourite menswear shop this Thursday - but I don't think they'd want me crapping all over the place would you?

I think of you each time I take a crap.... and count my blessings. On the other hand this body is celebrating being alive and treasuring the time it has on this tiny planet.

Your beautifully written reports are inspiring, shocking and informative. How blessed you are to have the wonderful Ric at your side, or should I say 'anus.'
All love and healing wishes to you dear friend
Martin xxx

*

Oh Nigel!!!

I so feel for you and your arse, why oh why does anybody have to go through such discomfort. I just don't know what to write apart from how brave you are and how I so appreciate all your descriptions.

I read each week twice as to make sure I don't miss any detail.

Thank god it all sounds as if you will be fine at the end of all this hell. Keep going and stay positive, you are so strong with it all I am completely amazed.

Sending you huge hugs and kisses Eunice xxx

*

Hi Nigel,

What a f....... awful week! Jesus. Thank God for the lovely Ric and for your ability to take each moment as it comes. And thank the Lord that you have a sense of humour throughout all this....and I don't mean ha ha, but the ability to experience this all and still be present and be very much You.

To be honest as gory as this is I do believe that sharing this is a gift. Thank you Mr. H. That's because sometimes we all become squeamish as to what it is to be human. I know I do. This is just telling it straight. Flipping hell I am just relieved that you have been spared a second chemo clobber. Reading this week's update has bought me out in a cold sweat and I'm willing the next Radiotherapy sessions to go easy on your poor regions. I don't want them hurting anymore. What a rollercoaster.

I'm willing your recovery and easing up of pain every night. Love to you Ann xx

*

Remind me not to sit next to you on the bus! Hehe!

I know this is a real physical and emotional roller coaster. I enjoy/value your storytelling. Thank god that in a few weeks, you will be in real recovery mode, and recovering from a disease that would have caused months of suffering and decline.

I feel your anguish and discomfort but celebrate your survival, and as I said before I cheer the army of strangers who did the science to make this happen for you.

Keep getting better, the world needs you... And who gives a shit about shits. We are all human; shits are brown and a bit smelly - so fucking what.

Life and love are all that matters!

What a journey, what a challenge. Thanks for be willing to share.

This chapter for me has some of your best writing, it is more sparse, more focused and so the narrative skips along. And of course the intimacy of the details is uncomfortable but humane and illuminating.

Love to you and Ric - Alan

*

Oh my god Nigel, this is as they say, 'some heavy shit'. I am really looking forward to seeing you both, IS it still ok to come? After reading your diary - it seems important to check again. Let me know as soon as you can - cos if I'm coming - it's tomorrow at 2:30 at Bury St Edmunds

Lots of love

Margot

WEEK FIVE - GANT ARE PANTS!

28th July

This coming week – 5.5 starting Monday 28 July - is just one more mountain to climb and one more river to cross – perhaps.

I go to Hamburg twice a year for one of my clients and it is a standing joke with my colleagues when we fly in and out of Hamburg Airport – there is a very convenient Gant outlet on the way to and from our arrival/departure gate. Usually, the flight home on a Friday evening, whether we fly BA or Lufthansa, is delayed, which gives me the perfect opportunity to drop in and replenish my underwear collection, in my view the most comfortable underwear ever! They are cotton, snug, support me in all the right places and come in multi-coloured packs. They are not cheap! But recently they have proved their worth and I am of a mind to write to Gant and tell them they have an added marketing opportunity. They are perfect as incontinence pants! (Details provided on request.)

This week has been the weirdest, most discombobulating week so far. There have been excellent highs and worrying lows and it has taught me to be absolutely in the moment and in touch with my natural rhythms - or else. As I wrote in last week's post came to last Monday with some trepidation and reluctance in the inevitable knowledge that there will be a decline in my fairly steady reaction to the radiotherapy. I did relish in the added knowledge that the second chemo was not going to happen – despite a momentary scare.

From Monday to Wednesday as the daily zap accumulated in my body, I had to integrate a mixture of stinging, burning, hot glass shard evacuations, interspersed with wallowing for a moments ease in a warm salt bath and the soothing cooling effect of the silver cream twice daily applied by my "reluctant carer".

I steeled myself every day for the unexpected and somehow got through the night with my hourly trips to my potty! Yet I gathered a sense of achievement every day as I counted down to the final treatment on 30 July. This was to be the second week of five in a row and I was unsure how even my so-called resilience was going to cope. Any time I was in doubt or fear I forced myself to focus on the five senses one by one to stay in the absolute present and to deal with whatever was going on with courage, tenacity, frustration, despair and yes to ensure that I was enjoying and celebrating the waves of ease and pleasure when I was not in pain.

I had a treat on Wednesday afternoon. I picked up Margot from Bury St Edmunds station and brought her home for a 24-hour visit. Margot lives in Auckland, and we met in 1988 where I led the first Creativity workshop there, The Mastery, and she now was on her way to a Group Psychotherapist's conference in Lisbon.

We enjoyed catching up after a 7 or 8 year gap. Yet even in our catch-up conversations the confusions penetrated. The daily news of the devastation, despair and destruction in Gaza infiltrated our consciousness and pulled me away from my own situation. The President of her pending conference is an Israeli and she was preparing for her group of 400 eminent psychotherapists to be debating the current situation. There were people suffering enormous painful losses and hardship as the conflict persisted and it made no sense to me how a few can inflict so much on others. Whichever side you are on, even if there are sides, the human condition is one thing and no-one seems to be considering the insects, the birds, the animals and other beings all caught up in this nightmare. Perhaps if the warring factions could all take a moment, stop, breathe and concentrate on their own five senses – they may come to their senses! But we are all fallible, I guess. She went off, both replenished by the hours in our peaceful surroundings but no clearer about what we could do as individuals to impact on Gaza.

With this in the back of my mind, we approached the final Rad Review with Dr Wilson.

We are now familiar with each other and as Ric and I enter his consulting room I indicate that I have something important to tell him that is not just about my medical situation. He unwittingly and conveniently asks about Dr Jephcott. "When did you last see her?" "Not since the first alarming consultation we had with her on May 23rd," says Ric. "Yes," I say. "In fact, that is the other thing that I would like to discuss please if it is appropriate. But shall we address the usual medical situation first?"

I go through the increasing effects of incontinence and more frequent bouts of neuropathy and how we are dealing with the accumulating impact of the radiotherapy burning my tender skin. All of which is no surprise to him and compassionately almost dismisses it with, 'to be expected' and 'you are at the height of the treatment regime now and the discomfort will continue for the next 10 days or so.' We have a detailed discussion about the use of the silver cream, and he contradicts the advice given by the radiography team and when challenged he says – "Well, I am only the Doctor they are more experienced in that area than I am." He does however suggest I include the 'more homeopathic approach' of taking additional Vitamin B. We agree that we will meet again three weeks after the last zap – around August 21st. "Just so I can check that everything is going according to plan and that your healing is progressing."

I bring up the enormous impact on us of the first consultation with Dr Jephcott. I explain that I realise Monday's clinic must be high pressure and difficult days for medical staff and patients alike and in that first and incredibly important meeting the Doctor has to deliver bad and unexpected news to a patient – it tests everyone's capacity to stay conscious and present.

With as much caring, empathy and understanding as I could muster, I did say that I was particularly alarmed with Dr Jephcott's communication style and how she handled that particular moment. She presented us with the facts and then without much pause for us to digest those facts she rattled through the possible and devastating list of side effects if I was to follow her considered treatment plan – and ended with an implied threat that if I didn't there would be even more dire and serious consequences.

Dr Wilson took in this information as best he could and, still calmly, he began to defend the situation. He described what we already knew that they were under enormous pressure and suffered compassion fatigue at the end of the day and he had to restore his spirits with a bottle of wine. He added that Dr Jephcott was a respected and valuable doctor and team member and in fact her eye for detail and programme planning was an enormous asset. He also rather sheepishly admitted that this was not the first time he had had this kind of feedback about her delivery style – which other people seemed to like.

It was therefore pointless to continue the discussion and I felt we had made our point and as a medical doctor he was of course the expert but as a team leader he was lacking. I made a note to self with my training cap on and spotted an opportunity to be followed up at a later date. We parted amicably.

My system by now was a little out of kilter, having had its rhythm upset by a delay due to this lengthy meeting. I also had to pick up more silver cream from the dispensary with a further 25-minute delay as Ric went to mess up the flat to make our presence felt. Finally, we had to get petrol otherwise we would not get back to Lawshall.

The consequence was that I went unconscious and did not heed the warning signs as we were driving past Cambridge Airport on our homeward journey – an unusual route – and lo and behold the call of nature descended in a flash and I said to Ric "Oh dear, I'm in trouble." He knew immediately what I meant, and I found a small layby where I pulled in with no time to scape to the side of the road and let rip - thereby testing Gant pants.

WEEK FIVE - RESPONSES

28th July

Hi Nigel,

Thank God for the Gants. A blooming blessing! Like the picture of you in your towel skirt...I'm not sure it will catch on though this season.

Counting down for you through the next few days.

This is such an amazingly painful thing to receive. To know how much pain you are in the midst of. However it is also uplifting and inspiring as its comforting to know that just breaking things down into those pain free moments and using the senses during the painful ones keeps us able to cope and get through.

I love the quote about how we are all so busy consuming and doing that we aren't even aware of being.

Willing that there will be moments of relief during the next week.

Counting down the moments. Love. Ann x

*

Just read week 5 - much lighter I detect, particularly the Gant references. But no song this week. (I can't say I'm sorry - singing isn't my natural talent!!)

Good luck on the continued climb back to full health.

John

29th July

Poem for the day after tomorrow by anon:

If life seems at its lowest ebb,
Because a day's gone wrong.
Let not your heart be troubled,
For a new day soon will dawn
And we can never be quite sure,
Just what it has in store.
Since each one is so different,
Than the one just gone before
As it penetrates the darkness,
With its soft and tranquil beams.
It calms even the most restless soul,
And brings new hopes and dreams
So when a day's been troubled,
And the night is dark and long.
Lift up your fallen spirits,
For a new day soon will dawn

30th July

Dear Nigel,
I am so impressed by your strength. Both in your own process and at the same time look at the process from the side.
Just to take the opportunity to give the doctor feedback is not an easy thing. I can understand they need a deep communication training to understand how terrifying it is for a person to be delivered hard information.

I am thinking of you, and I send you all my good and best thoughts and feelings.

Your friend
Lena

30th July

Dear Nigel,
I always thought it was going to get harder before it got better and I think your latest journal reflects that, so my feelings are absolutely with you.

Michael.

31st July

Hi Nige

I'm working backwards as I've just read Week 5.
I have observed you as a Gant man, by your pants, in working with you, (as in American
'Pants'). I'm a Gant girl too, although not pants. Might have to try em.

Thank you for the snapshot into your life, which you would never know from your work emails. Thanks for reminding me of the brilliance of Alan Watts too.

The Bristol Palestine group have 'occupied' the BBC on Whiteladies Road. They've covered the outside of the building with banners and posters and have an info table And have been holding a vigil for over a week - makes me proud to live here today!

Namaste
Susie

*

Dear Nigel

Great to get your recent No 5 missive and lovely to see you both outside your cottage.

Writing this from a little bar in Plestin, North Brittany - where I have managed to connect to wi-fi - rather a difficult thing to do in this rather remote area.

We are coming to the end of our almost two week holiday and come home late on Friday - it's been good to be out in the countryside and the weather has been pretty good for this rainy area - but we have both had bad backs! As mine has got better Michael has got one. I think this rather shows the rather stressed state we came to Brittany with.

Have felt very sad at the death of Robin Williams and the thought that life is so fragile and hard to live at times - even to someone with so much talent and a family life too. Reading Ruby Wax's book on depression and mindfulness at the moment and happy that I feel so much calmer these days - although it has taken a lot of years and fear can still well up when I get overwhelmed or shocked.

Your No 5 missive really gets across how on the edge it felt about getting to your consultant but fortunately you managed it, and it sounds like you are really well supported by her - how important to have another 'arm' of help alongside the hospital.

Signs are you are recovering well.

Much love from us both,

C and M

WEEK SIX

4 August 2014

Imagine you are sitting in the back garden of our 400-year-old Suffolk Cottage, it is around 8.40, twilight is looming. In front of you there is the wildflower meadow bedraggled and waiting to be cut. In the distant next field cows are grazing their cut meadow. To your right climbing up the back wall of the cottage are multi-coloured sweet peas – their scent wafting over and eclipsing your apple juice or Becks. Next to the sweet peas, two evening primrose plants standing about three feet tall with many stems holding tight buds and many flowers already bloomed and gone.

As the light fades, one by one the buds transform. Little by little over about twenty minutes, some invisible force sends energy up the stem and fills each bud to stretch itself. Suddenly the sepals holding each delicate flower retract, snap open and hey presto – the flower begins to open revealing its pollen laden stamen and celebrates its pale-yellow beauty. Magically just as it gets dark, the dog star rises over a perfect new moon, the Pipistrelle bats begin to flip and swoop overhead and the evening primrose moth flutters, lands and drinks.

A summer idyll? A romantic fantasy? No - It is our new evening entertainment! Just as the bee orchid became my sentinel for the beginning of this journey, now the evening primrose with its delicate and delightful transformation has become my new totem.

Monday 4 August - Climbing down the mountain.

After the jubilation of completing my 28 radiotherapy sessions, almost intact last Wednesday, I find myself in a strange state of more confusion, frustration, impatience and facing the inevitability of change. And time passes in a mysterious haze.

As promised the last few days have been progressively more uncomfortable as my body absorbs and desperately tries to adjust to the changes of the last five and a half weeks of nuclear attack. It seems I have been fortunate in escaping some of the major side effects – e.g. nausea, diarrhoea and haemoglobin depletion. But I have suffered other common ailments such as incontinence, bowel disruption, bladder shrinkage and mostly chronic skin cracking and breaking, causing severe soreness and discomfort, sitting walking and lying. The unexpected and most surprising is neuropathy where intermittently I get tingling and numbness in my toes and legs and my lumber region fizzes!

I approached last Monday with even more mixed feelings than each previous week, knowing it was my last and also knowing it may be the worst. My resolve to continue "being in charge" persisted as I chose to drive myself the last three times to 'Cambridge Health City', but I did make one concession – I allowed Ric to accompany me just in case. Counting and monitoring each minute and second of each journey and treatment became an obsession. Staying in touch with my tumultuous feelings was paramount. I knew that I could become unaware at any moment and opt out and surrender not in a good way. So, it took enormous effort to manage myself on all levels and accept all the generosity that was offered.

What I have learned or been reminded of is that relationships are what makes my world go round. Friends. 'A friend in need is a friend indeed' has been tested many times over. And for me to constantly ask my friends and family for help and support has been a lesson in humility. And the response has been remarkable. In many and diverse ways people have come up trumps through their generosity of time, personal visits, sending gifts, cards, notes, cooking special food, massage, reflexology, cranial therapies, texts, jokes, rude pictures, comments on my posts and the sharing of their own past or current painful experiences. I have discovered a new level of intimacy and trust which has been enlightening and hugely supportive.

What I have also been reminded of is that climbing down a mountain can sometimes be more of a challenge than climbing up. One literally has to change one's view! On the ascent of course there is the dream, the hope, the vision, the adrenalin and the drive to reach the top to see the stunning view or even just to say, "I did it". And often the reward is resting on the top and eating the prepared picnic while basking in the glow of satisfaction. But I once heard that most accidents happen when descending. People can become careless and reckless, or their tiredness can overtake them and make them choose the wrong path, or they stumble and fall because they are not paying attention to each step in the rush to get down and back to base camp, the car, the bath or the shower or mostly in my case the tea shop! So, since last Wednesday I am being mindful of the constant changes in my physical, mental and emotional states. On Thursday evening, only about 30 hours since my final 'Timo' zap, I found myself saying to Ric "I have run out of ways of dealing with this discomfort. I don't know how to lie, or sit, or stand or walk or even breathe anymore!" Then I remind myself of the inscription on my silver 25th anniversary ring I wear: *"This too will change."* -

And this song:

Changes

I still don't know what I was waiting for
And my time was running wild
A million dead-end streets
Every time I thought I'd got it made
It seemed the taste was not so sweet
So I turned myself to face me
But I've never caught a glimpse
Of how the others must see the faker
I'm much too fast to take that test

Ch-ch-ch-ch-Changes (Turn and face the strain)
Ch-ch-Changes
Don't want to be a richer man
Ch-ch-ch-ch-Changes (Turn and face the strain)
Ch-ch-Changes
Just gonna have to be a different man
Time may change me
But I can't trace time

I watch the ripples change their size
But never leave the stream
Of warm impermanence and
So the days float through my eyes
But still the days seem the same
And these children that you spit on
As they try to change their worlds
Are immune to your consultations
They're quite aware of what they're going through

Ch-ch-ch-ch-Changes (Turn and face the strain)
Ch-ch-Changes
Don't tell them to grow up and out of it
Ch-ch-ch-ch-Changes (Turn and face the strain)
Ch-ch-Changes
Where's your shame
You've left us up to our necks in it
Time may change me
But you can't trace time

Strange fascination, fascinating me
Changes are taking the pace I'm going through

Ch-ch-ch-ch-Changes (Turn and face the strain)
Ch-ch-Changes
Oh, look out you rock 'n rollers
Ch-ch-ch-ch-Changes (Turn and face the strain)
Ch-ch-Changes
Pretty soon you're gonna get a little older Time may change me
But I can't trace time

WEEK SIX - RESPONSES

31st July

YIPPEE! Yesterday I had my final radiotherapy session, and I am now in my three/four week recovery period at home.

IF any of you fancy a day out in gorgeous Suffolk - now is the time. I can promise you a delicious home grown lunch, fresh from the garden and I double promise you won't have to do any of the "nasty bits" as described in my recent posts.

SO if you fancy it...
Cheers, Nigel and Ric
Xxx

*

5th August

Hi Nod,

It was good to see you the other day, but I do wish I could have stayed longer. I love you guys and miss you both - I hope to come again very soon, without kids, cause I really need to catch up with you and other friends. Thanks a million for sending these! It's a hard read, but ultimately good to hear your story. 1 part read, 5 more to go, keep em coming!

Sending love and cuddles,

Seth xxx

*

What beautiful pictures and descriptions of the scene from your back garden. I remember it so well - easeful, relaxed times in gorgeous surroundings.

What an ascent it has been for you - and sounds as if you have walked the path, with all its tough terrain with courage and determination, doing what you can and accepting what you can't.

I am not surprised that your friends and family have come forth with their offerings of love and friendship and sounds as if the receiving of this has been the sweet nectar in a painful and challenging time.

May the descent bring stopping places to sit awhile and replenish, to enjoy the views with Ric, to look back over your shoulder and see how far you have come, and to be able to take the journey at your own pace.

Lots of love,
Terry xx

6th August

Nod,

It's great to hear you've come to the end of your treatments, and I hope with all my heart you're well on the road to a full recovery. As I mentioned in my text earlier today I'm really grateful you sent me this blog and that I could share in the journey you are making.

However, it has left me feeling a little inadequate and insensitive. With hindsight I guess it must have been about Easter that you called, and I was driving so you spoke to Suzanne.

Perhaps it was your intention to speak about your condition then or perhaps you just needed to reconnect with some people who have not featured in your life in recent years as they might have done. Either way, Suzanne and I failed to notice that anything was amiss, and I never called you back assuming from the conversation with Sue that all was well.

More recently though we came to visit you, still none the wiser, and I guess I must have, rather selfishly, gone on about my life and never left an opportunity for you speak of your own plight. It must have been hard to hold on to that but, as usual, you seemed interested and engaged so I still didn't notice anything was afoot. I'm sorry.

I'm not getting back to Suffolk as much as I'd like at the moment, but I am in the process of trying to buy a car, so impromptu visits should become more common. I'd love to get back and see you (hopefully Richard too next time) and will endeavour to do so as soon as I can.

In the meantime, I'm thinking of you often.

Love,
Matthew xx

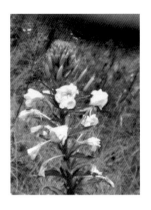
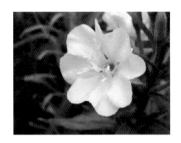

10th August

Nigel, how wonderful to imagine sitting with you & Richard sipping tea in the almost 400 year old garden of your Suffolk Cottage ~ but more than that, seeing you in the fading light, healthy and gaining energy and strength. Quite like you were when you were feeling the rhythm of your days and evenings. The way you were before you had to adjust to the rhythm of doctors & treatments, which you did brilliantly. And I remember the conversation we had about working together when you were here & I hope we can re-visit that conversation sometime soon.

Sending you love my friend,

Sal.

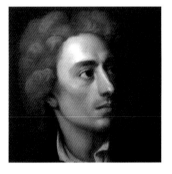

'Hope springs eternal in the human breast;
Man never is, but always to be blest.
The soul, uneasy, and confin'd from home,
Rests and expatiates in a life to come.'

Alexander Pope

94.

WEEK SEVEN - HOPE SPRINGS ETERNAL

11 August 2014

Today, as I approach the beginning of week eight and see eleven days drift into the dimming distance since my last radio zap, I have a huge amount of hope in my heart and body, with the occasional set back due primarily to my – impatience!

Last week saw two major turning points – number one a day trip to London, number two picking up the pace of my morning walk to almost normal speed. And an intimate third (!) Perhaps I will award a prize for an appropriate song this week????.

On Tuesday I fell in love. I was totally smitten. It encouraged my healing journey at a staggering rate. But on Monday 4th August evening between 9 and 11 it was a very different story. There was a long-term plan that once I had finished my regular Addenbrookes rigorous routine of daily radiotherapy, I would visit the Royal London Hospital for Integrated Medicine (RLHIM) and seek advice and guidance from the homeopathic approach. I had done my research and come up with Dr Sosie Kassab. Her CV was just the ticket, a sound background in regular medical oncology plus 25 years' experience of integrating the homeopathic methodology of looking at the complete patient picture and treating accordingly.

But to get there and to see her I had to climb Mount Everest, K9, Snowdon, Ben Nevis and any other mountain you could imagine in the space of 17 hours, checking outer garments, crampons, oxygen, fighting numbness and tingling in all parts of my anatomy, mind and emotions.

On Monday, as I was preparing to go to bed after a fairly positive day of rest and recuperation, good food and gentle loving care again from Ric, suddenly around 9 pm I went into what I consider now in retrospect was unconscious confusion, panic and fear.

My body turned somersaults that effected my mind and emotions, and I ended up on the precipice not knowing which way to turn, jump or fly.

The skin that had been healing relatively well suddenly erupted in dry itching and burning and internal pressure caused me to hover around the bathroom for ages not knowing if I was going to pass wind, do an enormous dump – or what. I ended up doing it all. Finally, Ric got hold of my feet and found a way literally to anchor me and I settled for the night. BUT in the morning as I went on my usual morning walk, the discomfort returned, which knocked my confidence. I didn't know if I was going to be able to sit in the car for a two-hour drive, sit in the hospital waiting room, see Dr Kassab and do the return journey in one piece. So how to approach this moment? – like climbing any mountain – have a clear view of the task at hand and do it step by step. I packed all the necessary materials, change of underwear, trousers, yoghurt pots to pee in, flannels, wet wipes, toilet roll, and a new addition – incontinence pants (just in case the Gants failed) - cushions and blankets to make me comfortable in the back seat. I felt like an incontinent 95-year-old. Minute by minute as the departure time of 11 am approached I oscillated wildly between "Yes I can" "No I can't" and "I bloody well will!" At 10.58 I said to Ric "OK let's go – but we may have to turn around at any time." Well – we did it. We arrived in Queen Square and even found a parking place without any incident or accident on the way. Ric, usually a hesitant London driver sailed through without a hitch. We approached RLHIM with a degree of achievement 40 minutes early, registered with the receptionist and waited.

A very different atmosphere from Addenbrookes. As soon as I entered, I felt humanity and care was number one on the agenda and people first seemed to be their ethos. We sat and made ourselves comfortable, Ric went to find some lunch for himself – I could not risk eating or drinking anything until our return journey, and we had reached the safety of the countryside again. We sat and made our list of questions for Dr Kassab.

As soon I saw her – that was it! A woman I am guessing in her mid-forties, about 5'9" tall, elegantly dressed in a 50's retro figure-hugging floral-patterned dress, her black and slightly greying hair swept into a sort of French roll, which set off her high cheek bones, strong jaw and pale blue eyes.

96.

She approached us and wondered which the patient was for a second. I introduced myself and Ric and she said, "OK, you look fairly relaxed sitting there, I have one patient with pins in at the moment and another one to see before you. I shall be about 25 minutes." "Have we met before?" "Only by e mail" I said. "Oh yes, I remember." And off she glided. I looked at Ric and we nodded. We both knew there was someone definitely at home!

While waiting we were sat in the perfect position to see the parade of the diversity of London patients on display. The hospital costume department had been really busy as people dressed in saris, hijabs, abayas, Kurtis, kaftans, shorts and tee shirts entered. More people wearing turbans and head gear of multi colours. The makeup and hairdressing department had also exceeded themselves as we saw incredible styles of swept up, swept back, curled around, over and under, tinted this, dyed that, eyes and lips accentuated in glorious Technicolor and various arrays as the multi cultured assembled.

"Ok – I'm ready. Follow me." Dr Kassab escorted us down the short corridor, picked up a leaflet from the dispenser outside her consulting room and invited us to sit. "What do you like to be called?" "Nigel." She looked directly into my eyes, and we began our instant love affair. Her manner was open, curious, and attentive and she seemed to listen with every pore open and with her heart on her sleeve there was instant rapport and intimacy. Her questioning was direct, relevant and acute without being at all threatening. With every answer I gave she gave a small grunt of acknowledgement. She referred to everything she recommended in the first person as if she also had experienced my condition. There was absolute clarity in her knowledge, and she never hesitated when she gave an opinion – yes, no, or maybe – which made me trust her 25 years of experience. She assured me that Addenbrookes had taken the right course of action and was keen to now add the holistic approach at the same time honouring the regular straight medical route. She was also keen not to raise false hopes or to misrepresent the value of homoeopathy. The outcome was for her to prescribe three things: mistletoe in drop form, which she says provides greater efficiency according to recent tests, some other drops to help my skin repair itself and a third set of drops to assist my incontinence.

"Now if I may, I am really curious to know about your cultural heritage? Kassab. Where does this come from?" "Iraq." "Oh, we have taken three or four steps into Iraq from Iran a couple of years ago," says Ric and relates the story - when we were in Southwest Iran we were sneaked across the armed border by three young guards who wanted a photo opportunity. The love match was complete.

And after 1 hour and fifteen minutes we were saying our goodbyes in the corridor when another level of conversation sprang up. She asked about my work and was intrigued and delighted when I told her of my theatre-based leadership work, and we shared another passion. I also noticed that there was a campaign on to help save the RLHIM from closure. So there and then I pledged allegiance to her cause, and we agreed to meet outside the consulting room at a later date to continue this conversation.

Literally reeling with pleasure Ric (as he was also rather taken with Sosie) and I made our way back to the car, navigated the growing London rush hour and reached the countryside border. I ate the pre-prepared snack Ric had provided and we enjoyed driving slowly back on the gently winding Essex and Suffolk country roads away from the scrabble and rabble.

Having completed this milestone, morning walking became easier as my skin healed, and my confidence returned. Each day I have upped my morning walk pace and enjoyed not suddenly having to duck behind a bush and get stung by nettles to discharge! The warm summer weather has added to my enjoyment, and I even basked in the occasional glow for a few minutes.

And speaking of hope springing eternal – well – one day something else sprang involuntarily – yes – an erection! ...

WEEK SEVEN - RESPONSES

11th August

Lovely writing. And there was quite a surprise at the end of that update! Glad to hear you're in working order.
One step (stiffie) at a time.

Mark

*

Ha-ha, for some strange reason I only read the last line so far... so... congratulations!!! :)

Seth

12th August

Dear Nigel & Ric

I have just had breakfast (chapatti, cauliflower and cabbage kedgeree, apple and apricot jam and chai) on a low table, humming fan, 30 degree heat and high humidity with a Buddhist monk and a Japanese academic (here collecting Hindi folk tales for a paper he will deliver in Japan in September).

Bit of a switch from the 5 star, glass fronted, Pullman Hotel in Gurgaon.

Enjoyed very much, week 7. It made me think of something from the wonderful movie The Lunchbox (Saw on plane over)

'The wrong train can take you to the right station'

Your accounts have to be published, they will give inspiration and practical guidance to others who follow.

The song......??? Well it has to be "HERE COMES THE SUN"

Because the opening guitar riff perfectly fits your account, as well as the lyrics.

Trust me I'm a DJ.
Susie xxx

*

Men get naughty at four O "40".......and the trend continues. Enjoy the tingling feeling :)

Love, Sanah

13th August

Hi, This all sounds so much better, so pleased.
And as for the erection, well about time!!!!
Much Love and enjoy Rowena and Jeroen visit.

Eunice x

*

Dearest Nod,

It's with both tears and laughter that I enjoy your progress reports. Think you should turn them into a book at some point! And I am SOOOOO glad that your manliness is stirring despite all the challenges. Isn't it lovely when you meet someone you can trust implicitly with your welfare.
Well done for getting there. And interesting about mistletoe drops!!

I know I have some information for you re: how to inhibit Angiogenesis. Here we go...

Angiogenesis is the natural process by which the body creates new blood supplies to particular areas to promote growth and healing. It helps with wound healing and also in women with foetal growth/menstruation.

Cancer cells, both primary and secondaries rely on it, negatively speaking, to provide new blood supply and hence food for a developing tumour.
A wonderful doctor Dr David Servan-Schreiber has written a book called 'anti-cancer, a new way of life. It is fairly scientific, but I have adopted a few of his diet recommendations which I wanted to share with you. Basically he is using certain foods as medicines:

Green Tea, pref. Japanese-A powerful antioxidant and detoxifier (activates enzymes in the liver that eliminate toxins. Steep 2 grams for 10 mins. 6 cups a day if you can.
Turmeric- a very powerful anti-inflammatory but needs to be taken with black pepper to be assimilated. Mix 1/4 tsp with good pinch of black pepper and 1/2 tsp olive oil, stir to a paste and eat alongside or mix with food.
Ginger-a powerful anti-inflammatory and anti-oxidant, more than Vit E Eat raw cooked or steeped as a tea.
Cruciform veg- Cabbage, sprouts, broccoli, cauli etc. Contain chemicals which can detoxify certain cancerous substances and they promote Apoptosis...suicide of cancer cells.

Onion family-Leeks onions garlic shallots chives. Contain chemicals that help to regulate blood sugar levels and hence reduce insulin secretion and IGF (insulin growth like factor) and hence the growth of cancer cells.
Orange fruit and veg including tomatoes-Contain Vit A and lycopene which stimulate the growth of immune cells and their ability to destroy cancer cells. Mushrooms also do this especially the more unusual ones.

Omega 3's - Long chain O 3's reduce inflammation and help to prevent metastasis. Oily fish especially small ones like sardines, flaxseed ground up. The important oils to use are linseed (flax) olive oil or canola oil. Other oils contain too much O 6 and therefore upset the delicate balance of 3/6/9.

Berries-ALL stimulate the mechanisms of elimination of carcinogenic substances and inhibit angiogenesis.

Citrus and pomegranate juice also good dietary additions
Other additions- Probiotics/Vitamin D foods rich in Selenium

Hope this is useful Nod. By the way are you about next Monday around lunch time. I am coming to a women's group reunion and would love to pop in.

Heaps of love. Lindsey

WEEK EIGHT - HERE WE ARE...

18 August 2014

You and I

Here we are on earth together,
It's you and I,
God has made us fall in love, it's true,
I've really found someone like you

Will it stay the love you feel for me,
Will it say that you will be by my side
To see me through,
Until my life is through

Well, in my mind, we can conquer the world,
In love you and I, you and I, you and I

I am glad at least in my life I found someone
That may not be here forever to see me through,
But I found strength in you.
I only pray that I have shown you a brighter day,
Because that is all that I am living for, you see,
Don't worry what happens to me
'Cause in my mind, you will stay here always
In love, you and I, you and I
You and I

Well, that is the song that I sang to and for my friend Ray Evans on 13th August 1999, the day before he died 15 years ago and at his funeral a week later.

It is this same song that I sang to you all as I walked along the long pebble and sand beach last weekend in Aldeburgh, to celebrate my growing wellness.

This Monday 18 August Ric and I drove to Cambridge and 'Health City' from our first weekend away in our favourite room in our favourite seaside Hotel, The Brudenell. We luxuriated for three full days in our deluxe sea view room, taking all our meals by room service so we could revel in the 2nd floor vista of the ever-changing sea and sky. The wind couldn't make up its mind in which direction to blow from or too – so much so that the flag outside our room ended up completely swirled and twirled around the flagpole in glorious confusion.

We had promised ourselves a bit of a break and change of scenery once I felt I was secure enough to leave the confines of my convalescent home in Lawshall Green. And of course, my reluctant carer needed a break from caring and cooking and all the intimate stuff he has been subjected to over the last four weeks. So, to celebrate my massive skin improvement and no longer a need for Ric to administer the various lotions and potions since last Wednesday and my ability to conduct my morning walk almost without incident, off we toddled on Friday with our metaphorical buckets and spades. It worked a treat; you know what they say about sea air – "it refreshes the parts other air cannot reach" (sic) and we tested it to its full and I am happy to announce that all parts are again in full working order. The various heavy-handed warnings of erectile dysfunction, dry ejaculation and loss of libido thankfully are not present in this survivor!

Since June 25th we have been completely concentrating firstly on my daily treatment and then on my daily recovery process and we noticed day by day the ups and downs of the cancer survivor process. Our creativity thankfully was also challenged and employed by working together on draft 6 of Ric's "Farm Play" which is very nearly completed.

The past seven weeks exactly matched and mapped the same time span 15 years ago when Hana, Matt and I were the chief carers to our dear friend Ray. He sadly did not survive the process, but he did teach us all how to face the end of life with spirit, passion, dignity and humour. So, in my mind I have been re-living those parallel weeks 15 years ago and calling upon his spirit to help guide me through. His soothing voice has often reverberated around my mind, body and spirit when I have needed extra support. So, it was with a real sense of gratitude that I walked along Aldeburgh beach and sang out strongly to thank him for all his excellent spiritual support. And it was also with gratitude that I sang it to each and every one of you who have also supported me in many, many ways. And it is each and every one of you that I love.

Back to this Monday and the drive to Addenbrookes 'Health City'. As we clocked up the 77 miles trundling along the A14 once again on a very familiar journey I also began to experience some familiar thoughts and feelings. It was only by staying very present and checking my physical sensations that I was able to gage my progress since my last visit there. I was a little trepidatious about whom we might be seen by, as it was the regular Monday colorectal clinic I was attending, and I was slightly fearful that I may encounter 'the enemy' – Dr Jephcott. I was concerned, if it was our luck to see her, about how I would behave and I began to practice some opening lines like, "Well this is a big surprise" to "I'm not sure this is appropriate, can I see another Doctor."

We arrived on time, registered, and was told with some certainty that they were on schedule and that I may even be seen slightly early. We settled in the larger waiting room, and I was almost immediately called – but only to be weighed. 70 kgs. I think I may have lost about 3 kgs in the process, but no one seems concerned. And when I asked if I needed to have my bloods taken, I was told, "If they need bloods, it will happen after you see the Doctor." So, we waited and Ric in his impatience to get home started twittering about nothing and whinging about everything, so I suggested he either shuts up, goes shopping or reads one of the delectable magazines.

Having discovered my reading glasses, he plumped for one of the books in the waiting room library. As we waited far longer than anticipated I noticed he read the first chapter and then the last and just as I was about to comment I noticed… her. My stomach turned a big somersault, and I tapped Ric on the shoulder and said, "Look who it is!" He didn't quite catch on and by the time he had re-focused she was out of sight. "Oh dear" I said, "looks like our luck has run out." 10 minutes later I approached the receptionist again and remarked that I was now over 30 minutes late for my appointment; she rang the consulting rooms and said, "There are three ahead of you and all doctors are there in the clinic, so it shouldn't be long now."

Almost as soon as I settled again, I was called. We were taken into the consulting room suite where we had our initial horrendous consultation with Dr Jephcott. I began to feel decidedly twitchy, by now sure that we were going to repeat the experience. BUT as chance (or probably design) had it, we had a very warm welcome from Dr David Noble who gave us both a hearty and warm handed handshake saying, "Very nice to see you again, please take a seat and we can see how you are progressing." With great relief I reminded him of the last time we encountered each other the day when the clinic was over-full, and he kindly came off his ward duties to check up on me because I had questions about the second proposed chemo treatment. "Oh yes" he said, "that was not a good day, and I was very sorry to keep you waiting amid all the confusion." "Anyway, how are you today?"

I noticed that he wasn't the "tall, dark and handsome" man of the first impression but rather thinning dark hair that would fit a Jewish kippah perfectly. And the more he listened the more Jewish he became. Sadly, under these hurried circumstances there was not time for he and Ric to share their common cultural heritage.

However, I went through my diminishing list of current side effects, skin healing well, neuropathy less irritating, more bladder and bowel control with fewer accidents. BUT a persistent internal ache and discomfort with the occasional sharp shooting pain and still sandpaper-like burning when passing motions.

"All this is to be expected at this still relatively early stage of your recovery. Let me have a look." He was very satisfied with what he saw and noticed that the skin healing process was well on target and remarked that yes, even though the anus itself was still a little raw it should be settling down in the next week or so.

Then we started our questions. "What do you recommend we do next to hasten the healing and when will I know if I have made a full recovery?" He confirmed that the muscles will need significant re-training and the recommended pelvic floor exercises would certainly help to regain control. This may take some time, months and even years, for the neural pathways to be completely re-educated. "You may never be the same again, so it is all about managing your situation carefully."

We talked about my visit to RLHIM and Dr Sosie Kassab which brought him on to the question of diet and still recommending a low fibre option as much as possible. And finally, I asked, "When do I expect my next internal examination?" "Now I think would not be a good time as we would probably scrape you off the roof! So, I suggest in six weeks' time when I expect everything to have settled down." "And is it a EUA?" "No that won't be necessary." "And what might you be looking for exactly?" "Well in your low-risk case we expect to find that the lesions will have healed and there may be some residual scar tissue and to the experienced finger we can ascertain that in a few seconds." "OK, thanks and if I get an inexperienced finger?" "Well in that case and if there is any doubt then a more experienced finger will explore!" "Mmmm – and will this be the same day or later?" "The same day." "Well then if I can have any sway in the matter may I request the experienced finger first please?" As you can imagine we are having this as an extremely serious conversation but at the same time our collective smile creases in our faces are beginning to be visible! We fix a date, 29th September six weeks from now and he confirms that all being well (which he expects), the next CT scan will be fixed for around the 25th July 2015, with quarterly check-ups 'til then.

Ric asked the final killer recurring question: "And Nigel's proposed USA trip in 2 weeks – what is your view?" "No problem, you will run a higher risk of DVT (deep vein thrombosis) but as long as you stay active on the flight – take a one-off dose of aspirin and decline alcohol and drink plenty of water to keep flushing." When I say I have the privilege of flying flatbed business class he said, "Well it is a pleasure I am yet to experience, but that will certainly help a great deal especially if you keep flexing your ankles and shins to activate the blood pump."

With a little urgency and without being rude he excused himself, wished us well and set off for his next patient.

Here we are, on earth together it's you and I…. and I have eternal gratitude.

WEEK EIGHT - RESPONSES

Dearest Niggly,

It's our last but one day here in France and great to hear this latest instalment. It sounds like you are on the upward healing curve, and it is so good to hear that!

Yes Ray has been present with me too. Albert is getting to know him a little too because he is in the home videos of some of our coop parties from the 80s which will be part of Alberts next film piece Another Utopia.

Great to know that your libido is still strong and all in working order there!

Will give a call when I am back next week.

Lots of love, Rob

*

Dearest Nige,

This is a very wonderful report, and I can't tell you how glad I am that you have such incredible powers of healing – body/mind/spirit all seems to be doing the job so very well thanks to your awareness. I remember you singing to Ray at his memorial. As I just read the words, the whole scene came flooding back and then a string of memories of him at his finest. What a dear man and spiritual teacher for many of us, in all his whole-ness.

I fly off to the States in a couple of hours. A week of work and then a week of family visits. Looking forward although a little reluctant as ever to leave the veg patch at this time of year!

LOVE and huge hugs to you both, Mag

*

Dear, dear, dear Nigel and Ric.

My eyes are filled with tears of joy.
I am so happy for both of you, and Nigel I knew that you are a fighter and you have shown the world and yourself that.

Thank you for opening your heart with your pen. I am looking so much forward to see you later this autumn in London.

Some news.... Last week I bought a flat in Palma. You are so welcome next year to visit me. 3 bedrooms... large terrace

Best from your friend

Lena

*

This is such a vivid walk into your world. Thank you. I'm so glad you didn't get the Doctor that was so lacking in compassion. I'm glad some healing is starting and I'm wishing ya love in that continuing.

That hotel by the sea sounded brilliant.. I could see you walking/singing on the beach!!

Ann xx

*

Just read your story from an 18th century colonial home in down east Maine, overlooking a large wild meadow with glimpses of the sea in the distance. I brought my mother here, 95 years young, or as she'd be sure to point out, 95-and-a-half now, and my increasingly ancient beloved dog, so the fragility and preciousness of life is as inescapable as the tides along the beach.

Every year in mid-August, whether I consciously remember at first or not, I wake up with a profound ache, a body memory for our dear friend Ray. This year was no different. How glad I am to know he was with you on this journey Nigel, and how glad I am to hear how you have passed through the eye of this storm and are healing so fully. Sending you and Ric all my love, and you too Sally -- thank you both for invoking our Ray's honey-tongued words and wisdom. Love, Matt

*

Well my dear old friend, this all sounds very encouraging.

What a time you've had, both of you I'm delighted that you seem to be emerging from this situation with your humanity intact and your sense of Gratitude paramount. How wonderful to revisit Ray's episode and gain from that.

He was a wonderful person too, just like you.

Isn't simply being alive truly amazing?!

All success with the USA trip and fly high all the way there and back, Because we all love you dearly. Martin XXX

*

Dear, dear Ray, such sweet, sweet friendship you and he shared. These moments in life are so full of pain and the sweetness of friendship, loved ones and humanity.

I am so pleased Nigel that you are recovering well - with all your determination and ability to ride the turbulent waves. May the storm continue to subside, and the waves gently lap and soothe.

I am looking forward to seeing you tomorrow and giving you a gentle hug. Please send my love to Ric.

Lots of love,
Terry xx

*

Thank you for your thoughtful and thought provoking letters Nigel, I hope they helped you as much as they helped me to understand what you have been going through. Tough times. As an (ex)-medic and currently in drug development, it is always good to get a reminder about what it is like to be on the receiving end of some of these harsher treatments.

Maybe I will see you in SSF in Sept.

Have a good and uneventful flight and a safe landing.

Take care, Alissa

WEEK NINE - UP, UP AND AWAY

Would you like to ride in my beautiful balloon?
Would you like to glide in my beautiful balloon?
We could float among the stars together, you and I
For we can fly, we can fly
Up, up and away
My beautiful, my beautiful balloon

The world's a nicer place in my beautiful balloon
It wears a nicer face in my beautiful balloon
We can sing a song and sail along the silver sky
Suspended under a twilight canopy
We'll search the clouds for a star to guide us
If by some chance you find yourself loving me
We'll find a cloud to hid us, keep the moon beside us

Love is waiting there in my beautiful balloon
Way up in the air in my beautiful balloon
If you'll hold my hand we'll chase your dream across the sky
For we can fly, we can fly
Up, up and away
My beautiful, my beautiful balloon

Saturday 30 August - on board Virgin Atlantic VS19
bound for San Francisco!

Well, I made it! But not in a balloon!

113.

This has been one of my long-term, carefully planned and risk-assessed goals. I am in seat A1 – which seems very fitting in the circumstances, and I realise how privileged I am to be here. On the top deck – just behind the pilots (and adjacent to the toilets!). I have been visualising with a strong and intended determination of being here today. It signifies a degree of confidence, willingness, risk and trust. It feels like a reward, but begs the question – why should I be rewarded when many in a similar situation like mine would not be? So, I do not take it for granted, and give myself and Ric, the medical team, my supporters and carers, my family and friends a big pat on the back. Phew.

As I sprawl on my flatbed, I muse about the last 12 days which have been eventful since my last visit to 'Health City' and my future finger up the bum conversation with Dr Noble.

Step one: The first test to meet my intended goal was attending Georg's (Ric's brother-in-law) 80th birthday celebrations. This involved a two and a half hour each way car journey, sitting through an hour's concert, afternoon tea, a speech about his life, a slideshow created by his children in his honour, then the return journey. All this I would normally take in my stride. But in my current situation we had to think it through extremely carefully. As well as considering the journey in my recovering condition, the celebrations also coincided with - The Big Finish! Ric had got to the point of no return with "Farm Play". He had worked meticulously scene by scene reviewing, cutting, editing, and focusing as per Rob's (his dramaturge) request and was tantalisingly close to the end of the final review: the two last scenes where the drama literally reaches its climax.

SO, there was the big decision to make. Can we risk the journey not only for me but also for him? It could be that we upset his equilibrium, and he blows the whole play. Conundrum. Proposed solution: he does his usual Wednesday writing routine – 09.30 to 14.30. I do my usual routine of walking, gentle gardening and some MLA consultancy (including coaching calls to the San Francisco team in preparation for the event I am now flying to conduct).

He would then work his usual morning routine and we are there ready for the 3pm afternoon concert in the Long Room of the Mansion where he spent some early childhood years. A delicate balance indeed. Will it work?

It worked a dream - despite his anxiety of breaking the flow and the danger of him being distracted by the grand gathering and the tantalising pull of wanting to mix and mingle all day with his gorgeous sister, Angela, brother-in-law, nephews, nieces, great nephews, great nieces and various old family friends, plus my anxiety of making the journey intact, and managing my possible sudden bathroom dashes. Georg chose a rich programme including a stunning Dvorak quartet, led by his amazing niece Shereen. All 40+ guests were enraptured by the quality of playing and listening in the room as well as being struck by the additional "spiritual attendance" of Ric's mother who we felt was observing and appreciating this unique and wonderful gathering in her favourite room in the Mansion. We all adjourned to Angela and Georg's home within walking distance to a traditional afternoon tea set out on their lawn in a perfect English garden with perfect dubious English afternoon weather! Mission accomplished. Ric managed his writing (under severe concentration strain), I managed my sensitive system, and the family managed an excellent afternoon celebrating a milestone birthday for an honoured member.

And that was only one momentous occasion of a series of steps on the road to get me literally here on this flight. Not surprisingly we both took the next day off! Ric's brain was overtaxed with the extra concentration strain and my system, even though it had performed well, needed 24 hours of stability before further challenges. We also realised that we were entering the August bank holiday weekend and even though Rob was not expecting Ric's script on Monday we realised we had an extra day of grace for Ric to complete and for us to thoroughly check and proofread before hitting the send button on Monday night at 22.07. Our parallel challenges had both reached their crescendos!

Step two: Practice bike ride up and down the lane succeeded without either falling off or any undue pain and discomfort. I had been rigorously practicing my pelvic floor exercises in tandem (pun?) with building up my diminished Gluteus Maximus. (Maximums?)

Step three: My independent re-entry into the business world was a daunting challenge for Wednesday. As it happens my last job just before treatment started was with 26 young highflyers on the Capgemini Accelerate Leadership programme in Paris (nice!). Three MLA colleagues and I had scored the highest in any development programme they had experienced (even nicer!) so when it came to the follow-up for the same team being planned for November, we were encouraged to pitch for the work. We did and won (nicer and nicer) and we are now in the final design stages for the pop up restaurant challenge. I had dramatically declared my situation in the final few minutes of the Paris programme, so everyone knew I was about to have a health sabbatical. Therefore, it was with a degree of anxiety and trepidation that I set off on Wednesday to London on my first solo mission with Capgemini. I had weighed up the risks and benefits, planned the journey, which was a familiar one, booked myself a first-class train ticket and set off. Such is the state of the nation, I can only conduct a journey if I know exactly where I am going, where the obstacles might be and, most importantly, to know all the toilet stop possibilities. I had pre-warned Sally at Capgemini that I needed to have close proximity to the conveniences and that I may at any point, even mid-sentence, duck out of the meeting! Ric had added to my carefully thought through plan by offering to taxi me to the closest train station, Sudbury, which would shorten my car journey as well as my long walk from car park to station platform to train with its obvious lack of toilet dangers. You see what my life now centres around? ... We set off as planned to reach Sudbury station in good time for me to pick up my automatic pre-paid ticket. I knew as well as there being a toilet on the far end of the train there were also two at the station where I needed to change to the main line. So far so good.

First obstacle – the automatic ticket machine was "not in service", secondly the expected train toilet was "out of order", and the third obstacle I encountered was that BOTH toilets at the exchange station were engaged! EEEEEEEEEEEEEK. Fortunately, I had done my preparation pre-journey poo and pees and very fortunately could last until the train pulled into Liverpool Street station where I used the working toilet. Hooray!

With added confidence I aborted my planned 10 minute taxi ride to Holborn Viaduct and jumped (possibly foolishly) on to the tube for a three stop ride, climbed the escalator at Chancery Lane, walked 250 yards down the road and ducked into Starbucks toilet just ahead of a City Sprint courier who indicated in no uncertain terms with dramatic body language that he was in desperate need – but I insisted my need was greater than his! – He forgave me when I mentioned the c word (as in cancer). I was welcomed with warmth and affection by Sally at Capgemini, and she showed me that the nearest conveniences were indeed 'very convenient'. Without incident we conducted a very successful planning meeting and we all left relieved – in the right way.

I then strolled fairly confidently up High Holborn to my next meeting at the Kingsway Hall Hotel, found the perfect table in a discreet area within striking distance of the - you've guessed it - nearest toilet! Three other MLA colleagues and I conducted another successful meeting, and I navigated my way back to an earlier than expected return train to Colchester where darling husband, writer and nearly-retired-reluctant-carer met me and drove me to our blissful home.

Step four: Day off! At home – no challenges but a delightful visit from one of my nieces and her partner. Followed by a longer bike ride around the Lawshall/Chadacre circle that I had not been on since the middle of June. Nice! The harvest was in, and the farmers were ploughing, harrowing and even setting spring wheat in a cacophony of crows and seagull cries. More stamina-building and more power to my gluteus maximums! We ended the day with a very early night and neck massage for Ric to ensure he caught up with some well-deserved sleep and I could re-pay him for the countless massages he had given me.

Step five: 'What is Gravitas? – 'Can we define it for ourselves? Do we have it? How can we improve it - in us and each other? And can we then help find a toolkit to offer to our clients?' - These were the questions and challenges that 10 Associates at MLA grappled with on Friday – my second (internal) business day.

All good questions. And an excellent process to help us sharpen up, share our experiences, give each other some specific (and sometimes challenging) feedback. And for me, another way to test my stamina and capability before embarking on this journey. All objectives were fulfilled, all challenges were overcome, and I travelled to Michael and Carol's home for a well-deserved evening with tried, tested and trusted old friends who gave me warm and generous hospitality and we chewed the cud on many of our varied and shared life issues.

WEEK NINE - RESPONSES

25th August

I'm very glad to hear your news and enjoyed your description - thank goodness for a sense of humour, as well as such a friend to share the experience and help you through. All set for the US, then? Those flatbeds looked delicious on my flights, as I looked over longingly from the economy sardine can seats!

Love, Brian

*

UP, up and away indeed. I am so pleased that you have managed to achieve what you set out to do Nigel. No mean feat! Have a great week and hopefully a really good sleep on your flatbed home! It was lovely to see you last week.

Love Terry

*

Good luck on the journey.
However, your Latin needs polishing. The plural for buttocks is gluteus maxibums!!

Clive and Sue xx

*

Hi, - Hi Flyer!!

You did it!!! San Fran! O my word. Well I must say you are one determined human being. What an achievement. Looks like you have paced yourself just right to get to this spot.

So respectful of your ability to get the support you need so you can continue in the way you want.

Hope the flat bed bought some joy and that the trip keeps adding to your ability to cope with anything.

Wishing you sound sleeps beneath your foreign sheets.

 Love, Pain in the Neck Ann.

WEEK TEN AND ELEVEN - BACK ON THE ROAD AGAIN

15th September

This has been an encouraging, confidence-building, scary, emotional roller-coaster two-week ride.

First job. San Francisco.

After all the planning, persistence, and patience the dawn rose on my first delivery day at Genentech. I had enjoyed two whole days acclimatising. I woke at 5.45 to the sound of the old trams' bells dinging and the cries of the sleepless seagulls and even the first blast of the Oakland Ferry horn as it docked and disgorged its full load. People dashing off with backpacks, bikes, tricycles and even briefcases on their regular way to work.

Feeling under some pressure – after all they had flown me over at enormous expense, paid for two extra hotel nights and set up high expectations that I will create some magic – no wonder I was feeling nervous about how to approach my first of three days! I had ordered a light room service breakfast, or thought I had! Within five or six minutes of rising, my first call to the bathroom to unload last night's delicious organic veggie burger that I shared with Karen the head of Genentech Global Oncology Leadership Team. We had a good catch up.

And just as I had finished my toilet and preparing to go for my morning walk along the waterfront I stopped in confusion as I needed some laundry doing but found no laundry bag in the cupboard, so I rang down for one to be sent up. Now what to do?

Walk, shit more, change or what? The time was ticking by, and I decided to forego my walk and wait for the valet to bring the laundry bag – I needed to have more clean underwear just in case and my 6.30 room service light breakfast would arrive any minute. I changed out of my dirty clothes put them in the laundry bag just in time and as the knock on the door came, I simultaneously received a text from Ric. I handed my laundry to the valet then read "Have a brilliant day one, I will be thinking of you." I burst into tears and replied: "Thanks, this message made me cry. Such a big step and I'm a bit scared." Then another knock on my door and my light breakfast arrived – but not so light and very expensive - $60 worth of granola with yogurt, fruit with yogurt, apple juice, coffee and pastries. I sighed and signed. I selected the granola with yogurt, the juice and one pastry and left a big note for the maid, 'Please leave and I will eat later' – hoping she read English. Had my shower, checked that I was safe to dress and tentatively walked down the corridor, got the lift, the doorman found me a cab as I had a bag full of props for the workshop and didn't want to risk the walk - and off I went. I continued our text conversation - "OK in the cab now, a short ride into the known unknown…" He said, "My love and strength are with you." And it made me cry even more! The Cab driver asked if I was OK. "Please don't worry. Thanks." And I stepped out of the cab into the grand entrance to Parc55, my heart beating fast and my bottom tingling with anxiety.

Having checked the venue out on Sunday and done the eleven block walk several times, I knew exactly where to go – up two flights of escalators to 4th floor where the Gents was waiting patiently for me on the left. For once I didn't need to use them! I made my way to the meeting rooms where the full team had already assembled – took a very deep breath - and began.

Three whole days passed where my attention was not entirely on myself for a change – and what a relief. I was there to help them become a more cohesive team – a distinct and highly experienced room full of scientists with Doctorates and highly tuned technical skills. I had to be on my toes. I rested and basked in the glorious balmy evenings and watched the Ferry traffic come and go and the seagulls squawk and wheel.

At 3 pm on Thursday I left them to it, jumped into my taxi and rode off into the golden afternoon sun to the San Francisco Airport Virgin lounge, looking forward to my luxury flat bed and an easy and satisfied journey home. PHEW!

My mind and body whirred and purred as we crossed the Atlantic, I declined dinner and reclined immediately. Becky my attendant respectfully left me in peace as I settled down to a half-sleep doze for 6 hours. I managed my toilet anxiety through the night, and she brought me a light breakfast before we landed. There was an easy passage through customs, my bag was waiting, and I visited the toilet again for security before jumping into my pre-arranged car for a direct ride home to Lawshall. Ric was away on a family conference, so I had some hours alone to prepare for job two!

Second job. Bonn.

Having revelled in my achievement of a three-day intensive ACE Teams building event, my next challenge was as Keynote Speaker at a DT (Deutsche Telekom) gathering for The Talent Conference - 350 high performing executives who were waiting to be inspired! I had called my session "On the Edge" and had created an interactive session based on R.I.S.K. Responsibility. Integrity. Status. Knowledge. I certainly felt right on the edge, not entirely knowing how my mind body and spirit were going to react to this one.

48 hours of delicious relaxation in warm September sunshine at home alone while my recently retired reluctant carer was away had set me up for this solo challenge. I drove to Stansted this time and took a small un-flatbed seat on an hour's flight to Cologne, then a 30-minute taxi ride to the Meridien Hotel in Bonn and bedded down for the night.

This time I was even more nervous because I was not so familiar with the journey or the hotel. But all went smoothly, my time at home and in the garden had done the trick and I was rested and ready to go. Also, I did not have an early start on Monday so I could relax.

I heard other presentations, observed the Marketplace activities, and got to know some of my audience before my slot at 4.30. My theme was "On the Edge" – they were being asked to think out of the box as they navigated their way through an ambitious career path at DT and the conference was set up to give them many opportunities of making new connections and increasing their skill set. I asked if they could partner with me and play. We were asking them to be Choosers not Victims. They proved to be an extremely willing and playful audience and at the end of the one-hour session they rose to their feet. (Er, not just to leave the building!)

Home again.

Proud and satisfied and in need of the next three days before going off on Friday to an internal MLA Company Day. We had big discussions around Women in Leadership which was challenging for us all. Then on Saturday Ric and I were guests of honour (we are the Founders) at the Green Light Trust 25th anniversary celebrations where we were both asked to speak. We spoke, then cut the 25th anniversary cake and left with a strong sense of enormous achievement and release, having passed the banner over as planned to the next generation who were already doing things differently but still following our guiding principles of Inspire. Engage. Empower. To "Bring people and Nature Together."

The last two weeks have indeed been eventful, and my healing continues, with some ups and downs – not surprising with the challenges I set myself. But I have learned as long as I plan thoroughly, stay alert, stay very present and ask for and accept help, then I am still progressing. My body and its various functions are gradually being re-trained. I am constantly aware that life is a gift, that we cannot take anything for granted and to live each day fully.

My next milestone as some of you may remember is an important one. September 29th I will have the dubious pleasure of, I hope, the experienced finger examination!

You will hear from me after that.

Well, I'm so tired of crying
But I'm out on the road again
I'm on the road again
Well, I'm so tired of crying
But I'm out on the road again
I'm on the road again
But I ain't going down
That long old lonesome road
All by myself

WEEK TEN AND ELEVEN - RESPONSES

Dearest Nigel,
A VERY wonderful and inspiring report. You have triumphed during these weeks, and I am so happy for you! We are lucky to have work that we really love and believe in, and I can imagine just how satisfying it is to navigate all your changes and to manage getting out there and giving to so many, as you always have.
Many, many congrats my dear friend.

LOVE and huge hugs, Mag

*
Just read this - OMG what a re-entry back to work!
I knew each event but reading them together like this it is quite extraordinary.

You are certainly living each moment...and more some!

Lots of love xx Terry

*
As I haven't seen another weekly episode since you were outbound to the States, I trust that you are well on the road to recovery after you're really difficult times. But you seem to have coped very well with the help of your emails. Your periodicals have been very interesting and no doubt an important part of your strategy for recovery - good for you, it's a brave step to have taken, but I have to say that I would not have been so keen to broadcast similarly!

Nevertheless as long as it assists you in your fight, let it go on for as long as you need it to provide support. I trust you will soon be back to 100% fitness - you certainly deserve it after your horrid times.

All the best, Norman

WEEK THIRTEEN AND FOURTEEN - THE EXPERIENCED FINGER

1st October

The moment you have all been waiting for arrives!

Since my last post I have been relaxing mostly at home enjoying the luxury of this glorious September – officially declared as the driest since records began in 1910 – after the wettest August. I wonder if something strange is happening with our climate… And Ric has been - wait for it – working on draft 7.5! He had some excellent notes and further challenges to perform on "Farm Play" which we hope will be the very final version. Rob has asked him to do the 'lean, lean, lean' version and delete yet another 8 pages! When Ric read the comments, he said it felt like an amputation. But on reflection he now understands what Rob is after and is doing his best with enormous internal wrangling to incorporate these new ideas. Yet another deadline has been set for this coming Friday 3 October.

We have also been delighted to host more friends and family at Farm Cottage – Ric's cousins and family – 9 of them – descended en masse for a sumptuous Sunday lunch, accompanied by hay meadow races and blackberry picking. And a gentle visit from Sophie and her son Chris who travelled 17 hours on the train (and back) from Wick in Northern Scotland. There is something hugely fulfilling and nourishing about being grounded at home that brings the world to our doorstep.

And so. Yesterday I got up at 4.45 to be met with dense fog. Sophie and Chris needed to be on the first train out of Sudbury at 05.30 in order for them to get the connections via London, Edinburgh, Inverness and Thurso to arrive home at 22.11.

We had a very quick cuppa and set off for the 20-minute drive to the station. It was quite hairy and because I have been driving the same road since 1976, I was able to guess the direction correctly when my vision was completely impaired as we hit a complete blanket of fog (and almost a lorry that was on the wrong side of the road) and arrived just in time to see the train trundling into the station. I packed them off and Sophie was to spend her 50th birthday all day on the journey. I returned at a gentler pace and curled up in bed again with Ric for a couple of hours before my second start of the day around 08.30.

Of course, my mind was on the 15.40 appointment. Many text messages pinged into my phone - people sending me their warm thoughts and wishes. I noticed I was feeling a little pressured to produce good news, not only for Ric and I but for all of you too! My heart was beating a little faster than usual and my tummy was churning a little more than normal – and not just due to the delicious Indian dinner we had on Sunday night.

Finally, 14.30 arrived and Ric and I jumped into the car to meet our fate. His mind was whirring with his cuts and my mind was whirring with what we might find at 'Health City'. I have noticed that many of my symptoms have settled down: no more endless internal throbbing and no short, sharp stabs of pain. Even my sudden dashes are more and more under my control, and I experience a mere stinging sensation when passing a motion which only lasts for five minutes or so. And yet a lingering question mark over "Is everything going according to plan?"

'Health City' loomed large rather too quickly, we parked and walked the same airless corridors with the similar sights of people in various wheelchairs, still hard to distinguish between the well and ill. Checked into the not so full waiting room with the same blue plastic/leather chairs, but no familiar faces this time. must be in another cycle now. People waiting perhaps for their first consultation, just about to receive life-changing news or perhaps at the end of their cycle waiting to be given the all clear, or like me, caught somewhere in the no-man's land between.

Something had changed, I noticed. When we arrived at Addenbrookes I did not need a sudden dash to the toilet.

I couldn't risk a swift cuppa or to guzzle a quick dubious hospital sarnie just in case there was a long wait – even though I said to Ric I was feeling a little faint from hunger and thirst. There was a call from one of the receptionists to the assembled throng: "Come and help yourselves please. One of our young helpers has made a cake and would like to invite you to eat it." "Sorry, there are no plates, but I have a pile of tissues." No one moved. "Go on and grab a bit." I said to Ric. "I can't have any, but you could start the ball rolling." He did. And tentatively one or two other brave souls broke down their shy barriers and approached the desk. "Mmmm. It's a bit dry." He reported to the receptionist when she asked. "Oh well, at least it's free."

"Nigel Hughes?" "Come and get weighed please." "71.8 – about 11st 4lbs in old money." "You've gained about half a stone since last time." "Good, thank you." And sat down to wait for... within minutes "Nigel Hughes?" It was the junior nurse calling, the one who had been unsure how to disconnect my PICC line the night I had such trouble with my chemotherapy automatic drip. "How are you?" she asked automatically. "Still alive thank you. And thank you for your care when I needed it." She gave me a slight nod of acknowledgement, not registering fully what I was referring to I think, showed us into our consulting room where we were to wait for the Doctor. A familiar space. A computer on the desk in the corner, 4 chairs, an examination couch and a carefully laid pair of blue plastic gloves, a kidney dish with a well-used tube of lubricating jelly! Not subtle at all! We waited for a few moments. We didn't have a list of prepared questions this time because we assumed it would all depend upon what the Doctor finds. As long as it wasn't Dr Jephcott I wasn't worried about who would do the necessary as it was clear that the experienced finger was required.

"Nigel Hughes?" "Hello I am Dr Paula." A rather short and stout figure appeared at the doorway. "May I come in?" she said in a deep resonant voice in rather broken English. "Oh hello, I am Nigel, and this is Ric." She had a bit of trouble closing the door and rather shyly sat in the corner chair by the computer. She was wearing a blue garment – looking a little like a uniform and a prominent badge pinned to her chest. Dr Paula di Nardo – Senior Clinical Fellow. I was a little surprised. Is this the experienced finger or is this a precursor to it?

"OK. How are you?" again in heavily accented broken English and I assumed Italian. She sat very still with her full attention on my report. I noticed she cocked her head to the left as her rather short neck was getting a little squashed. "You are telling me all good news." She said when I had finished my rather perfunctory report back on my improved symptoms, still unsure if I was going to have to say all this again. "Well, I read your notes in your case file and all sounds like you are progressing very well." Long pause. I didn't know who was going to speak next. "Do you have, er, questions?" Oh. I thought, this is it. "Yes" Ric said, "I have a question." "Er yes" I said. "I have two things. Firstly, even though my symptoms are receding I am wondering if there is anything different, I should be doing now?" "Oh, that was not the question I was going to ask," says Ric, perhaps sensing my shock and I think trying to rescue me. "And, when we had our last conversation with Dr Noble, we discussed the matter of an internal examination this time." "Yes, I will do that now." "Er, well. I do not want to appear rude but when we discussed the internal examination with David, he said that an experienced finger would be able to tell straight away if things were alright. May I ask what level of experience you have as we have not met before?" "Oh, it's OK. I am er, new to this team, but I been working in this area, down there, since 2008 and I see and feel if everything is OK." "Er, OK?"

"Shall I lie here on the couch as usual?" "Oh yes. OK please." And she started to pull the curtain across to separate the couch from the chair that Ric was sitting in. "Oh, you don't need to worry about that – he has seen it all before." I joked. "Oh no, I pull curtain just in case someone comes in the door while, er, um, while I, er, examining you! I heard a rustle and a tug of the plastic gloves being pulled on. And I heard the lubricating jelly squirt as she applied it to the... The process began and although not entirely comfortable it was not as excruciatingly painful as I half expected. I did take a peek over my shoulder, and I caught her in full action, her rather beefy arms bare up to her biceps, digging for gold, her head poised at an alarming angle, and it felt like she was struggling a little to either see or feel what she needed to. She wrestled twice and satisfied, and probably to spare me any further discomfort, completed her task, zipped off her un-attractive blue plastic gloves with a squish and a pop and handed me some tissues.

"Yes, all is OK. It is er, all OK. It feels scar tissue is healing well. I, er, did not to get right up to top but I am happy that everything is er, OK." I noticed she made a swift and surreptitious glance at the clock on the wall. Time was pressing. We discussed that I would need a six week check up again and she would book me an MRI scan – either in six weeks or three weeks – we all got a little confused with the aftershock of the embarrassing and intimate moment we had just shared. She assured me though that everything was going well, and the MRI scan would confirm what the finger had felt. "Three weeks MRI scan and six weeks appointment." "I book the scan."

She managed her exit with grace, and I noticed that she shook her left hand quite vigorously as she walked back to the nerve centre office where, I assume, the team consults before and after each appointment.

Goldfinger

He's the man, the man with the Midas touch
A spider's touch
Such a cold finger
Beckons you to enter his web of sin
But don't go in

Golden words he will pour in your ear
But his lies can't disguise what you fear
For a golden girl knows when he's kissed her
It's the kiss of death …

From Mister Goldfinger
Pretty girl, beware of his heart of gold
This heart is cold
He loves only gold
Only gold
He loves gold

WEEK THIRTEEN AND FOURTEEN - RESPONSES

How can I listen to Shirley Bassey's classic Bond rendition again?

A rollercoaster read as always...and I do seriously appreciate you sending this. Sorry for not responding sooner because I know these instalments are more than that. They are riveting and true and very you.

Ann x

*

Dear Nigel – and Ric

Firstly – thank you so much for the extraordinary updates. I cannot quite reconcile the time between our lovely spring walk and now – the beginning of autumn; and I am sure that you must feel the same but to an excruciatingly magnified degree. I am so glad that the most recent visit to Health City went as well as all could hope for, and of course will continue to keep extremities crossed for the tests.

And another deadline?! Gardeners summer prune to restrict growth, and winter prune to promote growth; so these last summer prunes will hopefully be the final adjustments – I am just picturing Ric with his pen-scissors making final adjustments to a topiary world poised to come alive!

Apologies for the deafening silence from Lavenham; Robert has been working his socks off as this time of year demands, and I have just about managed to get life back under control despite a real 'dead dog bounce' which hit me a few months ago. So – an autumn walk in the diary would be such wonderful plan, keeping us in touch with the irrepressible though comforting march of the seasons!

I know that Robert is hoping to finish drilling second wheat's (and I also know I can use technical descriptions) this weekend; but how are you fixed for next weekend? Let us know when you are next free, and we will look forward to seeing you then.

Much love, Amanda

*

Responding to the question in your text...At the time, and reflecting on it since, I thought your energy was pitched absolutely to the size, nature and needs of the group over the two days. Although I had moments of thinking about this being your first theatre job back after treatment and wondering how that was for you, they were in advance, and I wasn't really conscious of it during the two days. You seemed every bit yourself.

Performance-wise, I thought you were absolutely on the money. I thought the gentle way you drew people to step further for themselves was great, and your assuredness when going to the risky areas with Sandra made it safe for her to do what was important for her.

Attitude - again, spot on.

I thoroughly enjoyed the two days with you, Nige, and continue to learn from and be impressed by you...even after all these years :-)

Love, P

*

Dearest Nigel,

Thank you for keeping me in the loop re your progress. I was glad of the photo because my girls gave me a hard time for not taking a photo of you!!
 I have enclosed a poem that I love and as I was reading it to my class the other day - you sprang into my mind.

I read a poem at the beginning of the day when I am teaching - to open the space - which respects the Māori custom of karakia (prayer) without compromising myself.

Arriving home was bliss. I love to go away, and I love to return home and feel my people.

I haven't been able to write before now - partly because I had 2 teaching weekends in a row - lots of preparation to do. But also because I have not found the words to answer your question about the conference. It was a powerful experience and I am happy to have been a part of it. The large group was awesome. It was horrible and beautiful - it was human beings at our worst and at our best. There were some very traumatised and frightened people present from Serbia, Albania and Kosovo, from Israel from Russia/Ukraine and people who were suffering in other ways- through financial difficulties - Greeks and Portuguese in particular. I felt my difference - the softness of the people in my country. Though there are terrible social problems in New Zealand there is still a softness.

The process in the large (400 people) group was very split - just like out in the world. The Israelis were frightened of being attacked in the group - and they were - there was a great deal of hot air about what is going on, gradually though the energy opened out and all the other nationalities with their combination of problems became more visible. It felt as if we started out each holding onto our identity in the nation to which we identified, and for some that was held more tightly than others. The Brits have an arrogance of their place in the world that they are barely aware of (I think). The session Thursday was the most amazing where it felt as if we opened into a community of citizens of the world, each of us an individual, and connected. I was hopeful that something positive would happen. And a petition came together a week or so later through many more difficult conversations over the forum (our way of all staying connected as an organisation) - and where there is ongoing dialogue about the issues that are current.

So dear Nigel, its back to my ordinary life again now for a while. I hope your recovery improves exponentially.

Lots of love
Margot

*

Ooooh, great cheek-movement!! Congrats. I finally finished reading your weekly musings... thanks so much, it was everything - funny, sad, painful - but ultimately I'm happy to read it and share your journey a little. Keep up the amazing work :)

Love, Seth Xxxx

*

Look forward to seeing you Nigel. I am a bit behind coming back from holiday so must catch up on your story! Sounds like everything is going very well which is absolutely great! What's the purpose of your visit next week? Maybe we could grab some coffee? Carmen

*

Wowwww wowwww wowwwww handsome!!! Back in action :)
Truly a historic moment. So now I really do get an inspiration from you to get a bike (it'll help me lose some weight too ;)) hahahaha...

Take care of yourself! Hope you're feeling better now.

Give my love and regards to Ric. Loads of Love Jigyasa

*

Back on yer bike. How fabulous - a real test of your healing!
You're an inspiration to us all.

Brian x

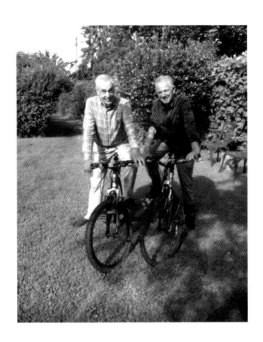

Yay! Back on your bike - and the incredible feat of riding upside down - how on earth do you do it? Or is it like that coz you are in the UK, and I am in NZ? I have loved reading your updates. Even if some of them have taken me to places I haven't necessarily wanted to go

Lots of love to you and Ric. Xxxx Josie

*

Great to see.
 May your arse be forever pain free and may you peddle off into the sunset with the wonderful
'Reluctant Carer' by your side ❤❤❤ Martin xx

*

There's no stopping you is there?
 (Is there a song for this one :-))
 John x

THE EPILOGUE

WHAT DO YOU DO WHEN YOU HAVE RECOVERED FROM CANCER?

GO TO IRAN – but that is another story.....

AFTERWORD

Thank you for reading my story. That first visit to Iran was indeed the beginning of the rest of my life. And I'm glad to say I'm still here – but I won't go into that song!

Technically, after regular annual checkups for five years, I was 'released' by Addenbrookes. And I'm living without cancer. I have shared my intimate story with a friend who works in the pharmaceutical industry. After reading it she asked me two important questions:

Q 1. - "Did I push myself too hard to keep working?"

Answer. To respond in the vernacular of my original writing, this song springs to mind:

"Accentuate the positive.
Eliminate the negative.
Latch on to the affirmative - and don't mess with Mr in between."

By pushing myself to keep working motivated my mind, my body, and my spirit. My life is always full of my own projects and by supporting Ric in his writing kept nourishing our relations. By focusing on the positive, I gave myself new milestones, new challenges, and new experiences. By having a constant companion and an extra listening ear was essential. There was always far too much information given in a short space of time.

Q2. - "On reflection, ten years later, would you have done anything differently?"

Answer. Song: "I did it my way" hits the nail on the head.

And now the end is here
And so I face that final curtain
My friend I'll make it clear
I'll state my case, of which I'm certain
I've lived a life that's full
I travelled each and every highway
And more, much more
Than this, I did it my way
Regrets, I've had a few
But then again too few to mention
I did what I had to do
I saw it through without exemption
I planned each charted course
Each careful step along the byway
And more, much more than this
I did it, my way
Yes, there were times I'm sure you knew
When I bit off more than I could chew
But through it all, when there was doubt
I ate it up and spat it out
I faced it all and I stood tall and did it my way
For what is a man, what has he got?
If not himself then he has naught
Not to say the things he feels
And not the words of one who kneels
The record shows I took the blows and did it my way

Perhaps I could have pushed my GP after the original suspicions and exploration to refer me to a specialist sooner. Perhaps I should have cancelled my India trip. And, once I accepted the fact that it was squamous carcinoma, had the surgery and was informed 'he didn't remove all the lesions,' perhaps I could have asked the surgeon to go back in and finish the initial job! Perhaps I could have been more insistent with the MDT and refused the first so-damaging chemotherapy.

Perhaps, perhaps, perhaps now is not the question to ask. I did what I did. I faced my own mortality. I looked back at my life and achievements to date and discovered that, if this was the beginning of the end, that I was truly satisfied so far and would be content to move on. I HOPED that with the right treatment, support, fortitude – 'feeling the fear and doing it anyway'– that with a 60/40% full recovery I would pull through. Some of Frank Sinatra's song rang true.

And finally, what got me through all the stresses and strains was having the love and devotion of my "reluctant carer."

TOOLKIT

For patients, family and clinicians, some of my learnings and some helpful tips to aid and guide you on your own journey.

This TOOLKIT is in five parts:

1. THIS EXPERIENCE BELONGS TO YOU – Taking ownership of your diagnosis and treatment

2. BEND IT LIKE YOU – Using small acts of control to make a big difference

3. YOUR TREATMENT NEEDS YOU – Personal empowerment in the decision-making process

4. CHAOS IS OK – Coping mechanisms for when it all gets too much and making peace with the things you can't control

5. SEE IT YOUR WAY – Exploring VISUALISATION and COMMUNICATION techniques to ease your experience in a clinical setting

1. THIS EXPERIENCE BELONGS TO YOU

After diagnosis, things move fast. There can be a lot of new people, new spaces and new words, all coming into your life at a time of emotional uncertainty. Imagine starting a new job in a new place with new colleagues and having to make big, consequential decisions right away, when you have no experience in the area and aren't familiar with some of the language they use. Then imagine that at exactly the same time, you're dealing with one of the biggest personal upheavals of your life.

It's a lot. More than you can imagine. Except you don't have to imagine it. It's happening, and you didn't even apply for this job.

It might seem that there's very little about this situation that's within your control. This makes it all the more important to take charge of every small thing you can. Your patient journey, your treatment choices, your day to day experience in medical environments, your relationships with medical professionals, and most importantly, your relationship with yourself.
THESE ALL BELONG TO YOU.

You and your illness do not belong to anyone else. When you become a patient, you're slotted into a pattern of diagnosis and treatment - that system is there to SUPPORT YOU. Lean into it, lean on it, and remember, you're entitled to push back when it feels like it's leaning on you.

This isn't ingratitude or negative thinking. Standing on your own two feet and taking responsibility for your patient journey is one of the most powerful tools you can bring to your treatment. Never apologise for owning your experience. There's no right way to have cancer. You can have it your own way.

2. BEND IT LIKE – YOU!

You're going to encounter many things that are initially outside your control. The kind of things that feel like they belong to someone else - the character in a film who receives a diagnosis, the friend you supported through their illness, the person in an advert telling their story to shine a spotlight on a charity. Until these things feel like they belong to you, they're just labels, and labels can make us feel alien to our own selves.

The horrible thing about cancer is that it happens every day and your patient journey will be full of small, ordinary details. You can bend these to suit you. Even a tiny change can make you feel back in control and every moment of feeling like you is a small triumph. Gather as many as you can and make a collection.

Here's some things to think about. Practise doing the flip and doing things your way.

THE MEDICAL SYSTEM

The nurses and doctors you encounter are part of this system and move through its mechanisms every day. You are new to this system (even if you've got previous experience yourself or with a loved one). You aren't meant to understand how it works.

ASK QUESTIONS. GET EDUCATED. Asking questions is ok. Asking a lot of questions is ok. People won't always be able to anticipate what it is you don't understand or what worries you. It's ok to keep asking until you're comfortable with your level of knowledge. It's ok to come back and ask again if there's something you forgot the first time. It's also ok to leave some questions unasked. You might be ready to ask them in the future. You might not.

HOSPITAL ENVIRONMENTS

There's no getting away from it. Hospitals are clinical, impersonal environments. They're designed with our illnesses in mind, not our everyday selves. Every squeaky lino clad corridor, every wipe clean bed, every disposable gown reminds us that in here, we're patient first, person second.
Chairs can be uncomfortable, temperatures might vary wildly. Daylight can be limited and catering facilities can be less than ideal! Perhaps most significantly, personal space can feel like a luxury. You might spend time waiting alongside other patients and get glimpses into other people's journeys, whether you want to or not. It might be hard not to absorb some of their experience into yours. Then there's the challenge of being dropped into an intimate situation with a nurse or doctor you've only just met. Suddenly, the norm can seem anything but normal.

MAKE IT YOUR OWN. Maybe you can't change the space you're in but you can change how you live in it for the hours you're there. Take whatever you need with you. There's nothing the nurses and doctors haven't seen before, and if there is, congratulations on being unique!

Wear whatever makes you comfortable, as many layers as you want to accommodate temperature changes, anything that helps with getting changed or having to be partially undressed some of the time.

Bring any food and drink with you and eat it when you need to (as long as it fits with your treatment, of course).

Consider whether music or the spoken word might help with the time you spend alongside others. It's not antisocial. Do what you need to do FOR YOU.

Let the hospital hold your treatment experience for you. See if there's a sense of relief to be found when you walk out of the door at the end of your appointment. Perhaps spend a moment grounding yourself. Feeling the hospital behind you. Look up at the sky, take a deep breath and move away.

3. YOUR TREATMENT NEEDS YOU

TREATMENT OPTIONS AND PROCESSES
Here are three things that are all true:

1. Your treatment choices affect YOU
2. You're the one making the decisions
3. You're often the least informed person in the room

How do you reconcile all those things?

The most important thing to remember is that however difficult the decisions, MAKE THEM YOURS. Even if your options are very limited and the narrative in the room is going in only one direction – a particular treatment or timeline, for example – you are always entitled to MAKE THE CHOICE YOUR OWN. A decision to surrender a little of your control for a while is still a decision.

This is where you can build on all the other, smaller ways you've already begun to exercise control. You've found a way to navigate strange spaces and uncomfortable situations.

You're holding onto a sense of yourself despite the sometimes dehumanising nature of the system. You're asking as many questions as you need to feel comfortable and informed.

All this good work will empower you when you're in the room, making decisions about your treatment and the next weeks and months ahead. The medical professionals are the experts on your illness and treatment methods and you're the expert on your life as a whole. Bring the two together and you can design a treatment plan that feels like part of your life, rather than like its paving over it.

One thing it's hard to understand until you've been in there, advocating for yourself, is THE POWER OF THE ROOM. A consultant's office or treatment room can feel like it has natural laws of its own.

Once you step inside, it's easy to bend to their flow, or even find yourself feeling in thrall. YOU'RE NOT THE FIRST PERSON TO FEEL LIKE THIS. You might find your instincts asking you to push back, or you might welcome the comfort of feeling that someone else will take responsibility for your treatment for a while. YOU'RE NOT THE FIRST PERSON TO FEEL LIKE THIS EITHER.

Whatever you feel, the important thing to remember is that once you step outside the room, your perspective will inevitably shift a little bit. Something that makes sense in the room, considering your illness in isolation, might feel different when you return to the rest of your life. Perhaps even when you return to the waiting room. Take time to adjust. Consider what's happened. It's ok to reconsider a decision. It's also ok to sit and let any feelings of support you felt in the room really sink in, so that when you get up and walk out of the hospital, you carry them with you. You could find a place to just be and breathe. Or you could sit in your car and call a loved one before you drive home.

Another thing that's ok is to take the rest of your life with you when you step into the room. You might bring some questions with you that relate to how your illness will interact with the other things that make you you – your home life, your job, the things you do to unwind or enjoy your leisure time. Bringing questions with you will mean you'll leave with answers tailored to you and it will also communicate to the medical professionals around you that you want to be considered as a person not a patient. Taking control doesn't have to mean being confrontational or even assertive – you can exercise self-determination in whatever way feels comfortable and reflects who you are. And remember – even relinquishing a little of your autonomy for a while is still taking a decision. And a little bit of control can go a long way.

4. CHAOS IS OK

No matter how much work you do to take control where you can, your diagnosis will bring about big changes in your day to day life.

This happened without permission from you, without any choice made by you. In fact, unlike other unexpected upheavals, this time no-one made a decision. There's no-one to blame. No explanation. That can feel like chaos.
The path of a treatment journey can seem clouded with unknowns. You might get into an established rhythm, when faces and spaces start to become familiar, but your body and mind's responses to treatment day to day are impossible to totally control.

THIS IS OK. IT'S OK NOT TO FEEL OK.

A lot of the time, there are struggles and meta-struggles, layered one on top of the other. Today, you might not cope as well as you did yesterday. It might be frustrating or confusing, it might get you down. The next day you feel ok, it might be tempting to anticipate a negative experience in the future. Your mind and body aren't giving you the reliable responses that come more readily in everyday life and work. In the chaos of cancer, it can be hard to see what success would even look like day to day.

It's a meta-struggle to get through a struggle filled day, week, month, treatment diary. Tell yourself, it's ok. Feeling like this is not failure. You've got enough going on without feeling bad about feeling bad. If you feel brighter one day, embrace it, but don't be hard on yourself if that feeling doesn't last or isn't consistent. You don't have to embrace the chaos, but there are things you can do to help make the path a little clearer.

COMMUNICATE

It can be helpful to find a way to talk about what's happening to you, in any way that feels natural and comfortable. This might be keeping a diary, sending out regular updates to carefully chosen friends or family, sitting down with someone close for a chat in person or over the phone. It might be that you prefer to find someone anonymous to talk to, through a service like Maggie's.

You could also consider bringing someone with you to your appointments, to share the experience with you. This might not be the person you immediately think of. You could have a regular buddy or a series of people who come to support you. Or you might feel most comfortable attending appointments on your own. Whatever you choose, and the choices might change over time, be kind to yourself about them.

Finding a way to communicate the details of your treatment and your reaction to it, can be a useful way of relocating some of the burden of this experience beyond yourself. You don't have to be strong and carry everything inside. It can also be helpful as a way for you to process it. You could read back through a journal, receive responses to an email, hear your thoughts spoken back to your down the phone. As a patient, you can feel like Alice tumbling down the rabbit hole – a little unreal, a little like playing by someone else's rules. The sense of unreality can be incredibly lonely. REACH OUT. You're entitled to as much support as you need, and you're also entitled to refuse anything that doesn't feel right for you.

ROUTINE

Most of us rely on at least some sense of routine in our everyday lives. Work patterns might impose structure without us even giving it much thought. Home life is built on repeating the same comforting, familiar tasks in the same place at the same time, over and over, until we walk a well-trodden path through our homes and lives. That sense of empowerment, all without having to think.

It's possible to replicate some of this in the treatment journey. Take notice of the things that made a visit to the hospital a little bit easier and consciously seek them out the next time, and the time after that.

Did you sit by a window? Was there a painting on the wall of the corridor that caught your attention? Did you stop to say good morning to the volunteer by the front door or arrive early enough for a coffee before your appointment time?

Make a friend of these experiences. Repeat them until you've created your own well-trodden path through your time in the hospital. This is another way of making the journey yours. Different from every other patient who's walked through those doors. You're still you in here and this is a way of showing it to yourself. Nothing can take away the feeling of pausing for a moment or two to stand in front of a painting. That's your time.

You can even take this idea of familiarity into the treatment room. You might feel more comfortable choosing not to interact with the equipment and process, perhaps closing your eyes and clearing your mind. Or you might find that asking questions, looking around the room, holding and understanding the tools of your treatment can help to close the gap between you and what's happening to your body. Perhaps give it a try and if it helps, do it again the next day. And the next. Find whatever works for you and allow yourself to make it into a routine.

5. SEE IT YOUR WAY

Sometimes, no matter how hard you've worked at managing your responses to the strange new experiences, things simply get too much. You're sitting in the waiting room and every tick of the clock feels like it matches your heart jumping in your chest. You walk into the treatment room and every step feels like dragging yourself through a swamp. THIS IS OK. NO-ONE COPES ALL THE TIME.

It can be comforting to know you've got a coping mechanism or two in your back pocket, so that if panic does set in, you're ready for it.

VISUALISATION

One useful trick is visualisation. It's a word that gets thrown around a lot, it can sound trendy or complicated. But really it just means thinking about the things in your life that make you happy. Perhaps the things you're longing to get back to. It can be a person, a moment, a place, a time of day.

Close your eyes if you can and take your mind towards that thing, so that some of your focus drifts away from the immediate source of your panic or discomfort.

Think about the thing that makes you happy. It's as simple as that.

FIND A FRIENDLY FACE

Sometimes, it can be difficult to find a source of calm inside ourselves. Which means it's time to outsource it. See if there's a friendly face nearby – the medical professional administering your treatment, a volunteer on your ward or in your waiting room, the person behind the coffee counter or coming the other way down the corridor. You don't even have to speak. A moment of connection can be enough to help you find the ground beneath your feet again. Or perhaps there is someone you can talk to.

Tell your nurse or doctor you're feeling nervous, ask for a moment of pause, or let them know you'd like to exchange a few words to fill a silence while something else is happening. There are kind, compassionate people behind these uniforms, just like there's a person behind your identity as a patient. IT'S OK TO REACH OUT AND SEEK CONNECTION. IT'S OK TO ASK FOR HELP.

And finally, finally – have patience.

NORWEGIAN NYNORSK

PETER HALLARÅKER

NORWEGIAN NYNORSK

An Introduction for
Foreign Students

UNIVERSITETSFORLAGET

BERGEN · OSLO · STAVANGER · TROMSØ

Cover design: Harald Nystad

Distribution offices:

NORWAY
Universitetsforlaget
Postboks 2977, Tøyen
Oslo 6

UNITED KINGDOM
Global Book Resources Ltd.
109 Great Russell Street
London WC1B 3NA

UNITED STATES and CANADA
Columbia University Press
136 South Broadway
Irvington-on-Hudson
New York 10533

Printed in Norway by
Reklametrykk A.s., Bergen

Foreword

New Norwegian is a language of long traditions in Norway. It represents a development of the native language of the country that can be compared to the relationship between Modern English and Old English. It is 'New' Norwegian in the sense that it descends from the Old Norwegian language used by Norway's vikings and medieval kings.

Whatever its characteristics, New Norwegian is the modern expression of the Norwegian people that results from its uninterrupted use and development in Norway over a period of thousands of years. It is used in social, political and business activities in large parts of Norway today and is a good means of communication for all purposes.

Because of historical developments not totally dissimilar from those that affected the Czech or the Irish languages, New Norwegian (nynorsk) has only been an official language (riksspråk) of Norway since 1885. Despite this, no textbook has yet been written from which English-speaking peoples could learn the language.

The need for such a text was first felt amongst Norwegian-Americans who knew that their immigrant forefathers spoke Norwegian dialects and not Dano-Norwegian (bokmål), which until now has been the language presented as 'Norwegian' in lesson books for English-speaking peoples.

This book presents the basic phonological, morphological and syntactical structures of the language, along with a basic vocabulary for everyday speech. It covers three semesters of classroom instruction at the college level, but is designed so that it may be used for self-study.

Each lesson consists of four parts: A. A dialogue that is followed by questions. B. Grammar notes with exercises. C. Notes on pronunciation and spelling with suggestions for drills. D. A reading text. A separate alphabetical wordlist and an index of topics are presented at the end of the book. Both grammatical structures and new words are introduced gradually, thus giving the students an opportunity to concentrate on a few new items at a time.

Students who already know Dano-Norwegian, or a Norwegian dialect, may wish to concentrate on the reading texts in order to learn New Norwegian at an accelerated rate.

The spelling of the New Norwegian vocabulary follows the New Textbook Norm of 1959 (Ny læreboknormal), which regulated orthography as well as some genders, inflectional forms, etc. It represents the official New Norwegian language of today. This norm instituted a school textbook standard and a variety of optional forms, which are permitted only in written schoolwork.

The book presents the language in the setting of present-day Norway. In addition to teaching the language it is intended to give the students some insight into Norway, the Norwegians, their culture and the country's economic life.

I wish to thank the following institutions and persons who have helped me with the preparation of the book: Vinlands Mållag, Connecticut (an affiliate of Noregs Mållag, Oslo, Norway), for financial support; Møre og Romsdal distriktshøgskule, Volda, Norway, for giving me a leave of absence to work on this project; The University of Wisconsin, Madison, for giving me work space in both their offices and library. I am particularly grateful to my colleagues in the university's Scandinavian Department for valuable suggestions and encouragement, especially professors Harald S. Naess and Richard B. Vowles. Finally, I wish to thank Mr. James Knirk, Yale University, for reading the manuscript and suggesting changes of various kinds. Without the assistance of his high linguistic competence this book could not have been written. I, however, am responsible for any errors or shortcomings.

University of Wisconsin
Madison
June 1979

Peter Hallaråker

Table of Contents

8

9

10

Abbreviations, Signs, and Symbols

m.	masculine gender
f.	feminine gender
n.	neuter gender
sing.	singular
pl.	plural
dat.	dative case
def.form	definite form
adj.	adjective
adv.	adverb
pron.	pronoun
conj.	conjunction
prep.	preposition
v.	verb
imp.	imperative
interj.	interjection
smb.	somebody
smth.	something
cf.	compare
esp.	especially
/. . . ./	Phonemic transcription is put between slanted lines.
[. . .]	Phonetic transcription is put within square brackets.
'	The sign ' in front of a syllable indicates Toneme 1 plus stress.
''	The sign '' in front of a syllable indicates Toneme 2 plus stress.

Introduction

The Language Situation in Norway Today

Norway has two official languages even though the country has only four million inhabitants. The two are New Norwegian (nynorsk) and Dano-Norwegian (bokmål).

Both languages have equal official status, and all state documents and forms must be available in both. School children must learn to read and write both, and questions for any written examination in any public school, college or university must be presented in both languages.

In each governmental administrative area, however, the local council decides which language shall be used for public administration. The language to be used in each school district is decided by the vote of the parents of school children within that district. Textbooks are legally required to be available in both languages at the same time and for the same price.

Today New Norwegian is taught as the first language to just under one-fifth of the school children. The highest percentage reached was 34.1%, in 1944. The decrease since then is due in large part to post-World War II urbanization and centralization. The school strongholds of New Norwegian today (1977–1978) are the counties of Sogn og Fjordane, Møre og Romsdal, Hordaland, Rogaland, Oppland, Telemark, Nord-Trøndelag and Aust-Agder.

New Norwegian is used in the local press, particularly in Western Norway, and some national newspapers and periodicals include articles in it. The best publications in New Norwegian today are probably the biweekly *Dag og Tid* and the periodical *Syn og Segn*. A number of contemporary authors write in New Norwegian, and about 20% of all radio and TV programs are in it (although state regulations require 25%).

Bokmål, which is called Dano-Norwegian in English to denote its Danish origin, was very Danish until 1907. It is the written standard used by the majority of the people, particularly in the cities in both Western and Eastern Norway. It is the main language of the mass media, and the first language of most school children.

New Norwegian and Dano-Norwegian are very similar in structure and are mutually understandable. This fact often results in their mixed use by students. Another complicating factor is that both languages allow some spelling variants for textbook use, and additional optional forms for use in written schoolwork.

As far as the spoken language is concerned, the situation is even more complex. Most people speak rural dialects or non-standard urban dialects in day-to-day use, but often use a more standardized form of New Norwegian or Dano-Norwegian when speaking in public. The western dialects resemble written New Norwegian quite closely, whereas some eastern dialects are more similar to Dano-Norwegian in their vocabularies, though not always in their grammars.

The Norwegian government has for a long time been very active in the field of language planning. The basic idea behind the spelling reforms of 1907, 1917, 1938 and 1959 was to get rid of the Danish tradition of writing and to further the mutual approach of the two written languages on the basis of popular speech. In order to make the two standards as representative as possible of the spoken languages throughout the country, the above mentioned variants are allowed.

The once popular idea of gradually amalgamating the two languages into a 'United Norwegian' (samnorsk) has very few supporters today. The present governmental policy is to protect both languages against the increasing influence of foreign languages, particularly English. Most members of the Language Advisory Commission (Norsk språkråd), set up by Parliament in 1970, are loyal to this policy of implied peaceful coexistence. However, the policy does not seem very realistic in view of the facts of everyday life in Norway. The fact is that the Norwegian linguistic controversy is very much alive.

The Historic Development of New Norwegian

Norway was a sovereign state until 1380. Its written language, which is called Classical Old Norwegian, was in use from 1050 until 1350, by which time Norway was in marked economic and

13

political decline. An extensive body of literature was composed both in this language and in Old Icelandic, which was very similar.

From 1380 until 1814 Norway was united with Denmark and governed from Copenhagen. The Danish language gradually suppressed the Norwegian language and finally became the only written language within Norway. The single event that sped this change most was the Reformation, which was accepted in Denmark–Norway in 1537.

The change in the written language had little effect on most contemporary Norwegians. They were illiterate and continued to use the same language as their forefathers had used. As a result, the Norwegian tongue developed along the same Norwegian lines as before, without being influenced by Danish to any great extent.

After four centuries of national subordination, Norway got its own constitution on May 17, 1814. That same year it also got home rule under Sweden, which lasted until 1905, when the union was dissolved. Since then Norway has been an independent state, except for the years 1940–45 when it was occupied by Nazi Germany.

Soon after Norway gained home rule there were growing feelings in the country in favor of establishing a national Norwegian language. Many people considered a national Norwegian language as the most distinctive sign of Norwegian nationality and freedom. Two courses of achieving this goal manifested themselves. One way was to modify standard written Danish so that the new Norwegian standard coincided with the way in which Danish was mispronounced by those in Norway who used it as their mother tongue. The other way was to build a native written language from the dialects that descended from Old Norwegian.

The native language was formed around 1850 by the great linguist and poet *Ivar Aasen* (1813–96). It was called *landsmål* (changed in 1929 to *nynorsk*) meaning 'language of the countryside' or 'national language'. It won its first official recognition in 1885, when it was made an official language with the same status as Norway's state Danish.

Ivar Aasen was the self-educated son of a small farmer in Ørsta in Sunnmøre. At age 18 he became a public school teacher, and turned from farming to books for good. He began his linguistic career in 1837 when he investigated the Sunnmøre dialect.

The Royal Society of Scholars in Trondheim became interested in Aasen's dialect studies and offered him a scholarship if he would travel throughout the country, gather information about the differ-

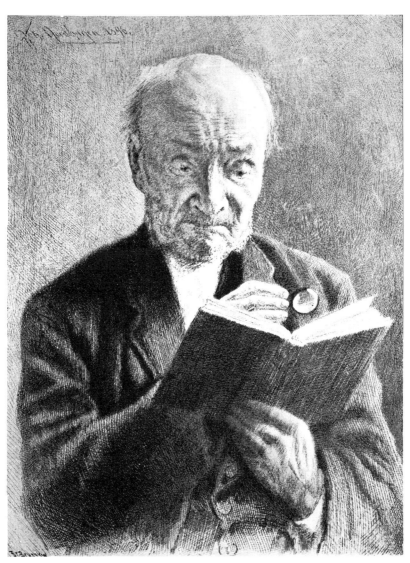

Ivar Aasen (1813–1896).

15

ent Norwegian dialects and then write a grammar and a dictionary on the basis of the information he collected.

Aasen accepted the offer and, in 1842, began five years of extensive field work in Norwegian dialects. He traveled through Western Norway, the Agder counties, Telemark, most of the valleys in Eastern Norway and some of the communities in the flatland districts there, and as far north as Helgeland, in what is now Nordland County. His results were published in *Grammar of the Norwegian Folk Language (Det norske Folkesprogs Grammatik)*, in 1848, and in *Dictionary of the Norwegian Folk Language (Ordbog over det norske Folkesprog)*, in 1850. Aasen was not the first to study dialect words and realize that they descended from Old Norwegian, but he was the first to demonstrate conclusively the connection between the Norwegian dialects and the language of the old sagas.

The idea of creating a native written language for Norway had been formulated before Aasen's time, but it was his genius that succeeded in carrying out the concept. In 1853, based on his own field work, he presented his first samples of a standard native language in a book called *Samples of the National Language in Norway (Prøver af Landsmaalet i Norge)*. Not until 1864, however, did he establish his norm definitely in *Norwegian Grammar (Norsk Grammatik)*, and his *Norwegian Dictionary (Norsk Ordbog)* followed in 1873.

The establishment of New Norwegian was not only felt to be a restoration of the Old Norwegian tradition of writing, but also as a democratic process that would make it easier for country people (then more than 90% of the population) to reach high positions in society. The democratic aspect has been stressed in recent years because it probably appeals to more people than the nationalistic one.

It was a great advantage for New Norwegian that Aasen was a poet. His little collection of verse called *Symra* (1863) clearly showed the poetic power of the language. Since then a large number of Norwegian authors have written in New Norwegian. These include such classic writers as Aasmund O. Vinje, Arne Garborg, Olav Duun, Tarjei Vesaas and young, contemporary writers such as Tor Obrestad, Einar Økland, Paal-Helge Haugen, Edvard Hoem, and Kjartan Fløgstad.

A long time before the establishment of New Norwegian as an official language, its supporters realized that the language question had become an important political issue. It was thus necessary to

16

organize in order to win new adherents and to pressure the political parties into taking clear positions about it. *Vestmannalaget* in Bergen and *Det Norske Samlaget* in Oslo were therefore established in 1868, and local groups gradually organized elsewhere for the same purpose. It was so important to publish newspapers, periodicals and books in New Norwegian that *Det Norske Samlaget* soon became a New Norwegian publishing house.

It was not until 1877 that the New Norwegian language movement got a common spokesman. In that year *Arne Garborg* (1851–1924) began to publish a New Norwegian newspaper called *Fedraheimen*, in which he used all his wit and intelligence to defend the new language. In 1894 *Fedraheimen* was succeeded by *Den 17de Mai*, which became the largest and most important mouthpiece the movement has yet had. *Den 17de Mai* ceased publication in 1935 because of internal disagreement, but the independent newspaper *Norsk Tidend* was started that year and is still printed in Oslo. Two other present-day New Norwegian newspapers are *Gula Tidend* and *Dag og Tid*, the latter of which basically follows the policy of *Noregs Mållag*, a national association of New Norwegian societies that was founded in 1906 and is today the main New Norwegian organization. All of the above mentioned newspapers seem to have two things in common: idealism and the struggle for survival.

In addition to building up a New Norwegian literature and a New Norwegian press, it was very important to get the language introduced into the schools. This is still a main cause for which the movement works.

In 1892 a law was passed that gave the different school districts the right to decide which language was to be used in their district. Especially after World War I, many school districts voted in favor of New Norwegian. A number of school teachers who had been inspired to work for the new language standard while in the teachers training colleges or the folk high schools *(folkehøgskular)* played an important role in the movement. The majority of them also voted for the Liberal Party *(Venstre)* at general elections, and it was *Venstre* that had passed the 1885 law that gave New Norwegian the same official status as Dano-Norwegian.

A chief characteristic of New Norwegian today is probably the widening of its base, a procedure which has taken it away from Aasen's norm. In order to make it more representative both of rural as well as of urban dialects throughout the whole country, a number of words and forms from Eastern Norway have been introduced.

17

Aasen's policy of lexical selection, which was puristic, has also been more or less discarded. These changes have made the two languages increasingly more alike, but have created unrest and bitterness in some groups.

The New Norwegian movement has often been described as a movement associated with Western Norway, rural culture, and nationalism. This is only partly true, and even less today than some years ago. The fact is that the movement is gaining ground both in Eastern Norway and Northern Norway, particularly among students. Many of them have been attracted by its ideas because they associate them with living in small communities. One way of keeping these communities alive is to fight for their cultural self-reliance. The preservation of local dialects is therefore basic. Students are aware of the suppression of spoken dialects, which may include their own, and they fight to improve their social status. They look upon the use of dialects as a human right since language is a part of one's individuality. New Norwegian, which is based on the dialects, is therefore preferred to Dano-Norwegian as their written language.

Sounds and Letters

The spoken standard of New Norwegian is not based on any particular dialect or group of dialects in a certain region of the country. It is very important to point out, however, that many variants of spoken New Norwegian can be heard in Norway today, ranging from what might be called 'regional standards' to a national standard. Below we will limit ourselves to the national standard.

In the *pronunciation* transcription, which is put within oblique lines, the letters of the Norwegian alphabet are used to represent their standard sounds. A colon indicates a long vowel. The nearest international sound symbol (IPA) is sometimes given; it is put within square brackets.

The Vowel Phonemes

New Norwegian has nine *monophthongs:* /i e æ a å o u y ø/, cf. the following series of words: /si:l/ *sil* m. 'filter' – /se:l/ *sel* n. 'cabin' – /sæ:l/ *sæl* adj. 'happy' – /sa:l/ *sal* m. 'hall' – /så:l/ *sål* f. 'soul' – /so:l/ *sol* f. 'sun' – /su:l/ *sul* f. 'collar for a swine' – /sy:l/ *syl* m. 'awl' – /sø:l/ *søl* n. 'anything wet'.

Three of the nine vowels are unfamiliar to you, namely /y ø å/, and each of the other six has its own pronunciation more or less different from the corresponding English one.

The nine vowels form a pattern as shown in the chart below.

	FRONT		CENTRAL		BACK	
	Unrounded	Rounded	Unrounded	Rounded	Unrounded	Rounded
HIGH	i	y		u		o
MID	e	ø				å
LOW	æ				a	

19

Quantity

All the vowels can appear as long or short. When a syllable is stressed, the vowel is long if it is followed by one consonant or none in writing, short if it is followed by two or more, e.g., /gu:l/ *gul* adj. 'yellow' (long vowel), but /gull/ *gull* n. 'gold' (short vowel). Although there are slight differences in vowel quality in such pairs, the relative difference in vowel quantity is considered the distinguishing feature. In unstressed syllables the vowel is always short.

Diphthongs are glides from one vowel to another. The following three diphthongs, /æu æi øy/, can be traced back to Old Norwegian, e.g., /æure/ *aure* m. 'trout' – /øyre/ *øyre* n. 'ear' – /æire/ *eire* v. 'become coated with verdigris'. The five diphthongs of foreign origin, /ai eu oi oy ui/, occur in a small number of words.

The Consonant Phonemes

New Norwegian has the following seventeen consonants: /p b t d k g f v s sj kj j h m n l r/. Examples of minimal pairs: /pall/ *pall* m. 'dais' – /ball/ *ball* m. 'ball'; /tæig/ *teig* m. 'piece of land' – /dæig/ *deig* m. 'dough'; /ka:r/ *kar* m. 'guy' – /ga:r/ *gard* m. 'farm'; /fi:n/ *fin* adj. 'fine' – /vi:n/ *vin* m. 'wine'; /sæi/ *sei* m. 'coalfish' – /sjæi/ *skei* f. 'spoon'; /kjæip/ *keip* m. 'rowlock' – /jæip/ *geip* m. 'grimace'; /ha:r/ *hard* adj. 'hard' – /ra:r/ *rar* adj. 'strange'; /må:/ *må* v. 'must' – /nå:/ *nå* v. 'reach'; /lå:s/ *lås* n. 'lock' – /rå:s/ *rås* f. 'path'.

The approximate phonetic values of all the consonants are shown in the chart below. The only consonant that may cause any great difficulty for you is the r-sound, which is pronounced by placing the tip of the tongue against the upper teeth or alveolar ridge and tapping it quickly. Instead of the fricative /kj/ and /j/, we often hear the corresponding affricates [cç] and [ɟj] in certain positions in certain areas, particularly in the western and midland regions of the country, e.g., in words like *sitja* v. 'sit' and *byggja* v. 'build'. The palato-alveolar consonant /sj/ is often pronounced as a sequence of two sounds in the same regions.

Tonemes

We have already mentioned that difference in quantity may have a distinguishing function in New Norwegian, cf. the pair of words /gu:l/ *gul* adj. 'yellow' – /gull/ *gull* n. 'gold'. Difference in stress does not have such a function, but difference in *word tone* or *word melody* may be linguistically relevant. Words containing one stressed syllable followed by one or more unstressed syllables have

Manner of Articulation

Place of Articulation

	Bilabial		Labiodental		Dental		Pal.-alv.	Palatal		Velar		Glottal
	Voice-less	Voiced	Voice-less	Voiced	Voice-less	Voiced	Voice-less	Voice-less	Voiced	Voice-less	Voiced	Voice-less
Plosives (Stops)	p	b			t	d				k	g	
Fricatives (Spirants)			f	v	s		sj	kj	j			h
Nasals		m				n						
Laterals.............						l						
Vibrants (Rolled)						r						

21

two different tone patterns, referred to as *Toneme 1* and *Toneme 2*. The sequence /soːla/, for example, means 'the sun' when it is pronounced with Toneme 1, but the place name *Sola* near Stavanger, if it is pronounced with Toneme 2. In very few cases, however, will this cause any misunderstanding, since the context will usually tell you which word is meant.

Toneme 1 is indicated in the phonemic transcription by the sign ' in front of the stressed syllable, e.g. /'soːla/, and Toneme 2 by the sign '' in front of the stressed syllable, e.g. /''soːla/.

The Alphabet

New Norwegian uses basically a phonemic spelling. The alphabet consists of 29 letters, the 26 letters of the English alphabet plus the three vowel letters æ, ø, and å (Æ Ø Å) at the end of the alphabet, in that order. In handwriting they look as follows: ∝, ∅, å. A capital is referred to as *stor* 'large', a small letter as *liten* 'small'. Each letter has its own name, which is used when you spell aloud a word or a name.

The letters *c*, *q*, *w*, *x*, and *z* occur only in foreign words and names.

All the 29 letters are listed below with an indication of their pronunciation:

A a	/aː/		K k	/kåː/		U u	/uː/
B b	/beː/		L l	/ell/		V v	/veː/
C c	/seː/		M m	/emm/		W w	/dåbbelveː/
D d	/deː/		N n	/enn/		X x	/eks/
E e	/eː/		O o	/oː/		Y y	/yː/
F f	/eff/		P p	/peː/		Z z	/sett/
G g	/geː/		Q q	/kuː/		Æ æ	/æː/
H h	/håː/		R r	/err/		Ø ø	/øː/
I i	/iː/		S s	/ess/		Å å	/åː/
J j	/jeː/ or /jådd/		T t	/teː/			

Even though New Norwegian uses basically a phonemic spelling, you will find many inconsistencies. The consonant /j/, for example, is written in many different ways: *j* in *ja* 'yes', *gj* in *gjest* 'guest', *hj* in *hjerne* 'brain', *lj* in *ljå* 'scythe', *g* in *gift* 'poison', 'married', *gyta* 'spawn', *geit* 'goat', and *gøyma* 'hide', to mention one of the most difficult cases. Any information about stress or word tone is left out, but quantity is indirectly represented in writing: A long vowel is followed by one consonant, whereas a short vowel is followed by two consonants or more.

1A Noreg

Noreg er eit land i Skandinavia. Bergen er ein by i Noreg. Bergen er
ein by på Vestlandet. Voss er ei bygd i Noreg. Voss er ei bygd på
Vestlandet. Tromsø er ein by i Nord-Noreg. Oslo er ein by på
Austlandet. Oslo er hovudstaden i Noreg. I Noreg bur det fire
millionar menneske.

NES	God dag.
ROY	God dag.
NES	Korleis står det til?
ROY	Berre bra, takk. Og korleis har du det?
NES	Takk, berre bra. – Du talar godt norsk. Er du nordmann?
ROY	Nei, eg er ikkje nordmann. Eg er amerikanar.
NES	Er mor di frå Noreg, kanskje?
ROY	Nei, men bestemor mi er norsk. Ho er fødd på Voss.
NES	Kvar er far din frå?
ROY	Han er frå Ohio.
NES	Forresten, eg heiter Per Nes. Kva heiter du?
ROY	Eg heiter Roy Eisel.
NES	Talar de norsk heime?
ROY	Nei, heime talar vi engelsk, men mor mi kan norsk.
NES	Talar ho nynorsk?
ROY	Ho talar dialekt, men skriv nynorsk.
NES	Kva gjer du i Noreg?
ROY	Eg studerer nynorsk.
NES	Eg må dessverre gå no. Ha det bra så lenge!
ROY	Ha det.

Noreg /"nå:reg/   Bergen /'bærgen/
er /æ:r/ – is   ein /æin/ – a, an
eit /æit/ – a, an   ein by – city
eit land – country   på – in, at, on
i – in   Vestlandet /"vestlande/

23

Voss /våss/
ei /æi/ – a, an
ei bygd – rural district or town
Tromsø /"tromsø/
Nord-Noreg /"no:r-nå:reg/
Oslo /"oslo/
Austlandet /"æustlande/
hovudstaden /"hå:vusta:den/
m. – the capital
bur /bu:r/ – live
det /de:/ – there, it
millionar /milli'o:nar/ m.pl. –
million(s)
menneske n.pl. – people
god dag /go 'da:g/ – 'good day',
hello, how do you do?
korleis /"korlæis/ – how
korleis står det til? /till/ – how
are you?
har /ha:r/ – have
du – you

korleis har du det? – how are
you?
og /å:g/ – and
takk – thanks, thank you
berre bra /"bærre/ – just fine
talar /"ta:lar/ – speak
godt /gått/ – well
norsk /nårsk/ – Norwegian
ho – she
ein nordmann /"no:rmann/ –
Norwegian
eg – I
ikkje /"ikjkje/ – not
ei mor /mo:r/ – mother
ei bestemor – grandmother
di – your
men /menn/ – but
frå – from
kanskje /"kansje/ – perhaps
ein far /fa:r/ – father
din /dinn/ – your

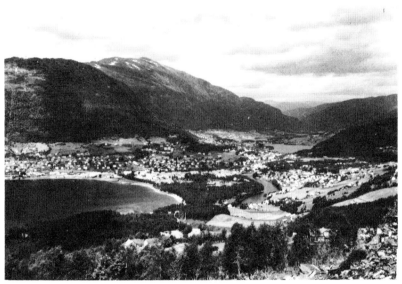

Fig. 1 *Voss er ei bygd på Vestlandet.*

fødd – born
er fødd – was born
forresten /få'resten/ – by the way
kvar /kva:r/ – where
kva – what
han /hann/ – he
vi – we
heiter /"hæiter/ – am, is, are called
eg heiter – my name is
kva heiter du? – what is your name?
de pl. – you
heime /"hæime/ – at home

mi – my
kan /kann/ – knows
nynorsk /"ny:nårsk/ – New Norwegian
skriv – writes
ein dialekt /dia'lekt/ – dialect
gjer /je:r/ – do
studerer /stu'de:rer/ – study
må – must
gå – go
dessverre /des'værre/ – unfortunately
no – now
ha det bra så lenge! – so long!
ha det – bye-bye

Spørsmål (Questions)

1. Er Bergen ein by? 2. Er Oslo ein by? 3. Er Voss ei bygd? 4. Er Tromsø ei bygd? 5. Er Noreg eit land? 6. Kvar bur Roy Eisel? 7. Kva gjer han i Noreg? 8. Kvar er han frå? 9. Talar mora nynorsk?

1B Grammar

1. The Indefinite Article

In nynorsk there are three genders. The indefinite article, *ein*, *ei*, or *eit*, which corresponds to English *a* (*an*), shows whether the noun is of the *masculine* (m.), *feminine* (f.), or *neuter* (n.) gender. The nouns in Lesson 1 can be put into three different groups according to the indefinite article associated with each of them:

ein by	ei bygd	eit land
ein hovudstad	ei mor	eit menneske
ein nordmann	ei bestemor	
ein amerikanar		
ein far		

We may refer to these three groups of nouns as *ein-nouns*, *ei-nouns*, or *eit-nouns*.

The indefinite article is mainly used as in English, but it is omitted in some cases where it is required in English.

25

1) It is omitted with unmodified nouns denoting a person's *trade, profession, nationality, rank, religion,* or *age,* after the verbs 'to be' or 'to become': Far min er forretningsmann. 'My father is a businessman.' Ivar Aasen var lingvist. 'Ivar Aasen was a linguist.' Per Nes er nordmann. 'Per Nes is a Norwegian.' Bror hans var kaptein i hæren. 'His brother was a captain in the army.' Han var protestant. 'He was a Protestant.' Som gut vart han send til sjøs. 'As a boy he was sent to sea.'
2) The indefinite article is used if the noun is preceded by a modifying adjective: Far min er ein god forretningsmann. 'My father is a good businessman.' It is omitted, however, if the adjective is just classifying: Han er katolsk biskop. 'He is a Catholic bishop.' Han er naturalisert amerikanar. 'He is a naturalized American.'

2. The Personal Pronouns. Subject Forms

1. Sing.	eg	I	
2. Sing.	du, De	you	
3. Sing.	han	he	
	ho	she	
	det	it	er, bur, har, heiter, talar, skriv, gjer, studerer
1. Pl.	vi	we	
2. Pl.	de, De	you	
3. Pl.	dei	they	

The capitalized form *De* is a formal form and is used only when addressing a person or a group of persons whom one might not address by first name. The forms *du/de* are used in all other circumstances.

3. The Present Tense

The present tense of any verb has only one form, and this form is independent of person and number. It ends in -ar, -er, -r, or has no ending, depending on the verb class to which it belongs. Examples: talar, heiter, bur, skriv.

4. Negation and Questions

Nynorsk has no equivalent to the English emphatic forms with the verb *to do* (do, does, did), which are often used in negated statements and questions, e.g., He does not know. Did you see him?

Sentences are negated by placing the negative adverb *ikkje* 'not' *after* the conjugated verb in a main clause, but *before* the conjugated verb in a subordinate clause: Eg er *ikkje* nordmann. Han talar *ikkje* norsk. Han seier at han *ikkje* er nordmann. 'He says that he is not a Norwegian.' Han seier at han *ikkje* talar norsk. 'He says that he does not speak Norwegian.'

Questions are formed in two ways. They begin with either:

1) The conjugated verb, which is followed by the subject (yes/no questions): Er du nordmann? Talar han norsk?, or

2) An interrogative *kven* 'who', *kva* 'what', *kvar* 'where', *kvifor* 'why', *når* 'when', followed by the conjugated verb, and then the subject: Kven er du? Kva heiter du? Kvar bur du? Kvifor talar du ikkje norsk? Når skriv du norsk? The interrogative itself may, however, be the subject of the clause: Kven kjem? 'Who comes? Who is coming?' Kven sa det? 'Who said so?'

When there is a compound tense (helping verb – main verb), the helping verb comes first or follows the interrogative: Vil han tala norsk? 'Does he want to speak Norwegian?' Kvifor må han gå? 'Why must he go?'

Oppgåver (Exercises)

1) Find and list the personal pronouns in the dialogue.
2) Find and list all the verbs in the present tense in the dialogue.
3) Make up a couple of sentences containing negation and questions.

1C Pronunciation/Spelling

The Rounded Vowels /å y ø/

The three rounded vowels /å y ø/ are unfamiliar to you, so you should study their articulation carefully and listen to them as often as you can.

Long /å/, IPA [o:], is a mid back rounded vowel fairly similar to o in *horn*, but closer than this. It is usually spelled å, but sometimes o. Examples: gå, må, på, Noreg.

Short /å/, IPA [ɔ], is a little more open and less rounded than long /å/. It is fairly similar to o in *horse*. It is usually spelled o, but sometimes å. Examples: godt, norsk, Voss, fått 'gotten', åtte 'eight'.

Both long and short /y/ have the same degree of opening as

nynorsk /i/, but are articulated with very rounded lips, like the u in French *lune*. Both variants are spelled y. Examples: by, ny (long); bygd, hytte 'cabin' (short).

Long /ø/, IPA [ø:], has the same degree of opening as nynorsk /e/, but it is articulated with very rounded lips, like the ö in German *Höhle* and the eu in French *deux*.

The short variant, IPA [œ], is more slack and open. Both sounds are spelled ø. Examples: snø 'snow', dør 'door' (long); född 'born', øks 'axe' (short).

Uttaleøving (Pronunciation Practice)
Drill on the long and short vowel sounds discussed above by saying aloud the following words several times: gå, må, på, Noreg; godt, norsk, Voss, fått, åtte; by, ny; bygd, hytte; snø, dør, född, øks.

1D Tusen fjordar og tusen fjell

Gamle Noreg, nørdst i grendom,
er vårt eige ættarland.
Der er hav, som heilt åt endom
leikar om den lange strand.
Der er vikar og vatn og øyar,
tusen fjordar og tusen fjell,
snøyder, der sjeldan snøen tøyar,
dalar, der fossen diger fell.

Frå Ivar Aasen (1813–96), *Gamle Noreg*.

tusen /'tu:sen/ – thousand
fjordar /"fjo:rar/ m.pl. – fjords
fjell n.pl. – mountains
gamle /"gamle/ – old
nørdst /nørst/ – northernmost
grendom /"grendom/ f.dat.pl. – neighborhoods
vårt /vårt/ – our
eige /"æige/ – own

ættarland /"ættarland/ n. – land of forefathers
ei ætt – family
der /dæ:r/ – there
hav n.pl. – oceans
som /såmm/ – that, which
heilt /hæilt/ – entirely, all the way
åt – to

endom /"endom/ m.dat.pl. – end

leikar /"læikar/ – play

om /omm/ – along

den /denn/ – the

lange /"lange/ – long

ei strand – beach

vikar /"vi:kar/ f.pl. – bays

vatn n.pl. – lakes

øyar /"øyar/ f.pl. – islands

snøyder /"snøyer/ f.pl. – desolate regions

der /dæ:r/ – where

snøen /'snø:en/ m. – the snow

sjeldan /"sjeldan/ – seldom

tøyar /"tøyar/ – thaws

der er snøyder der sjeldan snøen tøyar – there are desolate regions where the snow seldom thaws

dalar /"da:lar/ m.pl. – valleys

fossen /'fåssen/ m. – the waterfall

diger /'di:ger/ – big

fell – fall, falls

29

2A Ein norsk familie

Per Nes bur i Noreg. Han bur på Vestlandet. Han bur på Voss. Per
Nes har familie. Kona hans heiter Kari Nes. Per og Kari har to barn –
ein gut og ei jente. Sonen heiter Lars, og dottera heiter Brit. Lars og
Brit er sysken, og foreldra heiter Per og Kari.

NES	Lars, er du der?
LARS	Ja, her er eg.
NES	Er Brit der også?
LARS	Nei, ho er ikkje her. Ho er ute.
NES	Kvar er mor?
LARS	Ho er på eit møte.
NES	Når er middagen ferdig?
LARS	Eg veit ikkje.
NES	Kva har du der, Lars?
LARS	Det er ei ny bok.
NES	Har du avisa?
LARS	Nei, avisa har mor.
NES	Veit du ikkje kvar syster di er?
LARS	Nei, det gjer eg ikkje.
NES	Vil du laga middag til oss?
LARS	Nei, i dag kan du far laga middag.
NES	Ja vel. Då tek vi restar frå i går og varmar opp att.
LARS	Dersom mor ser det, vert ho sinna.
NES	Nei, mor seier ingenting for det.

Norsk ordtak: Hungeren er beste kokken.

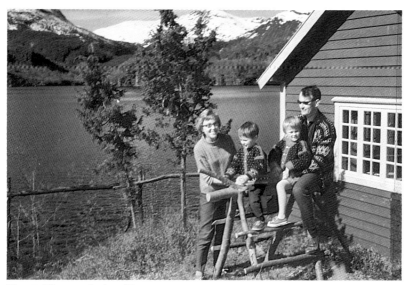

Fig. 2 Ein norsk familie.

Ein norsk familie

Per Nes	Kari Nes	Lars	Brit
ein mann	ei kvinne	ein gut	ei jente
ein far	ei mor	ein son	ei dotter
foreldre		ein bror	ei syster
			sysken

ein familie /fa'mi:lie/ – family
kona /"kå:na/ f. – (the) wife
hans /hans/ – his
Kari /"ka:ri/
to – two
barn /ba:rn/ n.pl. – children
ein gut – boy
ei jente /"jente/ – girl
sonen /'så:nen/ m. – the son
Lars /la:rs/
dottera /"dåttera/ f. – the
     daughter

sysken /"sysjen/ pl. – brothers
     and sisters, siblings
foreldra /får'eldra/ pl. – the par-
     ents
ja – yes
her /hæ:r/ – here
også /"åkså/ – also
ute /"u:te/ – out
møte /"mø:te/ – n. meeting
på eit møte – at a meeting
middagen /'middagen/ m. – the
     dinner

31

ferdig /"færdi/ – ready
veit /væit/ – know
eg veit ikkje – I don't know
ny – new
ei bok – book
avisa /a'vi:sa/ f. – the paper
ei syster /"syster/ f. – sister
nei, det gjer eg ikkje – no, I don't
vil /vill/ – will
laga /"la:ga/ – make
til /till/ – for, to
oss /åss/ – us
i dag – today
ja vel /ja 'vell/ – okay
då – then
tek – take
restar /"restar/ m.pl. – leftovers
i går /i 'gå:r/ – yesterday
varmar opp /"varmar 'åpp/ – warm up

att – again
dersom /'dæ:rsåm/ – if
ser – sees
vert /vert/ – becomes, gets
sinna /"sinna/ – angry
seier /"sæier/ – says
ingenting /"ingenting/ – nothing
for det /får 'de:/ – because of that
eit ordtak /"o:rta:k/ – proverb, saying
hungeren /'hongeren/ m. – the hunger
beste /"beste/ – best
kokken /'kåkken/ – the cook
ein mann – man
ei kvinne /"kvinne/ – woman
ein bror – brother

Spørsmål (Questions)
1. Er Per Nes ein mann? 2. Har Per Nes familie? 3. Kvar bur han? 4. Kva heiter kona hans? 5. Kven er Brit? 6. Kven er Lars? 7. Kvar er Brit? 8. Kven har avisa? 9. Kven lagar middag? 10. Korleis lagar Nes middag?

2B Grammar

1. Word Order

The basic rule for word order in *main clauses* is *verb second*. Exclamations (ja, nei, å) and conjunctions (og, men, for, eller) do not count.

Frequently the subject comes before the verb, but if the sentence is introduced by any other part of the sentence than the subject, e.g., an adverbial (an adverb, a prepositional phrase, a subordinate clause) or the object, the subject will follow directly after the verb. We call it 'normal word order' when the subject comes before the verb and 'inverted word order' when the subject follows the verb.

Below we will discuss the position of the *verb*, the *adverb*, and *unstressed pronouns* both in main clauses and subordinate clauses.

2. The Position of the Verb

In *main clauses* the subject comes before the verb, unless the clause is introduced by some other part of the sentence than the subject. Any other part of the sentence is emphasized by placing it first. Notice that yes/no questions are introduced by the verb (Er du frå Noreg? Bur du i Noreg?), and the same is the case with a main clause following 'direct speech' («Du talar godt norsk,» seier han).

Normal word order:

Subject	Verb	Other parts of the sentence
Eg	heiter	Per.
Eg	er	frå Noreg.
Du	talar	godt norsk.
Han	bur	på Voss.
Mor	har	avisa.
Far	lagar	middag.
Mor	vert	sinna, dersom ho ser det.

Inverted word order:

Other parts of the sentence	Verb	Subject	Other parts
Kva	heiter	du?	
	Er	du	frå Noreg?
Kvar	bur	du?	
	Bur	du	i Noreg?
På Voss	bur	eg.	
Der	bur	eg.	
Nei, avisa	har	mor.	
Middag	lagar	far.	
Dersom mor ser det,	vert	ho	sinna.
Då	vert	ho	sinna.

Subordinate clauses are usually introduced by subordinating conjunctions, relative pronouns, and relative adverbs. They have normal word order except when the conjunction is left out in a conditional clause. Compare the following sentences: Dersom mor ser det, vert ho sinna. Ser mor det, vert ho sinna.

Some common subordinating conjunctions are: *då* 'when' (single past event), *når* 'when' (referring to what usually happens or happened or what will happen in the future), *etter* 'after', *før* 'before', *medan* 'while', *sidan* 'since', *fordi* 'because', *dersom* 'if'.

33

The most common relative pronoun is *som* 'who, whom, which, that', and the most common relative adverb is *der* 'where'. The relative pronoun *som* is itself sometimes the subject of the clause.

Normal word order in subordinate clauses:

Conjunction	Subject	Verb	Other parts
Dersom ⊥ mor (son) som (Bygda) der ⊤ dei	mor dei	ser heiter bur,	det, ... Lars. . . . .

3. The Position of the Adverb

As stated in 1B4, the negative adverb *ikkje* comes *after* the conjugated verb (present tense, past tense, modal, other helping verb) in *main clauses*, but *before* the non-conjugated verb (present participle, past participle, infinitive). Examples: Han talar *ikkje* norsk. Han har *ikkje* tala norsk. 'He hasn't spoken Norwegian.' Han vil *ikkje* tala norsk. 'He doesn't want to speak Norwegian.'

Other adverbs that modify the whole sentence follow the same rule. The most common of them are: *alltid* 'always', *aldri* 'never', *kanskje* 'perhaps', *nettopp* 'just', *ofte* 'often', *sikkert* 'certainly', *nok* 'I guess, surely', *truleg* 'probably', *gjerne* 'gladly, usually, possibly'.

In *subordinate clauses* the adverb *ikkje* and other adverbs belonging to the same category (alltid, aldri, etc.) come immediately *before* the conjugated verb. Examples: Han seier at han *ikkje* talar norsk. Han seier at han *aldri* har tala norsk. Han seier at han *alltid* vil tala norsk.

4. The Position of Unstressed Pronouns

In *main clauses* unstressed pronouns normally intrude between a verb and *ikkje* or other adverbs of the same category, in *simple* tenses. In compound tenses, unstressed pronouns follow the verb forms, whereas the adverb comes between the two verb forms.

34

Examples:

Kona såg *han* ikkje.

Ho såg *han* aldrı.
Han såg *henne* ikkje.
Han såg *det* ofte.
But:
Kona har ikkje sett *han*.
Ho har aldri sett *han*.
Ho har ofte sett *det*.

His wife (literally: the wife) didn't see him.
She never saw him.
He didn't see her.
He often saw it.

His wife hasn't seen him.
She has never seen him.
She has often seen it.

Oppgåver (Exercises)

1) Identify sentences with inverted word order in the dialogue.
2) Comment on the placement of *ikkje* in the dialogue.
3) When does an unstressed pronoun intrude between a conjugated verb and *ikkje*?
4) Fill in the adverb *ikkje* in the following sentences:
   Eg heiter Per.
   Eg er frå Noreg.
   Du talar godt norsk.
   Han bur på Voss.
   Mor har avisa.
   Far lagar middag.
   Han vil laga middag til oss.
   Ho har tala dialekt.
   Han har tala nynorsk.
   Systera såg han.
   Broren såg det.
   Mora har sett det.
   Han seier at han vil tala nynorsk.
   Ho seier at ho vil laga middag.

2C Pronunciation/Spelling

The Rounded Vowels /o/ and /u/

Both long and short /o/, IPA [u:] and [u], are difficult to pronounce correctly, since they have no equivalents in English. The long variant reminds one of English *oo* in *fool*, but the tongue is more raised in the back, and the lips are more rounded. Examples: god, ho, mor. The short variant reminds one of English u in *full*, but is, in fact, closer to German u in *Buch*. Examples: om 'if', tomme 'inch', onkel 'uncle'. Neither long nor short /o/ ever have diphthongal pronunciation. Long /o/ is always spelled o, whereas short /o/ is also spelled u in some words, e.g. dum 'stupid', munk 'monk', tunge 'tongue'.

Both long and short /u/, IPA [ʉ:] and [ʉ], have a higher and more front articulation than the corresponding u in English *true*, but are somewhat similar to this sound. The short variant is a little lower and less tense than the long one. Both sounds are usually spelled u. Examples: du, bur, ute (long); buss 'bus', tull 'nonsense' (short).

Uttaleøving (Pronunciation Practice)
Drill on long and short /o/ and long and short /u/ by saying aloud the following words several times: god, ho, mor; om, tomme, onkel; du, bur, ute; buss, tull.

2D Kvar synest best om sine barn

Det var ein gong ein skyttar som var ute i skogen. Så møtte han myrsnipa.
«Kjære vene, skyt ikkje mine barn,» sa myrsnipa.
«Kva er det for nokre som er dine barn då?» spurde skyttaren.
«Dei venaste barna i skogen er mine!» svara ho.
«Eg får vel ikkje skyta dei då,» sa skyttaren.
Men då han kom attende, hadde han i handa eit heilt knippe myrsniper som han hadde skote.
«Au, au! Kvifor skaut du barna likevel då!» sa snipa.
«Var det dine barn dette?» spurde skyttaren, «eg skaut dei styggaste eg fann, eg.»
«Å ja,» svara snipa, «veit du ikkje at kvar synest best om sine barn?»

Norsk eventyr

kvar /kvaːr/ – everybody
synest om – likes
best – best
sine /"siːne/ pl. – their own
var /vaːr/ – was

det var ein gong – once upon a
  time
ein gong /gåŋg/ – once
ein skyttar /"sjyttar/ – hunter
skogen /"skoːgen/ m. – the woods

36

så – then
møtte /"møtte/ – met
myrsnipa /"my:rsni:pa/ f. – the
  sandpiper
kjære vene /"kjæ:re "ve:ne/ –
  (pretty) please
skyt /sjy:t/ imp. – shoot
mine /"mi:ne/ pl. – my
sa – said
kva er det for nokre som –
  which ones
å skyta /"sjy:ta/ – to shoot
dine /"di:ne/ pl. – your
spurde /"spurde/ – asked
skyttaren m. – the hunter
dei venaste /dæi "ve:naste/ –
  the most beautiful
svara /"sva:ra/ – answered
eg får vel – I suppose I better
då   when (single past event)
kom /kåmm/ – came
attende /at"ende/ – back
hadde /"hadde/ – had
handa /'handa/ f. – the hand,
  i.e., his hand

eit knippe /"knippe/ – bunch
heilt – whole
myrsniper f.pl. – sandpipers
hadde skote – had shot
au – exclamation: oh, ow
kvifor /'kvi:får/ – why
skaut /skæut/ – shot
likevel /like've:l/ – all the same
dette – this
var det dine barn dette? –
  were these your children?
dei styggaste /dæi "styggaste/ –
  the ugliest ones
eg skaut dei styggaste eg fann,
  eg – I did shoot the ugliest
  ones I found (eg is repeated
  for emphasis)
fann – found
veit du ikkje at – don't you
  know that
eit eventyr /"e:venty:r/ – folktale

37

3A Heime hjå familien Nes

Per Nes møter Roy Eisel på gata ein dag og bed han heim til seg. Roy kjem same kvelden.

FRU NES God kveld, og velkomen til oss!
ROY   God kveld, og takk for det!
FRU NES Ver så god og kom inn i stova! Per kjem snart.
ROY   Mange takk.
NES   Hallo igjen, og velkomen hit! Korleis går det med studiet?
ROY   Berre bra, takk. Eg går på folkehøgskulen i år, men neste år skal eg byrja på distriktshøgskulen i Volda.
NES   Det var interessant. Kvifor vil du dra til Volda og ikkje til Bergen t.d.?
ROY   Eg vil gjerne bu i eit nynorsk miljø.
NES   No ser eg at Kari har kveldsmaten ferdig. Ver så god!
ROY   Tusen takk. Dette ser norsk ut. Kva heiter dette?
FRU NES Dette er rømmegraut, spekemat og flatbrød, og det er god norsk mat. No må du berre forsyna deg.
– – –   (Litt seinare)
NES   No – liker du det?
ROY   Ja, det var godt, men noko uvanleg for meg.
FRU NES Vil du ha meir?
ROY   Nei, takk. No er eg godt forsynt. Tusen takk for maten. Og takk for i kveld. God natt.
NES   God natt.

Norsk ordtak: Maten er halve føda.

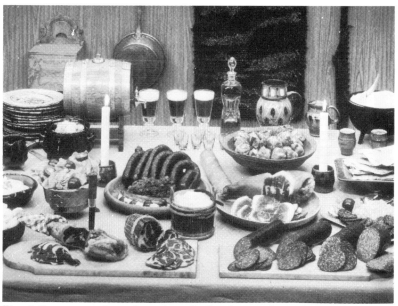

Fig. 3 *Rømmegraut, spekemat og flatbrød er god norsk mat.*

møter /"mø:ter/ – meets
gata /"ga:ta/ f. – the street
ein dag – one day
bed /be:/ – asks
heim /hæim/ – home
seg – himself
til seg – to himself, to his place
kjem /kje:m/ – comes
same /"sa:me/ – the same
kvelden /'kvelden/ m. – the evening
god kveld – good evening
velkomen /vel'kå:men/ – welcome
til oss – to us, to our place
takk – thank you
for det – for that
ver så god /'ve:r så 'go:/ – please
kom inn /kåmm'inn/ – come in
stova /"stå:va/ f. – the living room

snart – soon
mange takk – many thanks
maten /'ma:ten/ m. – the food
hallo /ha'lo:/ – hello
igjen /i'jenn/ – again
hit – here
med /me:/ – with
studiet /'stu:die/ n. – the study, i.e., your studies
går på /gå:r på:/ – go to
folkehøgskulen /"fålkehø:g-sku:len/ m. the folk high school
neste år /"neste 'å:r/ – next year
skal /skall/ – shall
byrja på /"byrja/ – begin at
distriktshøgskulen m. – the regional state college
interessant /intre'sant/ – interesting
dra til /dra:/ – go to

39

t.d. = til dømes – for example
eg vil gjerne – I would like to
miljø /mil'jø:/ n. – surroundings
ser /se:r/ – see
at /att/ – that
kveldsmaten /"kvelsma:ten/ m.
  – the supper
ser norsk ut – looks Norwegian
dette /"dette/ – this
rømmegraut /"rømmegræut/ m.
  – cream porridge
spekemat /"spe:kema:t/ m. –
  salt-cured meat
flatbrød /'flattbrø:/ n. – flatbread
det /de:/ – that
å forsyna seg med /får'sy:na/ –
  help oneself to
no må du berre forsyna deg –
  please help yourself

deg /de:g/ – you
litt seinare – a little later
liker /"li:ker/ – like
det var godt – it is good
uvanleg /u'va:nleg/ – unusual
meg /me:g/ – me
meir /mæir/ – more
vil du ha meir? – would you
  like to have more?
forsynt /får'sy:nt/ – full
god natt – good night
takk for maten – 'thank you for
  the food'
takk for i kveld – 'thank you for
  this evening'
god natt – good night
halve /"halve/ – half
føda /'fø:a/ f. – nourishment

Spørsmål (Questions)
1. Kven møter Per Nes på gata ein dag? 2. Kva seier Per Nes? 3. Når kjem Roy Eisel heim til Per Nes? 4. Kvar er fru Nes? 5. Kva skule går Roy på? 6. Kvifor vil han dra til Volda? 7. Kven lagar kveldsmat? 8. Liker han norsk mat? 9. Kva slags mat har dei? 10. Kva seier Roy då han går?

3B Grammar

1. Dette var godt, det var bra

In nynorsk the past tense is often used to express strong feeling even though one is referring to something occurring at the present time.

Examples:

Dette *var* godt.	This is good.
Dette *var* bra.	This is fine.
Dette *var* hyggeleg.	This is nice.
Det *var* bra.	That's fine.
Det *var* hyggeleg.	That's nice.
Det *var* synd!	That's too bad!

2. The Definite Article

The definite article (corresponding to *the* in English) is placed at the end of the noun. In the masculine singular it is -*en*, e.g., byen, hagen, 'the garden', in the feminine singular -*a*, e.g., bygda, leksa, and in the neuter singular -*et*, e.g., landet, eplet. Notice that the *t* in the neuter singular is silent: /'lande/, /''eple/.

The definite article. Basic pattern:

Masculine	ein by	byen	
	ein hage	hagen	– en
Feminine	ei bygd	bygda	
	ei lekse	leksa	– a
Neuter	eit land	landet	
	eit eple	eplet	– et

As can be seen from the examples above, a noun that ends in an unstressed -*e* drops this -*e* before the grammatical ending, e.g., ein hage – hagen, ei lekse – leksa, eit eple – eplet.

In the definite form plural, the corresponding endings are -*ane*, e.g., byane, hagane, -*ene*, e.g., bygdene, leksene, and -*a*, e.g., landa, epla.

The definite article is used in some cases where it is not used in English:

1. With abstract nouns used in a general sense: Ungdomen er ei herleg tid. 'Youth is a wonderful time.'
2. With names of seasons: Våren er vakker i Noreg. 'Spring is beautiful in Norway.'
3. With nouns denoting measure of time and quantity in a distributive sense: Han bur her to veker i året. 'He lives here two weeks a year.' Han tener 15 kroner timen. 'He earns 15 crowns per hour.'

3. The Infinitive

In dictionaries a *nynorsk* verb is usually listed with four forms: the infinitive, the present tense, the past tense, and the past participle. The infinitive is the form you will find listed as the first form, and the infinitive marker is *å*, which corresponds to English *to*. According to the *New Textbook Norm* of 1959, the infinitive may end in -*a* or -*e*. In this book all infinitives of two syllables or more

41

end in -*a*: å tala, å skriva. If we take away the ending -*a* (or -*e*) we get the *stem* of the verb: tal, skriv. Quite a number of verbs, however, are monosyllabic, and the infinitives of these verbs end in the vowel of the stem: å dra, å gå, å ha 'to have', å nå 'to reach', å ta 'to take'. For some of these there exist long variants that end in -*a*, e.g., å hava, å taka.

The infinitive is basically used as in English, i.e., together with the infinitive marker *å* and after modal helping verbs, e.g., Han liker å reisa 'to travel'. Eg må gå no. Vil du ha meir?

4. Å vera, å ha

As is the case in other languages, the verbs *å vera* 'to be' and *å ha* 'to have' have irregular forms:

Infinitive	Present	Past	Past participle
å vera	er	var	(har) vore
å ha	har	hadde	(har) hatt

5. Moods

The verb has three moods, namely the *indicative* mood, the *subjunctive* mood, and the *imperative* mood. The subjunctive mood has the same form as the infinitive with the ending -*e*, or has no ending, where the verb ends in the vowel of the stem. Today the use of the subjunctive mood is limited to high and religious style: «Leve kongen!» 'Long live the king!' Tru det den som kan! 'Believe it, if you can!'

The imperative is normally like the stem of the verb: Gå heim! 'Go home!' Kom hit! 'Come here!'

The indicative mood appears in various tenses in both the active and passive voices.

6. The Reflexive Pronouns

The reflexive pronouns are pronouns in the object form which refer to the subject of the clause in which they stand: Ho vaska seg. 'She washed herself.' Dei vaska seg. 'They washed themselves.'

The reflexive pronoun in the third person, singular and plural, is

42

seg, corresponding to English *himself, herself, itself, themselves.*
The English reflexive pronouns in the first and second persons
singular and plural – *myself, yourself, ourselves,* and *yourselves* –
are rendered by the respective personal pronouns *meg, deg* and
Dykk, oss, dykk and *Dykk.*

Pattern: å vaska seg

1. Eg vaskar meg. 2. Du vaskar deg. De vaskar Dykk (polite form).	I wash myself. You wash yourself. You wash yourself.

3. Han vaskar seg.
   Ho vaskar seg.
   Barnet vaskar seg.
	He washes himself.
	She washes herself.
	The child washes itself.

1. Vi vaskar oss. 2. De vaskar dykk. De vaskar Dykk (polite form).	We wash ourselves. You wash yourselves. You wash yourselves.
3. Dei vaskar seg.	They wash themselves.

The same pronouns are used after prepositions, where English
takes the personal pronouns:

Eg har pengar på meg.	I have money on me.
Har du pengar på deg?	Do you have money on you?
Han har pengar på seg.	He has money with him.
Dei har pengar på seg.	They have money with them.

In *nynorsk* there are many reflexive verbs which are not reflexive
in English. All reflexive verbs are listed with *seg* after the infinitive,
and they can be followed by an object or a preposition: å barbera seg
'to shave', å bry seg om 'to care for', å gifta seg med 'to marry smb.', å
sikra seg 'to secure', å ta på seg 'to undertake', å setja seg ned 'to sit
down', å forsyna seg 'to help oneself', å lika seg 'to like it'.
All the reflexive verbs follow the pattern given above as far as
pronouns are concerned.
The Norwegian word *sjølv*, pl. *sjølve*, corresponding to English
self, selves, is only used to stress that the action refers to one's own
person, not to others: Eg kan kle meg sjølv. 'I can dress myself.' Dei
kan kle seg sjølve. 'They can dress themselves.'

43

Oppgåver (Exercises)
1. Identify nouns in the definite form in Lessons 1–3.
2. Memorize all the forms of å vera and å ha given in 3B4.
3. Fill in the blanks with appropriate reflexive pronouns:
   a) Eg liker . . . . godt her.
   b) Ho liker . . . . godt her.
   c) Han forsyner . . . . godt.
   d) Dei vaskar . . . . på hendene.
   e) Du barberer . . . . ofte.
   f) Vi reiser . . . . frå bordet.
   g) No må de berre forsyna . . . .
   h) Dei forsyner . . . . alltid godt.
   i) Vi forsyner . . . . ofte.

4. Translate into nynorsk:
   a) We like it here.
   b) He often shaves.
   c) She cares for them.
   d) He is marrying her today.
   e) I can do it myself.

3C Pronunciation/Spelling

The Unrounded Vowels /i e æ/

Long /i/ is close to English ee in see. Short /i/ is a little higher than English i in sit. Both sounds are spelled i. Examples: bil 'car', smil 'smile' (long); til, vil (short).

Long /e/ is about like é in French café, or ee in German See, or the beginning of English a in name. It is spelled e. Examples: deg, meg, ser.

Short /e/ is a little lower, and is also spelled e in most cases. In speech it is often pronounced the same as /æ/. Examples: dette, kveld, men.

Long /æ/ is like English a in bad. Before /r/ it is spelled æ, but sometimes e. Examples: hær 'army', lærar 'teacher', her 'here', der 'there'. Short /æ/ has the same articulation as long /æ/, and is like English a in mat. It is spelled both æ and e. Examples: færre 'fewer', væske 'liquid', ferdig, verre 'worse'.

Uttaleøving (Pronunciation Practice)
Drill on /i e æ/ by saying aloud the following words several times:

44

bil, smil; til, vil; deg, meg, ser; dette, kveld, men; hær, lærar, her, der; færre, væske, ferdig, verre.

3D Gjertrudsfuglen

I dei gode gamle dagane då Vårherre og St. Peter gjekk og vandra her på jorda, kom dei ein gong inn til ei kone som sat og baka. Ho heitte Gjertrud, og hadde ei raud lue på hovudet.

Dei hadde gått lenge og var svoltne begge, og så bad Vårherre så vent om ei lefse å smaka på.

Ja, det skulle han få. Men eit lite emne tok ho og kjevla ut; likevel vart det så stort at det fylte heile bakeplata. Nei, så vart den lefsa for stor; den kunne han ikkje få.

Ho tok eit endå mindre emne; men då ho hadde baka det ut og lagt det på plata, vart den lefsa òg for stor. Han kunne ikkje få den heller.

Tredje gongen tok ho eit endå mindre emne, men den gongen òg vart lefsa altfor stor.

«Så har eg ikkje noko å gje dykk», sa Gjertrud. «Lefsene vert for store alle saman.»

Då vart Vårherre sinna og sa: «Fordi du er så gjerrig, skal du få den straffa at du skal verta til ein fugl, og ta di tørre føde mellom bork og ved og ikkje få noko å drikka oftare enn kvar gong det regnar.»

Og straks vart ho til gjertrudsfuglen, og flaug frå bakstebordet opp gjennom pipa.

Norsk eventyr

gjertrudsfuglen /''jærtrusfuglen/
– the black woodpecker
Vårherre /vår''hærre/ – Our
Lord
St. /sankt/ – Saint
gjekk /jekk/ – went
vandra /''vandra/ – walked
gjekk og vandra – were walking
på jorda /'jo:ra/ – on earth
ei kone /''kå:ne/ – woman
sat – sat
baka /''ba:ka/ – baked
sat og baka – was baking
heitte – was called; (her) name was

Gjertrud /''jærtru/
raud – red
ei lue /''lu:e/ – cap
hovudet /''hå:vude/ n. – the head, i.e., her head
hadde gått – had walked
lenge /''lenge/ – for a long time
svoltne /''svåltne/ – hungry
begge /''begge/ – both of them
bad om /'ba: om/ – asked for
så vent /ve:nt/ – so nicely
ei lefse /''lefse/ – kind of soft flatbread, buttered and served folded or rolled
å smaka på /''sma:ka/ – taste

45

skulle /"skulle/ – should
men /menn/ – but
å få – to get
eit emne /"emne/ – bit of dough
lite /"li:te/ – small
tok – took
kjevla ut /kjevla 'u:t/ – rolled
out with a rolling pin
vart /vart/ – became, was
så stort at – so big that
fylte /"fylte/ – filled
bakeplata /"ba:kepla:ta/ f. – the
baking sheet
den /denn/ – that one
for stor /får 'sto:r/ – too big
kunne /"kunne/ – could
endå mindre /"endå 'mindre/ –
even smaller
òg /å:g/ – also, too
hadde baka – had baked
hadde lagt – had laid
heller /'heller/ – either (after
negation)
tredje – third
altfor /'altfår/ – too
så – then
ikkje noko – not anything
å gje /je:/ – to give
dykk pron. (object form) – you

lefsene f.pl. – the bread
vert /vert/ – become, get
alle saman /"alle 'sa:man/ – all
of them
fordi /får'di:/ – because
gjerrig /"jærri/ – stingy
den straffa /'straffa/ f. – the
punishment
å verta til /"verta/ – to become
ein fugl – bird
ta – take
tørre /"tørre/ – dry
føde /"fø:e/ f. – food
mellom /"mellom/ – between
bork /bårk/ m. – bark
ved /ve:/ m. – wood
å drikka /"drikka/ – to drink
oftare /"åftare/ – more often
enn /enn/ – than
kvar gong – each time
det regnar /"regnar/ – it rains
straks /straks/ – immediately
flaug /flæug/ – flew
bakstebordet /"bakstebo:re/ n. –
the baking table
opp /åpp/ – up
gjennom /"jennom/ – through
pipa /"pi:pa/ f. – the chimney

4A På postkontoret

Roy Eisel går og leitar etter eit postkontor. Han stoggar ein mann på gata og spør etter vegen.

ROY	Orsak, kan De seia meg vegen til postkontoret?
MANNEN	Ja, det er rett fram attmed den raude bilen der.
ROY	Er det på høgre eller venstre sida av gata?
MANNEN	Det er første gata til høgre. Du ser skiltet der.
ROY	Tusen takk.
MANNEN	Ver så god ... Det var ein høfleg ung mann.
(På postkontoret)	
ROY	God dag. Eg heiter Roy Eisel og går på folkehøgskulen her. Er det eit brev eller ein pakke til meg frå USA?
EKSPEDITØREN	Nei, det kom ingenting med posten i dag. Var det eit rekommandert brev?
ROY	Ja, det var det. Eg ventar ein sjekk heimanfrå.
EKSPEDITØREN	Kan du ikkje låna litt pengar hjå ein kamerat?
ROY	Eg har alt lånt to hundre kroner, men eg vil gjerne betala dei attende så snart eg kan.
EKSPEDITØREN	Ja, eg forstår.
ROY	Kor mykje er portoen til USA no?
EKSPEDITØREN	For vanlege brev er portoen to kroner og femti øre, og for brevkort ei krone og femti øre. .
ROY	Ver så snill og gje meg nokre frimerke.
EKSPEDITØREN	Her er ei blokk på ti stykke. Det vert tolv kroner og femti øre.
ROY	Ja, eg kjøper den. (Han betaler.) – Ha det.
EKSPEDITØREN	Ha det. Men gløym ikkje pengane dine!

Norsk ordtak: For pengar får ein alt utan godt vêr.

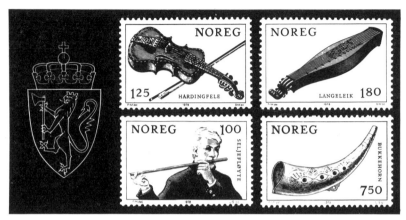

Fig. 4 Det norske riksvåpenet – Nynorske frimerke.

går og leitar etter (å leita etter) –
  is looking for
stoggar /"ståggar/ – stops
spør etter /'spø:r etter/ – asks for
postkontoret /'påstkonto:re/ n. –
  the post office
orsak /"å:rsa:k/ – excuse me
å seia /"sæia/ – to say, to tell
vegen /'ve:gen/ m. – the way
kan De seia meg vegen til – can
  you tell me the way to
rett fram /'rett 'framm/ –
  straight ahead
attmed – close by, near
raude /"ræue/ def.form – red
bilen – the car
på høgre sida /"hø:gre "si:a/ –
  on the right-hand side
på venstre /"venstre/ sida – on
  the left-hand side
av – of
første /"første/ – first
til høgre – to the right
skiltet /'sjilte/ n. – the sign
ver så god – you're welcome

høfleg /"høfleg/ – polite
ung /ong/ – young
eller /'eller/ – or
eit brev /bre:v/ – letter
ein pakke /"pakke/ – parcel
ekspeditøren /ekspedi'tø:ren/ –
  the clerk
ingenting /"ingenting/ – nothing
posten /'påsten/ – the mail
rekommandert /rekoman'de:rt/ –
  registered
ja, det var det – yes, it is
ventar /"ventar/ – expect
ein sjekk /sjekk/ – check
heimanfrå /"hæimanfrå/ – from
  home
å låna hjå /"lå:na jå:/ – to borrow from
litt /litt/ – some
pengar /"pengar/ m.pl. – money
ein kamerat /kame'ra:t/ – friend
har lånt – have borrowed
alt – already
hundre /"hundre/ – hundred

kroner /"kro:ner/ f.pl. – crowns; the crown is the monetary unit of Norway

å betala attende /be'ta:la at-"ende/ – to pay back

så snart eg kan – as soon as I can

eg forstår /får'stå:r/ – I see, understand

kor mykje er /kor "my:kje 'æ:r/ – how much is

portoen /'portoen/ m. – the postage

vanlege /"va:nlege/ – ordinary

femti /'femti/ – fifty

øre /"ø:re/ n.pl. – the smallest monetary unit; 100 øre = 1 krone

brevkort /"bre:vkort/ n.pl. – postcards

ei – one

ver så snill – please

nokre /"nåkre/ – some

frimerke /'fri:mærke/ n.pl. – stamps

ei blokk på /blåkk/ – book of ti – ten

tolv /tåll/ – twelve

stykke /"stykke/ n.pl. – copies, ones (often untranslated)

kjøper /"kjø:per/ – buy

å gløyma /"gløyma/ – to forget

gløym ikkje – don't forget

ein får /få:r/ – one gets

alt – everything

utan /"u:tan/ – except

godt vêr /'gått 'væ:r/ – good weather

Spørsmål (Questions)

1. Kva går Roy Eisel og leitar etter? 2. Kven stoggar han på gata? 3. Kva spør han etter? 4. Kvar ligg postkontoret? 5. Er det på høgre eller venstre sida av gata? 6. Kva seier Roy på postkontoret? 7. Kva ventar han heimanfrå? 8. Kvifor vil han ikkje låna pengar hjå ein kamerat? 9. Kor mykje er portoen for brev til USA? 10. Kva kjøper Roy på postkontoret?

4B Grammar

1. The Inflection of Nouns

As you can see from the previous lessons, a noun may appear in one of the following forms: indefinite singular, definite singular, indefinite plural, and definite plural. Each gender has its own set of endings: ein-nouns: -en, -ar, -ane; ei-nouns: -a, -er, -ene; eit-nouns: -et, no ending, -a.

49

The inflection of nouns. Basic pattern:

	Singular		Plural	
	Indefinite form	Definite form	Indefinite form	Definite form
Masculine	ein by	byen -en	byar -ar	byane -ane
Feminine	ei bygd	bygda -a	bygder -er	bygdene -ene
Neuter	eit land	landet -et	land no ending	landa -a

Notice that the ending -et is pronounced /e/.

There are some exceptions to the basic pattern given above, and we will mention the most important ones:

Masculine Nouns (ein-nouns)

A small group of masculine nouns take the endings -er and -ene in the plural. This applies to: 1) nouns ending in -nad (ein søknad 'application' – søknaden – søknader – søknadene); 2) loan words ending in -a (ein sofa – sofaen – sofaer – sofaene); 3) nouns with a vowel shift in the plural (ein son – sonen – søner – sønene), and 4) a small group that took similar endings in Old Norwegian (ein gjest 'guest' – gjesten – gjester – gjestene).

Feminine Nouns (ei-nouns)

A small group of feminine nouns take the endings -ar and -ane in the plural. This applies to: 1) nouns ending in -ing (ei hending 'event' – hendinga – hendingar – hendingane); 2) a small group that originally took the endings -ar and -ane (ei øy 'island' – øya – øyar – øyane).

Neuter Nouns (eit-nouns)

Some loanwords endring in -ium have irregular inflection (eit studium 'study' – studiet – studium – studia), and some foreign words ending in -um have kept the foreign ending (eit faktum 'fact' – faktumet – fakta – fakta).

Contracted Forms

Some of the nouns of the masculine, feminine, and neuter gender ending in -el, -en, -er, -al, -ar, and -ul have contracted forms.

50

Dictionaries will give complete information about these words. Here are some examples:

ein himmel 'sky' – himmelen – himlar – himlane
eit våpen 'weapon' – våpenet – våpen – våpna
ei hulder 'mountain nymph' – huldra – huldrer – huldrene
ein apal 'apple tree' – apalen – aplar – aplane
ein sommar 'summer' – sommaren – somrar – somrane
ein jøkul 'glacier' – jøkulen – jøklar – jøklane

2. Cases

Old Norwegian had four cases: nominative, genitive, dative, and accusative. Apart from the personal pronouns, which have both subject forms and object forms (see 6B3), nynorsk has only two cases, nominative and genitive. The genitive is formed by adding -s to the nominative both in the indefinite and definite form, singular and plural. The s-genitive, however, is very often replaced by a prepositional phrase, as is done in English:

gutens far – far til guten 'the father of the boy'
husets eigar – eigaren av huset 'the owner of the house'

Notice that no apostrophe is written between the noun and the ending -s.

3. The Numerals. Cardinal Numbers

0	1	2	3	4
null /null/	ein (ei, eitt)	to /to:/	tre /tre:/	fire /"fi:re/

5	6	7	8	9
fem /femm/	seks /seks/	sju /sju:/	åtte /"åtte/	ni /ni:/

10	11	12	13
ti /ti:/	elleve /"elleve/	tolv /tåll/	tretten /"tretten/

14	15	16
fjorten /"fjorten/	femten /"femten/	seksten /"seksten/

17	18	19
sytten /"sytten/	atten /"atten/	nitten /"nitten/

20	21	22
tjue /"kju:e/	tjueein /kju:e'æin/	tjueto /kju:e'to:/

51

The cardinal numbers are the numbers we use when counting : ein, to, tre, etc. The cardinal number ein is inflected in gender, and has three forms: ein, ei, or eitt, depending on the noun it qualifies, e.g., Han har ein båt 'boat' (ikkje to). Han har ei bok 'book' (ikkje to). Han har eitt blad 'newspaper' (ikkje to).

Some arithmetic

2 + 3 =   5 To pluss tre er fem.
6 − 4 =   2 Seks minus fire er to.
2 × 5 = 10 To gonger fem er ti.
8 : 2 := 4 Åtte delt på to er fire.

Oppgåver (Exercises)

1. Identify the nouns in the dialogue and list each noun with its four forms: the indefinite and definite singular forms, and the indefinite and definite plural forms, e.g., ei lekse – leksa – lekser – leksene.
2. Memorize the numbers from 1 to 29.
3. Translate into *nynorsk*:
   a) They have an office on the left-hand side of the main street.
   b) He is expecting two letters and three parcels from home.
   c) She has borrowed some money from a friend.
   d) Give me some stamps, please.

4C Pronunciation/Spelling

The Unrounded Vowel /a/

Long /a/ is similar to English a in *father*, and short /a/ is almost like English u in *cut*. Both sounds are spelled a. Examples; ha, sa, far (long); han, kan, mann (short).

Notice that vowel length is indirectly shown in spelling. One writes only one consonant letter after a long vowel, and two consonant letters after a short stressed vowel: gul /gu:l/ 'yellow', gull /gull/ 'gold'.

One exception is m, which is never doubled at the end of a word, even if the vowel is short and stressed: kam /kamm/ 'comb', lam /lamm/ 'lamb'.

Final l and n are not doubled in modal auxiliaries or pronouns: skal /skall/, vil /vill/, den /denn/, kan /kann/.

Find words in the dialogue that contain long or short /a/ and practice pronouncing them.

4D Nynorske frimerke

I Noreg kom det første frimerket i bruk 1. januar 1855. Det var laga i berre eitt verde (4 skilling), og det hadde det norske riksvåpenet til emblem. Teksten var på norsk-dansk, som var skriftspråket i Noreg på den tida.

Det første frimerket med det nynorske landsnamnet NOREG var Garborg-serien i 1951 (25 øre, 45 øre, 80 øre) til minne om Arne Garborgs fødsel hundre år før.

I 1963 vart namnet NOREG brukt på ny på to frimerke til minne om Ivar Aasens fødsel i 1813, og i 1964 på to frimerke til minne om den første folkehøgskulen i Noreg, som vart grunnlagd i 1864.

I 1968 kom det også to frimerke med NOREG på, og det var til minne om A.O. Vinjes fødsel i 1818, og i 1977 kom det to med motiv frå fisket langs kysten.

6. oktober 1978 gav Postverket ut fire nye frimerke med det nynorske namnet på landet. På kvart av dei er det eit bilete av eit typisk norsk folkemusikk-instrument. Det gjeld følgjande frimerke:

100 øre, grønt – Seljefløyte 'willow pipe'
125 øre, raudt – Hardingfele (a Norwegian variant of the violin)
180 øre, blått – Langeleik 'Norwegian zither'
750 øre, oliven – Bukkehorn 'ram's horn'

i bruk /bru:k/ – in use
januar /janu'a:r/ – January
var laga /''la:ga/ – was made
eitt /æitt/ – one
eit verde /''væ:re/ – value
ein skilling /'sjilling/ – obsolete coin
eit riksvåpen /'riksvå:pen/ – national coat of arms
eit emblem /em'ble:m/ – emblem
ein tekst – text

eit skriftspråk /'skriftsprå:k/ – written language
på den tida /'ti:a/ – at that time
eit landsnamn /'lansnamn/ – name of a country
Arne Garborg /''ga:rbårg/ – famous *nynorsk* writer
ein serie /'se:rie/ – series
til minne om – in memory of
ein fødsel /'føtsel/ – birth
vart brukt – was used
på ny – again

53

Ivar Aasen /'å:sen/ – famous linguist and poet

vart grunnlagd – was established

A. O. Vinje /''vinje/ – well-known nynorsk writer

eit motiv /mo'ti:v/ – subject

eit fiske /''fiske/ – fishing

langs – along

ein kyst /kjyst/ – coast

oktober /ok'to:ber/ – October

gav ut – issued

Postverket /'påstværke/ – the Postal Service

på kvart av dei – on each of them

eit bilete /''bi:lete/ – picture

typisk /'ty:pisk/ – typical

folkemusikk /''fålkemusikk/ m. – folk music

eit instrument /instru'ment/ – instrument

det gjeld følgjande – they are the following

grønt /grø:nt/ n.sing. – green

raudt /ræutt/ n.sing. – red

blått n.sing. – blue

oliven /o'li:ven/ – olive

1855 /attenfemti'femm/

1951 /nittenfemti'æin/

1963 /nittenseksti'tre:/

1813 /atten''trætten/

1964 /nittenseksti''fi:re/

1864 /attenseksti''fi:re/

1968 /nittenseksti''åtte/

1818 /atten''atten/

1977 /nittensytti'sju:/

1978 /nittensytti''åtte/

5A På kafeteria

Roy Eisel og Per Nes går inn på ein kafeteria for å eta.

NES   Her er eit ledig bord og to gode stolar. – Kva skal vi ha, ein varmrett eller smørbrød?

ROY   Eg vil berre ha eit par gode smørbrød og ein kopp kaffi. Vi får middag på skulen i kveld.

NES   Eg har lyst på kjøtkaker med kokte poteter og ferske grønsaker. Kjøtkakene er alltid gode her.

ROY   Eg tek to smørbrød med egg og tomat. – Skal du ha noko å drikka til maten?

NES   Ja, men berre eit glas vatn.

ROY   (Roy kjem med maten.) Her er knivar, gaflar og skeier. – Kva for faste måltid har de heime hjå dykk? Eg forstår at det er ulikt frå familie til familie.

NES   Til vanleg har vi frukost i 7-tida. Då et vi eit par brødskiver med pålegg og gjerne eit kokt egg. Pålegget er som regel brun eller kvit ost, syltety og kjøtpålegg, og vi drikk mjølk og kaffi til maten.

ROY   Kva et de midt på dagen då?

NES   Dei fleste har med seg eit par skiver på jobben, men eg kjøper av og til ein billeg rett på ein kafeteria. Middag plar vi ha i 4-tida, men somme et middag midt på dagen og kveldsmat i 8-tida. Middagen er eit stort måltid med kjøt eller fisk, grønsaker, suppe og dessert. Vi drikk kaldt vatn til maten, for det norske vatnet er reint og godt.

ROY   Drikk de aldri kaffi til middagen slik som i USA?

NES   Nei, vi tek heller ein kopp kaffi etterpå.

ROY   Dette var godt.

NES   Ja, maten er god og rimeleg her. – Nei, no må eg gå. Ha det bra så lenge!

ROY   Ha det.

Mat og matskikkar i Noreg

Tid	Måltidet heiter	Vi et
i 7-tida	frukost	eit kokt egg, brødskiver med pålegg (ost, syltety, kjøt); mjølk, te eller kaffi
i 12-tida	føremiddagsmat (lunsj)	eit par brødskiver med pålegg; kaffi eller te
i 4-tida	middag	kjøt eller fisk, kokte poteter, grønsaker, suppe, dessert; vatn, saft eller øl
i 6-tida	kaffi ·	kaffi og småkaker
i 8-tida	kveldsmat	smørbrød eller ein varmrett
Hugs: Alle seier «Takk for maten» etter eit måltid.		

Norsk ordtak: Sterkt øl gjer store ord.

ein kafeteria /kafe'te:ria/ – cafeteria
for å eta /''e:ta/ – (in order) to eat
eit bord /bo:r/ – table
ledig /''le:di/ – vacant
ein stol – chair
ein rett – course, dish
varm – warm, hot
eit smørbrød /''smø:rbrø:/ – sandwich (open-faced)
eit par – a couple of
ein kopp kaffi – a cup of coffee
på skulen /''sku:len/ – at school
i kveld – tonight
eg har lyst på – I want, feel like
ei kjøtkake /''kjø:tka:ke/ – meat patty (meatball)
ei potet /po'te:t/ – potato
ferske /''færske/ pl. – fresh
grønsaker /''grønnsa:ker/ pl. – vegetables
alltid /'allti:/ – always
tek – take

eit egg – egg
ein tomat /to'ma:t/ – tomato
noko /''nå:ko/ – something
til maten – with the food
eit glas vatn – a glass of water
ein kniv – knife
ein gaffel /'gaffel/ – fork
ei skei /sjæi/ – spoon
kva for – which
faste /''faste/ pl. – regular
eit måltid /''må:lti:/ – meal
ulikt /''u:likt/ n. sing. – different
frå familie til familie – from one family to another
til vanleg – usually
i 7-tida /i 'sju:ti:a/ – about 7 o'clock
et – eat
ei brødskive /''brø:sji:ve/ – slice of bread
eit pålegg /''på:legg/ – anything laid or spread on buttered bread to make eit smørbrød
gjerne – possibly

56

eit kokt egg – a boiled egg
som regel /'re:gel/ – as a rule
brun – brown
kvit – white
ein ost – cheese
syltety /"syltety:/ n. – jam
eit kjøtpålegg – meat slice topping for bread
drikk – drink
mjølk f. – milk
kaffi /"kaffi/ m. – coffee
midt /mitt/ på dagen – in the
middle of the day
dei fleste /"fleste/ – most people
har med seg – take, bring
ei skive /"sji:ve/ – slice of bread
ein jobb /jåbb/ – job
på jobben – at work
av og til – now and then
billeg /"billeg/ – cheap
vi plar ha – we usually have
somme /"somme/ – some people

kveldsmat /"kvelsma:t/ m. –
supper
kjøt n. – meat
fisk m. – fish
ei suppe /"suppe/ – soup
ein dessert /de'sæ:r/ – dessert
kaldt /kalt/ n.sing. – cold
for /fårr/ – for, because
reint /ræint/ n.sing. – clean
aldri /"aldri/ – never
slik som i – as in
heller /'heller/ – rather
etterpå /"etterpå:/ – afterwards
rimeleg /"ri:meleg/ – reasonable, inexpensive
ein matskikk /"ma:tsjikk/ – eating custom
saft f. – juice
hugs – remember
øl /ø:l/ n. – beer
småkaker /"små:ka:ker/ f.pl. –
cookies
sterkt /stærkt/ n.sing. – strong

Samtaleøving (Conversation Practice)
Improvise a conversation in class where you make use of text 5A.

5B Grammar

1. Ein kopp kaffi 'a cup of coffee'

When a noun indicates a certain unit of quantity of a following
noun, the two nouns are joined directly without any preposition
between them in *nynorsk*.

Examples:

ein kopp kaffi	a cup of coffee
ein liter mjølk	a liter of milk
eit glas vatn	a glass of water
eit glas øl	a glass of beer
eit par skiver	a couple of sandwiches
eit kilo poteter	a kilo of potatoes

57

2. The Agreement of Adjectives. The Indefinite Form

We have already used adjectives in a number of sentences, e.g., norsk, lang, sinna, god, stor, raud, etc.

The adjective has an *indefinite form* and a *definite form*. The *indefinite form* agrees in gender and number with the noun or pronoun it modifies, but has only two possible endings. The ending -t, as a rule, is added in the neuter singular, and the ending -e is added in the plural, regardless of gender. In the masculine and feminine singular, no ending is used.

The indefinite form. Basic pattern:

Masculine	ein fin (pretty) by	No ending
Feminine	ei fin bygd	
Neuter	eit fint land	-t
Plural, all genders	fine byar, bygder, land	-e

The indefinite form is used in the following cases: 1) when the adjective stands alone before a noun: godt vêr, roleg sjø 'quiet sea'; 2) when it is preceded by the indefinite article or an indefinite pronoun: ein fin by, ingen fin by 'no pretty city'; 3) when it is used after the verb 'to be' or 'to become': Byen er fin. Landet er fint. Bygdene er fine.

Exceptions from the Basic Pattern

Many adjectives do not take the ending -t in the neuter. The most important groups are: 1) those already ending in -t: ein svart gut 'black boy', eit svart land, ein steinut åker 'stony field', eit steinut land; 2) adjectives of more than one syllable ending in -sk, and all adjectives ending in -sk denoting nationality: ein historisk person, eit historisk slag 'battle', ein norsk gut, eit norsk språk, but: fersk fisk, ferskt kjøt, friskt barn 'healthy child'; 3) adjectives ending in -ig, -ug, or -leg: Arbeidet er ferdig. Det er eit vitug svar. 'That's a sensible answer.' Mannen er farleg 'dangerous'; 4) some adjectives ending in -a, -o, -u, and -y, most of them monosyllables; bra 'fine', tru 'faithful', slu 'cunning', edru 'sober', sky 'shy'.

Adjectives ending in a stressed vowel or a diphthong get -tt in the neuter: ein ny bil – eit nytt hus, ein blå dress 'blue suit' – eit blått plagg 'garment', ein brei veg 'wide road' – eit breitt felt 'wide area'.

58

Adjectives ending in -en, keep this ending both in the masculine and the feminine singular, but take the ending -e in the neuter, and -ne in the plural. The same pattern also applies to all past participles ending in -en (strong verbs). See 1/B1.

Adjectives ending in -en:

Masculine	ein open båt	
Feminine	ei open dør	-en
Neuter	eit ope hus	-e
Plural, all genders	opne båtar, dører, hus	-ne

Like adjectives and past participles ending in -en, adjectives ending in -el and -er have contracted forms in the plural: ein open båt 'boat' – opne båtar, ein sjofel person 'contemptible person' – sjofle personar, ein diger hest 'big horse' – digre hestar.

The adjectives eigen 'own' and liten 'little, small' have feminine forms of their own, and liten has also an irregular form in the plural:

eigen båt	eiga bygd	eige land	eigne båtar, bygder, land
ein liten båt	ei lita bygd	eit lite land	små båtar, bygder, land

Normally the adjective agrees in gender and number with the subject when it follows the verb 'to be' or 'to become': Mannen var stor. Kona var lita. Studentane var norske. In some cases, however, there is no grammatical agreement between the subject and the adjective.

1) The adjective may be associated with another word than the grammatical subject, e.g., Ein heil dunge med høy var tørt alt. 'A whole pile of hay was already dry' (høy is an eit-noun).

2) If the subject is a noun in the indefinite form referring to a whole category or to a general activity, the predicative is often in the neuter form singular, even though the subject may be of another gender or number:
Kjøtkaker er godt. (Det er godt.) Mat er godt. (Det er godt.) Kroppsøving er helsesamt. 'Physical training is healthy.' Jakt er morosamt. 'Hunting is fun.' Ein ting er sikkert. 'One thing is sure.' Røyking forbode. 'No smoking.'

3. The Past Tense

In *nynorsk* there are two ways of forming the past tense, just as in English:

1) By adding the endings *-a, -de, -dde,* or *-te* to the verb stem: å kasta – kasta 'threw', å dømma – dømde 'judged', å tru – trudde 'believed', å tenkja – tenkte 'thought'. These verbs are called *weak verbs.*

2) By changing the vowel of the stem without adding any ending to it: å bita – beit 'bit', å bryta – braut 'broke', å finna – fann 'found', å lesa – las 'read'. These verbs are called *strong verbs.*

Oppgåver (Exercises)

Fill in the correct form of the adjective:

1. Han arbeider i eit . . . . hus (stor)
2. Dei har . . . . stolar (raud)
3. Båten var . . . . (lys)
4. Bygda var . . . . (fin)
5. Det er . . . . studentar i klassen (norsk)
6. Grønsakene var . . . . (fersk)
7. Jenta var . . . . (liten)
8. Kjøtkaker er . . . . (god)
9. Frimerket var . . . . (blå)
10. Dei hadde . . . . båtar (liten)
11. Han hadde . . . . hus (eigen)
12. Dei hadde . . . . dører (open)
13. Det var eit . . . . frimerke (norsk)

5C Pronunciation/Spelling

The Diphthongs /æi øy æu/

The *nynorsk* diphthongs /æi øy æu/ are different from the English diphthongs in *say, boy,* and *so.*

In Norwegian the second element of the diphthong is as prominent as the first one, whereas in English the first element is emphasized, and the second one is a consonantal glide.

The first element of /æi/ is close to /æ/, and it moves in the direction of /i/. This means that it starts with the mouth more open than English *ay* in *say* and ends after a quick upward glide in a clear Norwegian /i/. Examples: ei, dei, veit.

The first element of /øy/ is an open /ø/ that moves quickly in the direction of a clear /y/ (a slack or rounded /i/). Examples: øy 'island', fløyte 'cream', løysa 'untie'.

The first element of /æu/ is /æ/ or /ø/, and the diphthong ends in /u/. Examples: aust 'east', blaut 'soft', graut 'porridge'.

Uttaleøving (Pronunciation Practice)
Drill on the diphthongs /æi øy æu/ by saying aloud several times the following words: ei, dei, veit; øy, fløyte, løysa; aust, blaut, graut.

5D Nokre stubbar

Om tidløyse
– Kven var det du stod ute i tunet og prata med ein heil time?
– Det var fru Hagen. Ho hadde ikkje tid til å koma inn.

Falske pengar
Han Ola hadde fått fatt i ein tikroning som ikkje var ekte, og så var han innom krambua med han.
– Den kan du nok ikkje handla for. Han er falsk, sa handelsmannen.
– Eg veit det, men eg ville berre veksla han, svara Ola.

Lær å spela orgel til jul
«Lær å spela orgel til jul. Send oss 50 kroner», stod det i ei lysing. Ein mann sende 50 kroner, og ikkje lenge etter fekk han svar: «Takk for pengane. Gløym no ikkje å læra å spela orgel til jul.»

Det er skilnad på folk
Guten: «Du far, kva er skilnaden mellom ein generaldirektør og ein vanleg direktør?»
Faren: «Om lag 25 kilo, skulle eg tru.»

ein stubb – yarn, short tale
tidløyse /'ti:løyse/ f. – the state of being busy or occupied

stod /sto:/ – stood
prata /'pra:ta/ – talked
stod og prata – were talking

61

eit tun – yard (courtyard, farm yard)
ein time /"ti:me/ – hour
heil /hæil/ – whole
ho hadde ikkje tid til – she didn't have the time to
å koma inn /kå:ma 'inn/ – to come in
falsk – false, counterfeit
hadde fått fatt i – had gotten hold of
ein tikroning /"ti:kro:ning/ – ten crown bill
ekte /"ekte/ – real, genuine
ei krambu /"krambu:/ – general store
han – it (referring to the masculine noun tikroning)
å handla /"handla/ – to buy, to trade
du kan nok ikkje – I'm afraid you can't
den kan du nok ikkje handla for – I'm afraid you can't buy anything for that one (inverted word order)
den . . . for – for (with) that
ein handelsmann /'handels-mann/ – tradesman, merchant

eg ville berre – I only wanted to
å veksla /"veksla/ – to change
å læra /"læ:ra/ – to learn
å spela /"spe:la/ – to play
eit orgel /'årgel/ – organ
å spela orgel – to play the organ
til jul /ju:l/ – before Christmas
å senda /"senda/ – to send
stod det i – it said in
ei lysing /"ly:sing/ – advertisement
sende /"sende/ – sent
ikkje lenge etter – not long afterwards
fekk – got, received
eit svar – answer
ein skilnad /"sjilna/ – difference
folk /fålk/ – people
det er skilnad på folk – people are different
ein generaldirektør /gener'a:l-/ – managing director
ein direktør /direk'tø:r/ – director
om lag /om 'la:g/ – approximately
å tru – to think
skulle eg tru – I should think

6A I butikken

Kari Nes liker å gå i butikkar for å sjå på nye varer. Ein dag dreg ho inn til sentrum for å sjå på ein kjole.

EKSPEDITRISA Ver så god!
FRU NES   God dag. Eg vil gjerne sjå på ein kjole.
EKSPEDITRISA Kva slags kjole skal det vera?
FRU NES   Det skal vera ein fritidskjole.
EKSPEDITRISA Kor stor skal han vera?
FRU NES   Eg bruker førtito.
EKSPEDITRISA Vi har mange i den storleiken der borte.
FRU NES   Nei, dei kjolane kler meg ikkje. Dei gjer meg så gammal. – Har de ikkje andre modellar?
EKSPEDITRISA Jau, kom hit bort. Her har vi dei nye modellane.
FRU NES   Den raude vil eg gjerne prøva.
EKSPEDITRISA Ver så god. Prøverommet er rett til høgre.
FRU NES   Kva kostar denne kjolen?
EKSPEDITRISA Han kostar to hundre og åtti kroner.
FRU NES   Det vert for dyrt for meg.
EKSPEDITRISA Vi har nokre på utsal til eitt hundre og femti kroner. Vil du sjå på dei?
FRU NES   Ja, takk. Det vil eg gjerne.
EKSPEDITRISA Kvaliteten er god, men dei er ikkje på moten no.
FRU NES   Nei, denne fasongen liker eg ikkje og heller ikkje fargen. Eg tek den raude til to hundre og åtti kroner likevel.
EKSPEDITRISA Takk skal du ha. Eg skal pakka han inn til deg. – Vil du betala kontant, eller skal vi skriva det?
FRU NES   Kontant, takk.
EKSPEDITRISA Då får du tre prosent i rabatt. Ver gild og betal i kassen!

63

FRU NES   Ha det.
EKSPEDITRISA Ha det bra, og velkomen att.

Norsk ordtak: Klede skaper folk.

ein butikk /bu'tikk/ – store
å sjå på /'sjå: på/ – to look at
ei vare /"va:re/ – article, prod-
    uct
dreg – goes
eit sentrum /'sentrum/ – center
til sentrum – downtown
ein kjole /"kjo:le/ – dress
ei ekspeditrise /ekspedi'tri:se/ –
    saleswoman
kva slags – what kind of
kva slags kjole skal det vera? –
    what kind of dress are you
    looking for?
ein fritidskjole /'fri:ti:skjo:le/ –
    casual dress
stor – big, great
eg bruker førtito – I wear (use) 42
ein storleik /"sto:rlæik/ – size
mange /"mange/ – many
der borte – over there
dei kler meg ikkje – they don't
    suit me
dei gjer meg så gammal – they
    make me look so old
andre /"andre/ – other
ein modell /mo'dell/ – fashion,
    style
jau – yes (in answer to a ques-
    tion which contains a doubt
    or a negation)
hit bort – over here
å prøva /"prø:va/ – to try (on)
eit prøverom /"prø:veromm/ –
    fitting room
rett til høgre – straight ahead to
    the right

kva kostar denne kjolen? – how
    much is this dress?
dyr – expensive
åtti /'åtti/ – eighty
for dyrt – too expensive
eit utsal /'u:tsa:l/ – sale
på utsal – on sale
ein kvalitet /kvali'te:t/ – quality
ein mote /"mo:te/ – fashion,
    style
ikkje på moten – not in style
denne – this
ein fasong /fa'sång/ – fashion,
    cut, style
heller ikkje – not (either)
ein farge – color
ein kjole til to hundre – a dress
    for two hundred (crowns)
takk skal du ha – thank you
å pakka inn /pakka 'inn/ – to
    wrap up
kontant /kon'tant/ – cash
å skriva noko – to charge
    something
ein prosent /pro'sent/ – percent
ein rabatt /ra'batt/ – discount
ein kasse /"kasse/ – cash reg-
    ister
gild /jild/ – kind
ver gild og betal i kassen! –
    please pay at the cash reg-
    ister
velkomen att /vel'kå:men 'att/ –
    welcome back
klede /"kle:e/ n.pl. – clothes
skaper – make

64

1. Kvifor går Kari Nes ofte i butikkar? 2. Kva slags kjole kjøper ho?
3. Kva storleik bruker ho? 4. Kva farge har kjolen? 5. Kva kostar
han? 6. Kvar betaler ho? 7. Betaler ho kontant? 8. Får ho rabatt?
9. Kva seier ho då ho går? 10. Kva svarar ekspeditrisa?

6B Grammar

1. The Agreement of Adjectives. The Definite Form

The *definite form* of the adjective is the same form as the indefinite
form plural, i.e., it ends in -e. The only exception is *liten*, which has
the definite singular form *litle* or *vesle*.

The definite form. Basic pattern:

Masculine	den fine byen	
Feminine	den fine bygda	-e
Neuter	det fine landet	
Plural, all genders	dei fine byane, bygdene, landa	

As can be seen from the chart above, the definite article which is
used before a noun modified by an adjective is *den* in the
masculine and feminine singular, *det* in the neuter, and *dei* in the
plural. This article is often referred to as the *definite article of the
adjective*, since it is used before an adjective with a nominal
function or before an adjective modifying a noun, e.g., dei kvite 'the
white ones', dei svarte 'the black ones', den fine byen. You should
notice that both the definite article of the adjective (den, det, dei)
and the definite article of the noun (-en, -a, -et; -ane, -ene, -a) are, as
a rule, both used when an adjective is followed by a noun: den fine
byen, den fine bygda.

The definite form of the adjective is used in the following cases:
1) after the preposed definite article: den fine byen, dei fine landa;
2) after demonstrative pronouns (denne, dette, desse): denne fine
byen (this), desse fine bygdene (these); 3) after personal pronouns:
du vesle gut, eg arme 'poor' mann; 4) after possessive forms: vårt
fine land, Noregs fine kyst 'coast'.

Unlike English, the definite form preceded by the definite article

65

can be used as a noun without adding the word 'one' or 'ones': den fine 'the pretty one', dei vesle 'the small ones'.

Notice that adjectives and nouns denoting nationality or religion are not capitalized in nynorsk: norsk, nordmann, engelsk, protestant, katolikk.

2. The Numerals. Cardinal Numbers (continued)

30	40	50
tretti /'tretti/	førti /'førti/	femti /'femti/

60	70	80
seksti /'seksti/	sytti /'sytti/	åtti /'åtti/

90	100	101
nitti /'nitti/	hundre /''hundre/	hundreogein

123	1000
hundreogtjuetre	eitt tusen /'tu:sen/

3. The Personal Pronouns

We have already used most of the personal pronouns, and in 1B2 we have given a survey of the subject forms. In the chart below both subject and object forms are given.

The personal pronouns. Subject and object forms:

Person	Subject form		Object form	
1. Singular	eg	I	meg	me
2. Singular	du	you	deg	you
	De	you	Dykk	you
3. Singular	han	he	han/honom	him
	ho	she	henne/ho	her
	det	it	det	it
1. Plural	vi	we	oss	us
2. Plural	de	you	dykk	you
	De	you	Dykk	you
3. Plural	dei	they	dei	them

66

The subject form is used when the personal pronoun is the subject of the clause: Eg såg ein film. 'I saw a movie.' Dei bur i Bergen. 'They live in Bergen.'

The object form is used when the personal pronoun is the direct object or the indirect object of the clause, or when it is governed by a preposition: Hunden beit meg. 'The dog bit me.' Gje oss mat. 'Give us food.' Brevet var frå henne. 'The letter was from her.'

After the verb 'to be' and in comparison with the subject after the word *enn* 'than', the usage varies. It is considered grammatically correct to use the subject form in these cases: Det er eg. 'It is I.' Er det du? 'Is that you?' Or: Det er meg. Er det deg? Han er flinkare enn eg (er). 'He is cleverer than I.' Ho er yngre enn du (er). 'She is younger than you.' Or: Han er flinkare enn meg. Ho er yngre enn deg.

The personal pronouns *han* and *ho* refer to masculine and feminine nouns of all kinds, i.e., they refer to human beings, animals, and things:

Mannen kjem. *Han* kjem.
Hesten er svart. *Han* er svart. 'The horse is black. It is black.'
Vi måtte reparera radioen, for *han* var i ustand. 'We had to fix the radio, because it was out of order.'
Kona går. *Ho* går.
Geita er kvit. *Ho* er kvit. 'The goat is white. It is white.'
Boka var blå. *Ho* var blå. 'The book was blue. It was blue.'

The personal pronoun *det* /de:/ refers to nouns of the neuter gender:
Barnet var norsk. *Det* var norsk.
Dyret var grått. *Det* var grått. 'The animal was gray. It was gray.'
Brevet var raudt. *Det* var raudt. 'The letter was red. It was red.'

If we want to stress a masculine or feminine noun in the singular, we do not use *han* or *ho*, but the demonstrative pronoun *den* when referring to it: Tok du den nye bilen? 'Did you take the new car?' *Den* vil eg ha (see 15B1).

Oppgåver
1. Find all the adjectives in the dialogue and list them with their indefinite and definite form.
2. Count from 30 to 100.
3. Memorize all the personal pronouns.
4. Translate into *nynorsk*:
   a) What does the red dress cost?

b) The new fashions are here.
c) We like our pretty country.
d) The fresh ones are good.
e) Many Norwegians speak English.

6C Pronunciation/Spelling

The Fricative Consonants /kj/ *and* /sj/

The fricative consonant /kj/, IPA [ç], is a voiceless sound which is different from any English sound. It is similar to *ch* in German *ich*, and reminds one a little of English *h* in words like *huge, hue*, only stronger. It is articulated by raising the middle of the tongue towards the roof of the mouth so as to produce a very narrow passage.

In some western dialects it is replaced by an affricate [cç], which, therefore, is acceptable if you find it easier to pronounce that one. However, it must be clearly distinguished from /sj/, IPA [ʃ], which is about the same as *sh* in English *shilling*.

The consonant /kj/ is spelled in different ways: 1) *kj* in most words: kjole, kjerring 'old lady; housewife'; 2) *k* before *i, y, ei*, and *øy* in stressed syllables: kiste 'trunk', kyst, keisam 'boring', køyra 'drive'; 3) *tj* in some words: tjue, tjukk 'thick', tjuv 'thief'.

The consonant /sj/ is also represented in writing in different ways: 1) by *sj* in sjel 'soul', sjuk 'sick', sjø 'sea'; 2) by *sk* before *i, y, ei*, and *øy* in stressed syllables: ski, sky 'cloud', skei 'spoon', skøyte 'skate'; 3) by *skj*: skjorte 'shirt', skjor 'magpie', skjøna 'understand'.

Uttaleøving

Drill on /kj/ and /sj/ by saying aloud several times the following words: kiste, kyst, keisam, kjole; sjel, sjuk, ski, sky, skei, skjøna.

6D Snarkjøpsbutikkar og varehus

Det er mange butikkar i alle byar og tettstader i Noreg. Med handelslova i 1842 fekk ein full handelsfridom. I byane vart detaljhandelen og engros-handelen meir spesialisert, og på bygdene vart landhandelen ein viktig sosial institusjon ved sida av å vera handelsstad.

Framleis går mykje av handelen føre seg i små bedrifter, men

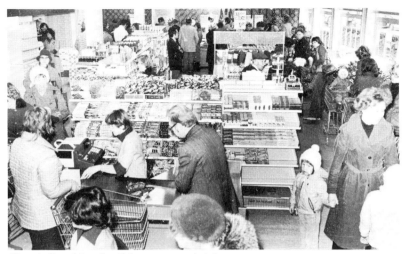

Fig. 6 *Snarkjøpsbutikkane er praktiske.*

utviklinga synest å gå i retning av store varehus og ulike former for kjedeforretningar, jamvel om mange er imot dette. Og talet på snarkjøpsbutikkar veks.

Butikkane plar opna klokka ni om morgonen, og dei stengjer klokka fem om ettermiddagen. På laurdagar stengjer dei klokka eitt, og dei er stengde på sundagar.

Snarkjøpsbutikkane er om lag som snarkjøpsbutikkar i andre land. Ein treng ikkje seia eit ord, men folk bruker å seia «Ver så god» når dei betaler.

Folk går ofte omkring og ser på varene, og ein ekspeditør eller ei ekspeditrise kjem gjerne bort og seier «Ver så god» eller «Får du?» Folk svarar «Eg berre ser, takk.»

Snarkjøpsbutikkane er mindre personlege enn den gamle landhandelen eller krambua, som dei sa. Krambulivet gav bygdesamfunnet noko av sitt særmerkte drag. Krambua var svært populær, og mange saknar henne. Men ho kjem nok ikkje attende meir.

ein snarkjøpsbutikk – self-service store
det er – there are
ein tettstad /'tettsta:/ – heavily populated area
ein handel /'handel/ – trade, commerce, business

ei lov /lå:v/ – law, regulation
ei handelslov – trade law
ein – one (indef. pronoun)
full – complete
ein fridom /'fri:dom/ – freedom
ein handelsfridom /'handels-/ – freedom of trade

69

ein detaljhandel /de'taljhandel/ – retail trade
ein engros-handel /an'gro:-/ – wholesale business
spesialisert /spesiali'se:rt/ – specialized
på bygdene – in the countryside
ein landhandel /"landhandel/ – general store
viktig /"vikti/ – important
sosial /sosi'a:l/ – social
ein institusjon /institu'sjo:n/ – institution
ved sida av – in addition to
ein handelsstad /'handels-/ – trading center, store
framleis /"framlæis/ – still
går føre seg – takes place
små pl. of liten – little, small
ei bedrift /be'drift/ – concern, company
ei utvikling /'u:tvikling/ – development
synest /"sy:nest/ – seems
ei retning /"retning/ – direction
eit varehus /"va:rehu:s/ – department store
ulik /"u:li:k/ – different, various
ei form /fårm/ – form
ei kjedeforretning /"kje:defåretning/ – chain store
jamvel om – even though
imot /i'mo:t/ – against
eit tal – number
veks – is increasing
å opna /"å:pna/ – to open
plar opna – usually opens
klokka ni /klåkka 'ni:/ – at 9 o'clock
ein morgon /"mårgon/ – morning

om morgonen – in the morning
stengjer /"stenjer/ – close
ein ettermiddag /"ettermiddag/ – afternoon
om ettermiddagen – in the afternoon
laurdag /'læurdag/ m. – Saturday
på laurdagar – on Saturdays
er stengde – are closed
sundag /'sundag/ m. – Sunday
på sundagar – on Sundays
treng – need
eit ord /o:r/ – word
folk bruker å seia – people usually say
går omkring – walk around
når – when (referring to what usually happens or happened or what will happen in the future, cf. då)
får du? – are you being helped?
mindre /'mindre/ – less
enn – than
krambulivet /"krambuli:ve/ – the 'krambu' culture
gav – gave
eit bygdesamfunn /"bygdesamfunn/ – rural community
særmerkt /"sæ:rmærkt/ – distinctive
sitt – its
eit drag – characteristic
svært /svæ:rt/ – very
populær /popu'læ:r/ – popular
saknar – miss
men ho kjem nok ikkje attende – but it won't come back, I guess

7A Hagen vår

Per og Kari Nes arbeider i hagen ein kveld då Roy kjem innom.

ROY   God kveld, og takk for sist!
FRU NES   God kveld, og sjølv takk for sist. Korleis går det?
ROY   Berre bra, takk. Nynorsk er lettare å forstå no. – De har
           ein fin hage.
NES   Ja. Kari liker godt å arbeida i hagen, og ho arbeider
           raskt og effektivt. Men hagen til grannen er nok finare.
           Dei har større tomt, men det er betre jord her.
ROY   Kor stor er denne tomta då?
NES   Ho er på om lag eitt mål, det vil seia eitt tusen
           kvadratmeter, altså ein firedel av ein 'acre'. Tomta til
           grannen er både større og dyrare.
FRU NES   Eg synest at vår tomt er både finast og best.
ROY   Kva heiter dei raude og gule plantene der?
FRU NES   Det er roser, og der borte har vi bærbuskar og frukttre.
ROY   Kva er namnet på grønsakene de dyrkar?
FRU NES   I grønsakhagen dyrkar vi poteter, kål, gulrøter, salat og
           andre grønsaker. Plommene veks godt, ser du, men
           epla treng vel varmare vêr for å modnast.
ROY   Arbeider aldri Lars og Brit i hagen?
NES   Nei, eg trur ikkje at dei liker hagearbeid. Dei har ikkje
           tid, seier dei. Dei må lesa lekser om kvelden.
ROY   Slår de graset med ljå eller plenklippar?
NES   Vi bruker plenklippar, for det er enklare og lettare.
ROY   Eg liker godt rosene.
NES   Ja, Kari steller fint med dei. Om vinteren dekkjer ho dei
           til med granbar, og ho klipper dei alltid til rett tid.

Norsk ordtak: Di mindre gras, di tyngre slått.

vår /vå:r/ – our
arbeider /"a:rbæier/ – are working
ein hage /"ha:ge/ – garden
kjem innom /kje:m "innom/ – drops by
takk for sist – 'thanks for last time'
sjølv takk for sist – the same to you
lettare /"lettare/ – easier
å forstå /får'stå:/ – to understand
å arbeida – to work
raskt – fast
effektivt /'effekti:ft/ – efficiently
ein granne /"granne/ – neighbor
finare /"fi:nare/ – nicer, prettier
er nok finare – is prettier, I guess
større /'større/ – larger
ei tomt – (building) lot
betre /'be:tre/ – better
ei jord /jo:r/ – soil
det vil seia = dvs. – that is, i.e.
ein kvadratmeter /kva'dra:t-me:ter/ – square meter
altså /'altså/ – that is
ein firedel /"fi:rede:l/ – one fourth
tomta til grannen – the lot of our neighbor
både /"bå:de/ . . . og /å:g/ – both . . . and
dyrare /"dy:rare/ – more expensive
eg synest at – I think that
finast – prettiest
gul /gu:l/ – yellow
ei plante /"plante/ – plant
ei rose /"ro:se/ – rose

ein bærbusk /"bæ:rbusk/ – berry bush
eit frukttre /'frukttre:/ – fruit tree
dyrkar /"dyrkar/ – grow
ein grønsakhage – (vegetable) garden
kål m. – cabbage
ei gulrot /"gu:lro:t/ pl. -røter – carrot
salat /sa'la:t/ m. – lettuce
ei plomme /"plomme/ – plum
veks godt – grow well
eit eple /"eple/ – apple
vel – probably
varmare /"varmare/ – warmer
å modnast – to ripen
eg trur ikkje at – I don't think that
eit hagearbeid – gardening
ei tid – time
å lesa /"le:sa/ – to read
ei lekse – homework, assignment
å lesa lekser – to do one's homework
om kvelden – in the evening
å slå graset – to cut grass
ein ljå /jå:/ – scythe
ein plen /ple:n/ – lawn
ein plenklippar – lawn mower
enklare /"enklare/ – simpler
å stella med – to take care of
ein vinter /'vinter/ – winter
om vinteren – in (the) winter
dekkjer dei til – covers them up
granbar /"gra:nba:r/ n.pl. – spruce twigs with needles
klipper – cuts
til rett tid – at the right time
di . . . di – the . . . the
tyngre /'tyngre/ – harder
ein slått – mowing

1. Kva seier Roy då han kjem? 2. Er nynorsk lett å forstå no? 3. Kva synest han om hagen til Per og Kari? 4. Kor stor er tomta til Per og Kari? 5. Kor stor er tomta til grannen? 6. Kva slags grønsaker dyrkar Per og Kari? 7. Har dei frukttre? 8. Kvifor veks ikkje epla så godt? 9. Kvifor arbeider ikkje Lars og Brit i hagen? 10. Slår dei graset med plenklippar? 11. Kva gjer Kari med rosene om vinteren? 12. Når klipper ho rosene?

7B Grammar

1. Eg trur (at), eg synest (at), eg tenkjer (at)

The English verb *think* is translated by four different verbs in *nynorsk*:

1) *å tru* is used when the speaker is expressing something he *believes* to be true. It can be translated with either 'think' or 'believe': Eg trur ikkje dei liker hagearbeid. 'I don't think they like gardening.'

2) *å synast* or *å tykkja* is used when the speaker is expressing a taste or an opinion. Eg synest *(at)* or eg tykkjer *(at)* can be translated either 'I think' or 'It is my opinion that . . .': Eg synest at vår tomt er finast. 'I think that our lot is the prettiest one.'

3) *å tenkja* is used when the speaker is expressing that thinking or consideration is taking place. Eg tenkjer can be translated either 'I am thinking', 'I am considering', or 'I am intending (to)': Eg har tenkt å skriva ein nynorsk grammatikk. 'I've thought about writing a *nynorsk* grammar.'

2. The Comparison of Adjectives

The comparison of adjectives is similar to the English system. The endings are -*are* in the comparative and -*ast* in the superlative. Adjectives ending in -*el*, -*en*, or -*er* have contracted forms both in the comparative and in the superlative.

The comparison of adjectives. Basic pattern:

Positive	Comparative		Superlative	
billeg 'cheap'	billegare		billegast	
dyr 'expensive'	dyrare		dyrast	
fin 'fine, pretty'	finare	-are	finast	-ast
enkel 'simple'	enklare		enklast	
open 'open'	opnare		opnast	
vakker 'beautiful'	vakrare		vakrast	

A small group of adjectives form the comparative and the superlative by adding respectively -re and -st together with a vowel shift. The stem vowels /a o u/ are changed to /e ø y/.

Pattern:

Positive	Comparative		Superlative	
lang 'long'	lengre		lengst	
stor 'large, big'	større		størst	
tung 'heavy'	tyngre	-re	tyngst	-st
ung 'young'	yngre		yngst	

The following adjectives form their comparatives and superlatives from another stem than the positive:

Positive	Comparative	Superlative
gammal 'old'	eldre	eldst
god 'good'	betre	best
liten 'small'	mindre	minst
mange 'many'	fleire	flest
mykje 'much'	meir	mest
vond 'bad'	verre	verst

Similar to English, a number of adjectives are compared by means of meir and mest (English more and most), particularly long adjectives and adjectives ending in -a, -sk, -en, -ut, and present and past participles. Examples:

74

Positive	Comparative	Superlative
sinna 'angry'	meir sinna	mest sinna
praktisk 'practical'	meir praktisk	mest praktisk
drukken 'drunk'	moir drukken	mest drukken
bakkut 'hilly'	meir bakkut	mest bakkut
strålande 'brilliant'	meir strålande	mest strålande
likt 'liked'	meir likt	mest likt

The comparative has only one form regardless of gender and number, e.g., ein dyrare bil, ei dyrare bok, eit dyrare hus, dyrare bilar, bøker, hus.

The superlative form is also independent of gender and number when it is used predicatively, but distinguishes between *indefinite* forms with no ending except for the superlative -*st* and *definite* forms ending in -e, e.g., Han er rikast. Ho er rikast. Det er rikast. Dei er rikast. But: Han er den rikaste. Ho er den rikaste. Det er det rikaste. Dei er dei rikaste.

Unlike English, the superlative is also used when two persons or things are compared, e.g., Ho er den eldste og den vakraste av dei to systrene. 'She is the older and the more beautiful of the two sisters.'

3. The Present Tense

As mentioned in 1B3 the present tense indicative in the active voice has only one form. It ends in -*ar*, -*er*, -*r*, or has no ending, depending on the verb class to which it belongs.

The present tense. Basic pattern:

Infinitive	Present tense		Verb class	
å kasta 'to throw'	kastar	-ar	Class 1	
å dømma 'to sentence'	dømmer	-er	Class 2	Weak verbs
å tru 'to believe'	trur	-r	Class 3	
å telja 'to count'	tel	–	Class 4	
å bita 'to bite'	bit			
å bryta 'to break'	bryt			
å finna 'to find'	finn	–		Strong verbs
å bera 'to carry'	ber			
å lesa 'to read'	les			
å fara 'to go'	fer			
å blåsa 'to blow'	blæs			

In nynorsk the present tense has different functions. The most important ones are as follows:

75

1) It is used about an action taking place in the present time. Examples: Eg går på skulen kvar dag. Eg les no. Ho et. It also renders the progressive forms in English (I am reading now. She is eating).
2) It is often used about a future action, particularly in connection with time phrases referring to the future: Eg kjem snart. Han byrjar neste år.
3) It is used about an action that is not limited in time: Månen går rundt jorda. 'The moon goes round the earth.' Lys er bølgjer. 'Light is waves.'

Notice that the progressive forms in English, which are expressed by a form of the verb 'to be' plus the present participle of the main verb, have no corresponding formation in *nynorsk*: Studentane sit på golvet. 'The students are sitting on the floor.' If we want to stress that an action is continuous, we sometimes express that by means of combination with the verbs *å sitja* 'to sit', *å stå* 'to stand', *å liggja* 'to lie', or *å halda på med* 'to be doing something': Han sit og les. 'He is reading.' Dei står og pratar. 'They are talking.' Ho ligg og les. 'She is reading.' Han held på med å skriva ei bok. 'He is writing a book.'

4. The Days of the Week

The days of the week are: måndag /'måndag/, tysdag /'ty:sdag/, onsdag /'onsdag/, torsdag /'to:rsdag/, fredag /'fre:dag/, laurdag /'læurdag/, and sundag /'sundag/.

Notice that the days of the week are not capitalized in *nynorsk*.

Oppgåver
1. Translate into *nynorsk*:
   a) What do you think of Kari Nes?
   b) Mr. Nes has thought of writing a grammar.
   c) He thinks that the children don't like gardening.
   d) I think he is a nice person.
2. Fill in the correct comparative or superlative form of the adjective:
   a) Det er . . . . her enn i byen.   (billeg)
   b) Lars er den . . . . av barna.   (vakker)
   c) Bussen er . . . . enn bilen.   (stor)
   d) Den . . . . : . . . . byen i Noreg er Oslo.   (stor)
   e) Det bur . . . . menneske i USA enn i Noreg.   (mange)
   f) Dei . . . . menneske er glade i naturen.   (mange)
   g) Ein lenestol er . . . . enn ein vanleg stol.   (tung)
   h) Lars er ikkje den . . . . av dei.   (tung)

i) Det er .... luft her enn i byen.   (god)
j) Brit er den .... jenta i bygda.   (god)
k) Oslo er .... enn Chicago.   (liten)
l) Det .... landet i Skandinavia er Danmark.   (liten)
m) Brit er .... enn Lars.   (gammal)
n) Brit er .... av dei.   (gammal)
o) Lars er .... enn Brit.   (ung)
p) Lars er .... av dei.   (ung)
q) Brit er .... enn Lars.   (praktisk)
r) Mora er .... av alle.   (praktisk)

7C Pronunciation/Spelling

The Vibrant Consonant /r/

In nynorsk /r/ is a dental or alveolar vibrant, i.e., with a number of quick taps or trills against the upper teeth or alveolar ridge. This so-called *rolled* /r/ is quite unlike the American /r/, but is similar to the trilled /r/ of Scotch or Italian.

The *rolled* /r/ is a most difficult consonant for American students and needs very much practice. If you have any trouble producing it, try starting from /p/, /t/, or /d/: *prr..., trr..., drr...*

Examples: bra, rett, far, er, for, talar.

7D Huset til familien Nes

Per og Kari Nes har eige hus, og dei er glade i huset sitt. Huset har ei golvflate på om lag eitt hundre kvadratmeter, og det er i to høgder. Lars og Brit har sine rom i første høgda, og foreldra har soverommet sitt i andre høgda.

Brit er to år eldre enn Lars, og derfor har ho det største rommet. Lars tykkjer det er urettferdig at den yngste alltid skal ha det minste rommet. Det ville vera rettare å trekkja lodd om romma, meiner han. Han er ofte inne på rommet til Brit, for der er det betre plass, og så er det ryddigare enn på hans rom. På rommet til Lars er det meir rotut.

I første høgda har dei eit lite TV-rom. Det er mindre enn rommet til Brit, men større enn rommet til Lars. Møblane på TV-rommet er enklare og lettare enn i stova oppe. Der er ein lett og enkel sofa, eit salongbord eller kaffibord, to lenestolar og to vanlege stolar. På veggen er det to lampettar, og i taket heng det ein taklampe med to lyspærer i. Dei har ikkje farge-TV, berre svart-kvitt.

I andre høgda er det to soverom, ei stove, eit kjøken, ein gang og eit bad. Til vanleg et dei i kjøkenet, for der er det god plass.

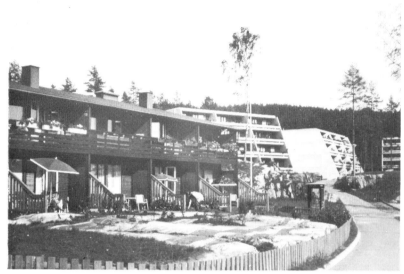

Fig. 7.1 *I dei store byane er tomtene dyrare enn på landet. Mange kjøper derfor mindre husvære 'apartments'.*

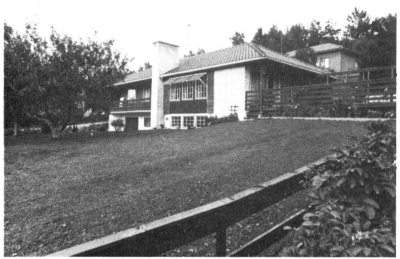

Fig. 7.2 *Per og Kari er glade i huset sitt.*

Komfyren, kjøleskapet, kjøkenbenken og vasken står på eine sida, og bordet og stolane på andre sida. Stova er god og romsleg, og dei har peis og tyngre møblar der. Om kvelden fyrer dei ofte på peisen og har det triveleg.

78

glad i – fond of
ei golvflate /''gålvfla:te/ – floor area
eit golv /gålv/   floor
ei høgd – story, floor
sine /''si:ne/ – their
eit soverom /''så:verom/ – bedroom
andre – second
eit år – year
eldre /'eldre/ – older
derfor /'dærfår/ – therefore
tykkjer – thinks
urettferdig /''u:rettfærdi/ – unfair
minst – smallest
rett – right
å trekkja lodd om – cast, draw lots for
å meina /''mæina/ – to think, to be of the opinion that
inne – in
ein plass – room, space
betre plass – more room
så – besides
ryddig – tidy
rotut /''ro:tut/ – disorderly, messy
enkel /'enkel/ – simple, plain
lett – light (in weight)
møblar /''mø:blar/ n.pl. – furniture
oppe /''oppe/ – upstairs

ein sofa /'so:fa/ – sofa
eit salongbord /sa'långbo:r/ – coffee table
ein peis – open fireplace
ein lenestol /''le:nesto:l/ – easy chair
ein vegg – wall
ein lampett /lam'pett/ – bracket lamp, sconce
eit tak – ceiling
å hanga /''hanga/ – to hang
ein taklampe /''ta:klampe/ – ceiling light
ei lyspære /''ly:spæ:re/ – light bulb
farge-TV – color TV
svart-kvitt – black and white
eit kjøken /'kjø:ken/ – kitchen
ein gang – hall, corridor
eit bad /ba:d/ – bathroom
god plass – plenty of room
ein komfyr /kom'fy:r/ – stove, range
eit kjøleskap /''kjø:leska:p/ – refrigerator
ein kjøkenbenk – kitchen counter
ein vask – sink, washbasin
romsleg /''romsleg/ – spacious
å fyra på /''fy:ra på/ – light a fire
å ha det triveleg – to enjoy oneself

79

8A Sundagstur

Det er sundag, og familien Nes vitjar foreldra til Per Nes. Dei har ein fin gard øvst i bygda. Brit og Lars liker seg godt hjå bestefar og bestemor. Det er god luft og roleg og fredeleg på garden. Dei spring omkring og ser på dyra og leikar seg i høyet på låven.

BARNA   Hei, bestefar! Hei, bestemor! Er tante Aslaug og onkel Olav heime?
BESTEMOR   Ja, tante Aslaug er i fjøset, og onkel Olav er borte på låven. Han skal ut med hesten ein tur.
ROY   God dag. Eg heiter Roy Eisel og er frå Amerika. – Ja, dette var ein fin gard. – Kor stor er han?
BESTEFAR   Garden er ikkje så veldig stor. Vi har om lag 40 dekar innmark, men det høyrer med litt skog, fjell og utmark til garden. Og så har vi ei seter oppe på fjellet. Vi ønskjer av og til at vi hadde ein storgard på Jæren eller Austlandet eller i Trøndelag. Der er gardane flate og store. Ja, dei er mest like store som gardane der du kjem frå.
ROY   Kan de leva av denne garden?
BESTEMOR   Det er knapt nok. I det siste har vi drive med litt fruktdyrking og grønsakdyrking for å greia oss.
ROY   De driv altså med fleire ting samstundes?
BESTEMOR   Ja, vi trur at det løner seg, og så er det tryggare, men vi må arbeida hardt heile året. I år har vi seks kyr, nokre geiter og eit par kalvar. Det er Olav som har odelsrett på garden, og han liker det best slik.
ROY   Nei, no må eg gå bort til dei andre. Takk for praten.
BESTEMOR   Sjølv takk.

Norsk ordtak: Ei lita kjerring gjer mykje medan ei stor snur seg.

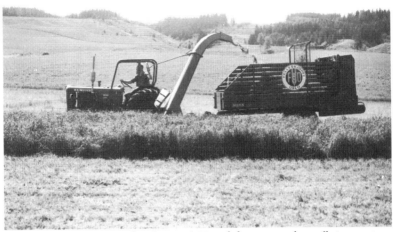

Fig. 8.1 *På Jæren, Austlandet og i Trøndelag er gardane flate og store.*

ein tur – trip
å vitja /"vikjkja/ – visit
ein gard /ga:r/ – farm
øvst – at the top
å lika seg – to like it
ein bestefar – grandfather
luft f. – air
fredeleg /"fre:deleg/ – calm,
  peaceful
å springa /"springa/ – to run
omkring /om'kring/ – about
eit dyr – animal
å leika seg – to play together
eit høy – hay
ein låve /"lå:ve/ – barn
hei /hæi/ – hi
ei tante /"tante/ – aunt
ein onkel /'onkel/ – uncle
eit fjøs – cow barn
han skal ut med hesten ein tur –
  he is taking the horse out for
  a walk

veldig /"veldi/ – very, terribly
eit dekar /'de:kar/ – decare
  (measure of land), ca. ¼ acre
ei innmark /"innmark/ – cultivated land
å høyra med til – to belong to
litt – a little, some
ein skog – woods
eit fjell – rocky upland
ei utmark /"u:tmark/ – uncultivated land, pasture
ei seter /'se:ter/ – (mountain)
  outfarm
å ønskja /"ønsja/ – to wish
flat – flat
mest like store som – almost as
  large as
der du kjem frå – where you
  come from
å leva av – to live off
knapt nok /'knapt 'nåkk/ – just
  barely, hardly enough

81

i det siste – during the last few years
å driva med – to be into, to be doing
ei fruktdyrking /'fruktdyrking/ – growing fruit
ei grønsakdyrking – truck-gardening, vegetable gardening
å greia seg – to get along
ein ting – thing
samstundes /''samstundes/ – simultaneously, at the same time
å løna seg – to pay, to be profitable
trygg – safe

å arbeida hardt – to work hard
ei ku, pl. kyr – cow
ei geit /jæit/ – goat
ein kalv – calf
ein odelsrett /'o:delsrett/ – allodial rights (form of property ownership acquired by a family to a farm held for at least 20 years, whereby the oldest son or daughter of the family has the right to redeem it within five years of sale)
ein prat – talk, chat
slik – in that way
ei kjerring – woman, wife
å snu seg – to turn around

Spørsmål

1. Kva dag vitjar familien Nes foreldra til Per Nes? 2. Kvar er garden? 3. Kor stor er garden? 4. Har dei seter? 5. Kva er ei seter? 6. Kva for dyr har dei på garden? 7. Kvifor liker Brit og Lars seg så godt hjå besteforeldra? 8. Kan dei leva av garden? 9. Kven har odelsrett? 10. Kvifor har ein odelsrett i Noreg?

8B Grammar

1. The Adverbials

An adverbial may be an adverb, a prepositional phrase, an adverbial clause, or the neuter form of the adjective ending in -t (fint, godt). An adverbial may modify a verb, an adjective, an adverb, or a whole sentence.

Examples:

Plommene veks *godt*. (verb) — The plums are growing well.

Garden er *svært* fin. (adjective) — The farm is very nice.

Ho skriv *uvanleg* godt. (adverb) — She writes exceptionally well.

Ho var *aldri* trøytt. — She was never tired.

82

In English, many adverbials end in -ly, e.g., certainly, formed from the adjective certain. The corresponding ending in nynorsk is -t, i.e., the neuter form of the adjective. If the -t is lost in the neuter, e.g., in adjectives ending in -ig, it is also lost when it has the function of an adverbial (ein veldig stor gard). Notice also that adjectives ending in -en (open, naken), take the ending -e in the neuter, and thus take the ending -e when they have an adverbial function: Han talar ope om alle ting. 'He speaks openly about everything.'

Adverbs have usually no inflection, but certain adverbs of place have two forms, one with no ending indicating motion, the other ending in -e indicating location at a place:

Motion			Location	
bort	(going) away		borte	away (at a place)
fram	(going) forward		framme	at a destination
heim	(going) home		heime	at home
inn	(going) in		inne	inside
ned	(going) down		nede	down (at)
opp	(going) up		oppe	up (on)
ut	(going) out		ute	outside

Notice that the two adverbs of motion, hit 'to here' and dit 'there, to that place', correspond to the two adverbs of location her 'here' and der 'there'.

Adverbs are compared in the same way as adjectives (see 7B2).

Summary:
1. The neuter form of adjectives = adverbs.
   Ho er fin. – Ho talar fint.
   Ein open mann. – Han talar ope.
2. Adverbs: ikkje 'not', aldri 'never', kanskje 'perhaps', ofte 'often', gjerne 'gladly', lenge 'long' (referring to time).
3. The comparison of adverbs = the comparison of adjectives.
   Ho talar fint. – Han talar finare. – Dei talar finast.

2. Possessive Relationships

In nynorsk possessive relationships are expressed in four different ways:

83

1) By means of a possessive adjective or pronoun: Han har bilen min. Huset er mitt.
2) By adding -s to the noun (the s-genitive): far – fars hatt 'hat', Vinje – Vinjes dikt 'poems'.
3) By using a compound, which often is a contracted s-genitive: vitskapens menn = vitskapsmenn 'scientists', bondens yrke = bondeyrket 'farming profession'.
4) By means of a prepositional phrase, corresponding to the use of phrases with *of* in English: gutens bil = bilen til guten, Vinjes dikt = dikta til Vinje (see 4B2).
5) By using the noun (usually in the definite form) followed by a form of *sin* (his, her, its, their, own): Eg såg guten sin bil, etc. Also: Kven sitt hus er dette?

3. The Possessive Pronouns and Adjectives

Each of the personal pronouns has a corresponding possessive form which denotes ownership.

The possessive pronouns. The first and second persons:

	Singular			Plural		
	eg	du	De	vi	de	De
Masculine	bilen min	din	Dykkar	vår	dykkar	Dykkar
Feminine	hytta mi	di	Dykkar	vår	dykkar	Dykkar
Neuter	huset mitt	ditt	Dykkar	vårt	dykkar	Dykkar
Plural, all genders	bilane, hyttene, husa mine	dine	Dykkar	våre	dykkar	Dykkar

It is very important to notice that the form of the possessive pronoun does not change according to its position in the sentence, as in English (cf. my, mine), but according to the type of noun it modifies or refers to. This is because the same *nynorsk* possessive form may function both as an adjective, used with nouns, and as a pronoun, used by itself. Compare the *nynorsk* and English possessive pronouns and adjectives in the following sentences:

Han har bilen *min*.   He has *my* car.
Bilen er *min*.   The car is *mine*.
Han har bilen *din*.   He has *your* car.

84

Bilen er *din*.
Han har bilen *vår*.
Bilen er *vår*.

The car is *yours*.
He has *our* car.
The car is *ours*.

When the possessive pronoun has the function of an adjective
and modifies a noun, it is usually placed *after* the noun it modifies:
Han har bilen min. Han har boka mi. If the possessive pronoun is
stressed, however, it is often placed before the noun it modifies:
Dette er *min* bil. Dette er *mi* bok. Dette er *mitt* hus.
If the possessive pronoun is placed after the noun, the definite
form of the noun is always used, whereas the indefinite form is used
if it is placed before the noun for emphasis: Han har *bilen* min. –
Dette er min *bil*. When speaking of relatives, however, the forms:
mor mi, bror min, etc. are usually used.
In the third person singular, the possessive pronouns are *sin (si,
sitt, sine)* and *hans* and *hennar*. In the third person plural, the forms
sin (si, sitt, sine) and *deira* are used.

The possessive pronouns. The third person:

	Singular			Plural	
	han/ho	han	ho	dei	
Masculine Feminine Neuter	bilen sin hytta si huset sitt	hans	hennar	sin si sitt	deira
Plural, all genders	bilane, hyttene, husa sine			sine	

The possessive pronoun *sin (si, sitt, sine)*, which varies in gender
and number like *min* and *din* (see above), renders *his, her, hers, its,
their*, and *theirs*. It refers to the subject of the clause in which it
occurs: Han tok fram bilen sin. Han gjekk til hytta si. Ho liker huset
sitt. Dei liker bilane sine. It is also used in the special possessive
form discussed on p. 84, e.g., Eg såg mannen sitt hus.
The possessive pronouns *hans* and *hennar* (his; her, hers) are
used when the pronoun does not refer to the subject of the clause:
Ho likte bilen hans. Ho likte hytta hans. Han likte huset hennar.
Han likte bøkene hennar. They are also used when they modify the
subject or refer to only part of the subject: Bilen hans var fin. Hytta

85

hans var dyr. Huset hennar var raudt. Bøkene hennar var dyre. Han og sonen hans gjekk til byen.

The possessive pronoun *deira* (their, theirs) is used in the third person plural. Like *hans* and *hennar*, *deira* is used when it does not refer to the subject of the clause or when it modifies the subject or refers to only part of the subject: Han likte bilen deira. Han likte hyttene deira. Bilen deira var fin. Hytta deira var dyr. Dei og dotter deira kjem snart.

In *nynorsk* the possessive is often left out when it seems unnecessary to indicate the owner. This is true whenever one talks about parts of the body after having mentioned the owner, or when one talks about clothing. The noun has then the definite form: Han rista på hovudet. 'He shook his head.' Eg brende meg på fingrane. 'I burned my fingers.' Han sat med hendene i lomma. 'He sat with his hands in his pockets.' The possessive is sometimes left out when referring to members of one's immediate family: Kona kjem snart. Or: Kona mi kjem snart.

Oppgåver

1. Identify the possessive pronouns in the poem *Blåmann* (8D).

2. Fill in the correct pronoun (personal or possessive) instead of the words within the parentheses: (Arne) sykla ein tur. Eg møtte (Aslaug). (Mennene) arbeidde hardt. Du kan få låna (boka). Vi prøvde å finna (hesten). Kona (til Olsen) har kjøpt bil. Dei møtte foreldra (til Kari). Vil du vera så gild å opna (brevet)? Eg bar (kofferten) for henne. Dotter (til fru Berg) skal senda (pakken). Med (gutane si) hjelp kom han opp att. Per Nes møtte sonen (til Per Nes) på stasjonen.

3. Translate into *nynorsk*:
   a) They have a very big farm.
   b) My father is not at home.
   c) She is going home next year.
   d) The plants are growing well.
   e) She writes beautifully.
   f) They speak openly about everything.
   g) He likes his new car.
   h) She saw his house.
   i) Her dress was very nice.
   j) She liked her cabin.
   k) He burned his fingers.

8C Pronunciation/Spelling

The Plosive Consonants /p b t d k g/

The plosives (stops) /p b t d k g/ are pronounced almost as in English. The dentals /t/ and /d/, however, are articulated by placing the tip of the tongue against the back of the teeth, while in English it touches the alveolar ridge. Words for practice: penn, ball, tal, dal 'valley', kar 'guy', gard.

8D Blåmann

Blåmann, Blåmann, bukken min,
tenk på vesle guten din!
Bjørnen med sin lodne fell
kan deg taka seint i kveld.

Gamle Lykle, moder di,
seint kom heim med bjølla si.
So ikring seg ho mund' sjå
liksom der var fåre på.

Det såg ut som der var naud,
kanskje no du ligger daud.
Tidt du dansa kringom meg,
mangt eg rødde då med deg.

Når eg låg som blind og dauv,
grov du på meg med di klauv.
Ja, du ville vekkja meg
opp til leiken din med deg.

Du var sprek og glad og god,
all min ros du vel forstod.
Tidt du veit eg sa til deg:
«Han veit meir enn mata seg.»

Blåmann, Blåmann, svar meg no!
Mekre med ditt kjende ljod!
Ikkje enno, Blåmann min,
må du døy frå guten din.

Av A. O. Vinje

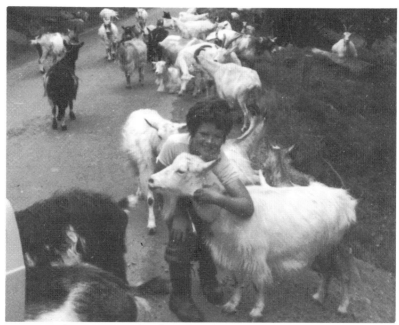

Fig. 8.2 *På somme vestlandsgardar driv dei med geiter.*

Aasmund Olavsson Vinje (1818–70) var husmannsson frå Vinje i Telemark. Han var den første diktaren etter Ivar Aasen som tok i bruk nynorsken (landsmålet). Vinje hadde skrive på dansk fram til 1858. Då bestemte han seg for at for framtida ville han berre bruka norsk mål. Eit norsk skriftspråk måtte koma som ei naturleg følgje av vår politiske fridom, meinte han.

ein bukk – billy goat, he-goat
ein bjørn – bear
loden /"lå:den/ – hairy
ein fell – fur, pelt
seint – late
i kveld – tonight
ei moder – old form of *mor*
ei bjølle /"bjølle/ – bell
ikring /i'kring/ – about
mund' = munde – past tense of
 å *muna*, will likely

liksom /'liksåm/ – as if
der var – there was
ein fåre /"få:re/ – danger
der var fåre på – it was dangerous
det såg ut som – it looked as if
ei naud /næu/ – difficulty, peril
der var naud – it was dangerous
ligger – lie, the modern form is
 ligg
daud /dæu/ – dead

88

tidt /titt/ – often
dansa /"dansa/ – past tense of å
 dansa, to dance
kringom /"kringom/ – round,
 about
mangt – many things, much
rødde /"rødde/ – past tense of å
 røda, to talk, to discuss
låg – past tense of å liggja, to lie
blind – blind
dauv /dæu/ – deaf
grov – past tense of å grava, to
 poke
ei klauv /klæu/ – hoof
å vekkja – to wake, awaken
ein leik – play, playing
sprek – active, vigorous
glad /gla:/ – happy
ros m. – praise
vel – well
forstod /får'sto:/ – past tense of
 å forstå, to understand
å mata seg – to feed oneself
å mekra /"mekra/ – to bleat
kjend – well-known
eit ljod /jo:/ – sound, voice
ikkje enno – not yet
å døy – to die
ein husmann /"hu:smann/ –
 tenant farmer, cottager

ein husmannsson – son of a
 husmann
Telemark /"te:lemark/ – county
 in southern Norway
ein diktar – poet, author
å ta i bruk – to take into use
hadde skrive – had written
på dansk – in Danish
fram til – until
bestemte /be'stemte/ – past tense
 of å bestemma, to decide, to
 determine
å bestemma seg for – to make
 up one's mind to
ei framtid /"framti:/ – future
for framtida – in the future
å bruka /"bru:ka/ – to use
eit mål – language
måtte /"måtte/ – past tense of å
 måtta, to have to
ei følgje /"følje/ – consequence
naturleg /na'tu:rleg/ – natural,
 logical
politisk /po'li:tisk/ – political
meinte – past tense of å meina,
 to think, be of the opinion
 that

9A Har du gjort leksa di?

Både Lars og Brit går i grunnskulen. Lars går siste året i barneskulen, og Brit går i åttande klassen i ungdomsskulen.

LÆRAREN	Men Brit! Har du ikkje gjort leksa di til i dag?
BRIT	Nei, eg har gløymt det.
LÆRAREN	Har du gløymt å gjera leksa di?
BRIT	Ja, det har eg. Vi har vore på tur, og så gløymde eg leksa.
LÆRAREN	Ja vel. – Ta fram blyant, viskelêr, linjal og skrivepapir. Vi skal ha ei lita oppgåve.
BRIT	Eg har heldigvis hugsa på å ta med skrivesakene.
LÆRAREN	Fint. – Har de lese i avisa om den nye skulen?
BRIT	Ja, vi har sett at han vert veldig dyr. Det stod i avisa for ei veke sidan.
LÆRAREN	Veit de kven som har teikna han?
BRIT	Nei, det har ingen fortalt oss, men eg trur at det er ein lokal arkitekt.
LÆRAREN	Ja, det er det. – No kan de skriva korleis de vil at ein ny skule skal sjå ut. Så kan de teikna både leikeplass, idrettsplass, hage, vegar, parkeringsplass og sjølve skulehuset. Etterpå skal vi samanlikna med arkitekten si teikning, som eg har fått ein kopi av.
BRIT	Det var interessant.
LÆRAREN	Hugs på å laga stort nok lærarrom. Hm.
BRIT	Det er viktigare med ein stor symjehall og ein fin gymnastikksal.
LÆRAREN	Har de tenkt på kven som skal betala alt dette?
BRIT	Kommunen!
LÆRAREN	Har de lært noko av denne oppgåva?
BRIT	Ja, dette var både interessant og lærerikt.

Moderne ordtak: Ein lærer så lenge ein har elevar.

90

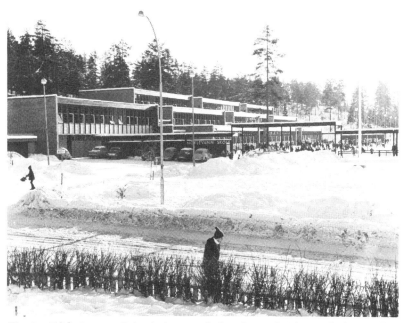

Fig. 9.1 *Både Lars og Brit går i grunnskulen. Lars går i barneskulen, og Brit går i ungdomsskulen.*

ein grunnskule /''grunnsku:le/ – 'basic school', i.e. a school providing the first nine years of basic education
ein barneskule /''ba:rnesku:le/ – elementary school
ein ungdomsskule /''ongdom-sku:le/ – junior high school
siste – last
ein klasse /''klasse/ – grade
gjort /jort/ – past participle of å *gjera*, to do
til i dag – for today
gløymt – past participle of å *gløyma*, to forget
ja, det har eg – yes, I have
på tur – on a trip
gløymde /''gløymde/ – past tense of å *gløyma*

ta fram imp. – take out
ein blyant /'bly:ant/ – pencil
eit viskelêr /''viskelæ:r/ – eraser
ein linjal /lin'ja:l/ – ruler
skrivepapir /''skri:vepapi:r/ – writing paper
ei oppgåve – exercise
heldigvis /''heldig'vi:s/ – fortunately
å hugsa på – to remember
å ta med – to bring
skrivesaker /''skri:vesa:ker/ f.pl. – writing materials
fint – fine
lese /''le:se/ – past participle of å *lesa*, to read
for . . . sidan – ago
teikna – past participle of å *teikna*, to design

91

ingen /"ingen/ – nobody
fortalt /får'talt/ – past participle
of å fortelja, to tell
lokal /lo'ka:l/ – local
ein arkitekt /arki'tekt/ – architect
ja, det er det – yes, it is
å sjå ut – to look like
ein leikeplass /læikeplass/ –
playground
både . . . og – both . . . and (can
be used with any number of
objects, not just two!)
ein idrettsplass /"i:drettsplass/
– athletic fields
ein veg – road
ein parkeringsplass /par'ke:-
ringsplass/ – parking lot
eit skulehus /"sku:lehu:s/ –
school building
sjølve skulehuset – the building
itself
å samanlikna /"sa:manlikna/ –
to compare
ei teikning – design, plan

fått – past participle of å få, to
get
ein kopi /ko'pi:/ – copy
stort nok – large enough
eit lærarrom /"læ:raromm/ –
teachers' common room,
lounge
ein symjehall /"symjehall/ –
swimming pool
ein gymnastikksal /gymnas-
'tikksa:l/ – gymnasium
tenkt – past participle of å
tenkja, to think
alt dette – all this
ein kommune /ko'mu:ne/ – municipality (city, town, or
village)
lært – past participle of å læra –
to learn
lærerik /"læ:reri:k/ – informative, instructive
ein lærer så lenge ein har elevar
– one learns as long as one
has pupils
ein elev /e'le:v/ – pupil, student

Spørsmål
1. Kva skule går Brit i? 2. Kva skule går Lars i? 3. Kva klasse går Brit
i? 4. Kva klasse går Lars i? 5. Kvifor har ikkje Brit gjort leksa si? 6.
Vert læraren sinna? 7. Kva oppgåve får dei? 8. Kven har teikna den
nye skulen? 9. Skal elevane teikna berre skulehuset? 10. Liker dei
denne oppgåva? 11. Kva er ein kommune? 12. Kva synest du om
ordtaket?

9B Grammar

1. The Present Perfect Tense

In nynorsk, as in English, the present perfect tense in the active
voice is formed by using the present tense of the verb å ha (har)
with the past participle of the main verb.

The present tense of å vera (er) can be used instead when the main verb is å verta, the synonymous å bli, or a verb denoting motion.

Examples:

Ho har gjort leksa.
Ho har gløymt det.
Dei har lese det i avisa.
Han har skrive det på tavla. He has written it on the board.
Ho har vorte sjuk. Or: Ho er vorten sjuk. She has been taken ill.
Han har gått. Or: Han er gått. He has left.

The present perfect tense is used about an action that took place in the past without referring to a definite point of time. If the action refers to a particular time or date, the past tense is used, e.g., Har du gjort leksene dine? Ja, dei gjorde eg i går.

The present perfect tense is otherwise used about an action that leads up to the present time (Han har vore lærar i 20 år), and about an action that takes place before another one in the future: Når du har gjort leksa di, kan du gå.

2. The Conjugation of å verta and å bli

Infinitive	Present	Past	Past Participle
å verta 'to become'	vert	vart	vorte
å bli	blir	blei	blitt

3. Kva er klokka? Or: Kor mykje er klokka?

Kl. 8.05 (8:05 AM): Ho er fem over åtte. Or: Ho er åtte null fem.
Kl. 20.05 (8:05 PM): Ho er fem over åtte. Or: Ho er tjue null fem.

As can be seen from the two examples mentioned above, there are two ways of telling the time in nynorsk. The former is used in informal conversation, whereas the latter is apparently becoming more and more usual in public administration, since no misunderstanding can occur when using the 24-hour system. Åtte null fem can only mean 8:05 AM, never 8:05 PM, which would be tjue null fem (20.05) in the 24-hour system.

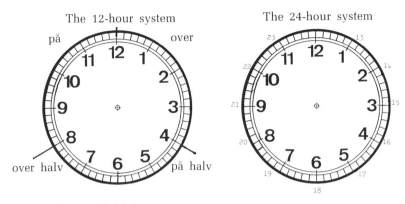

The 12-hour system

The 24-hour system

Fig. 9.2 *Kva er klokka?*

Examples

Kl. 8.10	Klokka (ho) er ti over åtte. Klokka (ho) er åtte ti.
8:10 AM	It is ten past eight.
Kl. 8.15	Ho er kvart over åtte. Ho er åtte femten.
8:15 AM	It is a quarter past eight.
Kl. 8.20	Ho er ti på halv ni. Ho er åtte tjue.
8:20 AM	It is twenty past eight.
Kl. 8.30	Ho er halv ni. Ho er åtte tretti.
8:30 AM	It is half past eight.
Kl. 8.40	Ho er ti over halv ni. Ho er åtte førti.
8:40 AM	It is twenty to nine.
Kl. 8.45	Ho er kvart på ni. Ho er åtte førtifem.
8:45 AM	It is a quarter to nine.
Kl. 9.00	Ho er ni (presis). Ho er ni null null.
9:00 AM	It is nine o'clock (sharp).
Kl. 20.00	Ho er åtte. Ho er tjue null null.
20:00 PM	It is eight o'clock.
Kl. 20.10	Ho er ti over åtte. Ho er tjue ti.
20:10 PM	It is ten past eight.

Kl. 1.00	Ho er eitt. Ho er ein null null.
1:00 AM	It is one o'clock.

Kl. 13.00	Ho er eitt. Ho er tretten null null.
1:00 PM	It is one o'clock.

The principal differences between the Norwegian system and the English system are:

1) The half hours are reckoned *before* the hour, not after as in English: *halv ni* = 8:30, half past eight.
2) Minutes (up to ten) are reckoned before and after the half hour intervals: *ti på halv ni* = 8:20, twenty past eight; *ti over halv ni* = 8:40, twenty to nine.
3) In the 24-hour system, which is used to give all public scheduled times, the minutes are always given after the hour: kl. 8.40 = åtte førti; 20.45 = tjue førtifem.

Notice that a period is placed between the hour and the minutes in *nynorsk*, not a colon as in English. It is also quite common to write four digits, e.g., kl. 0840, kl. 2045, etc.

Oppgåver

1. The present perfect is a compound tense. Fill in the past participle of a suitable main verb:
   a) Har du .... leksa di?
   b) Eg trur at han har .... i byen.
   c) Han har .... arbeidet sitt.
   d) Læraren er .... attende.
   e) Eleven har............. boka si.
   f) Dei har................ om den nye skulen.
   g) Brit har .... å gjera leksa si.
   h) Ho har .... oss det.
   i) Dei har................ korleis ein ny skule skal sjå ut.

2. Write out the following times, using both the 12-hour system and the 24-hour system: 9:12 AM, 10:20 AM, 11:25 PM, 1:05 PM, 1:17 PM, 1:35 PM, 5:03 PM.
3. Translate into *nynorsk*:
   a) Brit hasn't done her homework.
   b) She has forgotten to do it.
   c) She has remembered to bring her writing materials.

d) I think it is a local architect who has designed the new school.

e) I have read about it in the paper.

9C Pronunciation/Spelling

The Lateral Consonant /l/

The Norwegian lateral /l/ is "light" compared with English "dark" /l/, because the tongue is higher, flatter, and farther forward. It is articulated with the tongue against the inner edge of the upper teeth.

It is spelled *l*, but before *j* the *l* is silent, e.g., ljå 'scythe', å ljoma 'to resound, to echo'.

Words for practice: land, luft, leik, ball, hall, kalla, falla.

9D Skulesystemet i Noreg

Det er ni års skuleplikt i Noreg, og ein byrjar på skulen det året ein fyller sju år. Dei første seks åra går ein i *barneskulen*, og deretter tre

Barneskulen 7–13 år		1.–6. klasse Obligatoriske fag	Generell vurdering
Ungdomsskulen 13–16 år	Grunnskulen	7.–9. klasse Obligatoriske og valfrie fag	Eksamen Avgangsvitnemål
Den vidaregåande skulen 16–19 år		1.–3. klasse Mange linjer Obligatoriske og valfrie fag	Eksamen Avgangsvitnemål
Universitet og høgskular 19 år –		5–7 år 2–4 år	Eksamen Cand. mag. Cand. philol. Cand. med., etc.

Fig. 9.3 *Skulesystemet i Noreg.*

år i *ungdomsskulen.* I barneskulen har ein berre obligatoriske fag, men i ungdomsskulen har ein også valfrie fag.

Etter *grunnskulen,* som denne 9-årige skulen heiter, kjem *den vidaregåande skulen,* og den varer i tre år. Mange som har teke den vidaregåande skulen, byrjar å studera ved ein *høgskule* eller eit *universitet.*

Det er mange høgskular i Noreg, og det er fire universitet. Universitetet i Tromsø ligg i Nord-Noreg, Universitetet i Bergen ligg på Vestlandet, Universitetet i Trondheim ligg i Trøndelag, og Universitetet i Oslo ligg på Austlandet. Universitetet i Oslo er eldst og vart skipa i 1811.

På same måten som universiteta er høgskulane spreidde over heile landet, både lærarskulane, distriktshøgskulane og andre høgskular.

Det er billeg å studera i Noreg samanlikna med USA, for det er ingen skulepengar å betala, og alle studentar ved høgskular og universitet får rimelege lån i *Statens Lånekasse* for å dekkja utgiftene til husleige, mat, klede og bøker.

Ein av dei største vanskane studentane har, er å finna ein stad å bu, men no byggjer dei studentheimar ved alle høgskular og universitet.

Folkehøgskulane er private skular for vaksen ungdom.

eit skulesystem /"sku:lesyste:m/ – educational system
ei skuleplikt – compulsory school attendance
å fylla /"fylla/ – to complete
å fylla sju år – to turn seven
deretter /'dæ:retter/ – then, after that
obligatorisk /obliga'to:risk/ – compulsory
eit fag – subject
valfri /'va:lfri:/ – optional
eit valfritt fag – elective
-årig – year(s)
ein vidaregåande skule – senior high school, upper secondary school
å vara – to last
å ta(ka) (tek, tok, teke) – to take

ein høgskule /"hø:gsku:le/ – college
eit universitet /univærsi'te:t/ – university
vart skipa /"sji:pa/ – was established
ein måte /"må:te/ – way
på same måten som – in the same way as, like
spreidd – spread
ein lærarskule /"læ:rarsku:le/ – teachers training college, college of education
skulepengar /"sku:lepengar/ m.pl. – tuition
eit lån – loan
Statens Lånekasse – the State Loan Office
ei utgift /"u:tjift/ – expense

97

ei husleige /"huːslæige/ – rent
ein vanske /"vanske/ – difficulty
ein stad – place
å byggja – to build
ein studentheim /stu'denthæim/ – residence hall, dorm

privat /pri'vaːt/ – private
vaksen /"vaksen/ – grown-up
ein ungdom /"ongdom/ – young person

10A Hjå skulelækjaren

Lars har fått melding om at han skal møta hjå skulelækjaren for å
verta undersøkt.

LÆKJAREN	Vi må kontrollera om du er heilt frisk.
LARS	Eg har ikkje vore sjuk på lenge. Eg har berre vore forkjølt eit par gonger i vinter.
LÆKJAREN	Det er bra, men vi må undersøkja deg likevel. Lat oss byrja med hovudet. – Ser du godt? Høyrer du godt?
LARS	Ja, det har aldri vore noko i vegen med augo eller øyro mine, og eg har ikkje hol i tennene.
LÆKJAREN	Vil du gapa opp? Eg vil gjerne sjå ned i halsen din.
LARS	Eg har litt vondt på høgre sida.
LÆKJAREN	Ja, eg ser at du er litt tett i halsen og i nasen, men det er ingenting alvorleg. Plagar det deg?
LARS	Nei, ikkje mykje, men eg har ofte vondt i ryggen når eg sit lenge med leksene.
LÆKJAREN	Du må sitja med rett rygg og stø ryggen mot stolen, og så hjelper det godt å driva idrett.
LARS	Eg går mykje på ski om vinteren, og då vert eg betre.
LÆKJAREN	Vil du reisa deg opp slik at eg får sjå om ryggen din er skeiv? – Nei, dette ser bra ut. Armane og beina ser ut til å vera i orden også.
LARS	Ja, eg er i god form no. Det er berre to andre i klassen min som har betre kondisjon enn eg no. Vi trenar fast tre kveldar i veka.
LÆKJAREN	Ja, du er heilt frisk. Eg skal berre ta pulsen din og blodtrykket ditt. Til slutt skal vi ta eit par prøver – ei urinprøve og ei blodprøve.

Norsk ordtak: Ei god helse er meir enn rikdom.

99

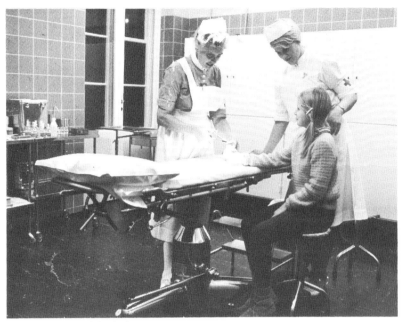

Fig. 10.1 *Hjå skulelækjaren.*

ein skulelækjar /"sku:lelæ:kjar/
 – school doctor
ei melding – notice, message,
 word
undersøkt – past participle of å
 undersøkja, to examine
å kontrollera /kontro'le:ra/ – to
 check, to control
om – if, whether
frisk – well, healthy, sound
sjuk – sick, ill
ikkje på lenge – not for a long
 time
å vera forkjølt – to have a cold
i vinter – this winter
å lata – to let
lat oss byrja med – let us start
 with
eit hovud /"hå:vu/ – head
å sjå (ser, såg, sett) – to see

å høyra (høyrer, høyrde, høyrt)
 – to hear
noko i vegen med – something
 wrong with
eit auga, pl. augo – eye
eit øyra, pl. øyro – ear
eit hol /hå:l/ – cavity
ei tann, pl. tenner – tooth
å gapa opp – to open one's
 mouth wide
ned – down
ein hals – throat
eg har vondt /vont/ i halsen – I
 have a sore throat
han er tett i halsen – he is
 congested
ein nase – nose
alvorleg /al'vå:rleg/ – serious
å plaga (plagar, plaga, plaga) –
 to bother

100

plagar det deg? – does it bother you?

ein rygg – back

eg har vondt i ryggen – I have a sore back

å sitja (sit, sat, sete) – to sit

rett rygg – straight back

med rett rygg – upright

å stø – to support

mot – against

å hjelpa (hjelper, hjelpte, hjelpt) – to help

det hjelper godt – it helps a lot

ein idrett /ˈiːdrett/ – athletics, sports

å driva idrett – to engage in athletic activities, sports

å gå (går, gjekk, gått) – to go

å gå på ski – to go skiing

å reisa seg opp – to get up, to stand up

slik at – so that

skeiv /sjæiv/ rygg – scoliosis, curvature of the spine, crooked back

ein arm – arm

eit bein – leg

i orden /ˈården/ – all right

eg er i god form – I am in good shape

å ha god kondisjon – to be in good shape

å trena (trenar, trena, trena) – to exercise

tre kveldar i veka – three times (evenings) a week

ein puls – pulse

eit blodtrykk /ˈbloːtrykk/ – blood pressure

til slutt – finally

ei prøve – test, sample

ei blodprøve – blood test

ei urinprøve /uˈriːnprøːve/ – specimen of urine

ei helse – health

ein rikdom /ˈriːkdom/ – wealth

Spørsmål

1. Kvar skal Lars møta? 2. Kvifor vil lækjaren undersøkja han? 3. Er Lars ofte forkjølt? 4. Har han vondt i halsen? 5. Er han tett i nasen? 6. Har han vondt i ryggen? 7. Har han skeiv rygg? 8. Kva seier lækjaren at han må gjera? 9. Driv Lars idrett? 10. Går han mykje på ski? 11. Har han betre kondisjon enn kameratane sine? 12. Kva slags prøver tek lækjaren til slutt?

10B Grammar

1. Some Irregular Nouns

ein feil 'mistake'	feilen	feil(ar)	feila(ne)
ein sko 'shoe'	skoen	skor	skorne
ein ting 'thing'	tingen	ting	tinga

101

ein bror 'brother'	broren	brør	brørne
ein far 'father'	faren	fedrar	fedrane
ein mann 'man'	mannen	menn	mennene
ein fot 'foot'	foten	føter	føtene
ein son 'son'	sonen	søner	sønene
ein bonde 'farmer'	bonden	bønder	bøndene
ei bok 'book'	boka	bøker	bøkene
ei natt 'night'	natta	netter	nettene
ei mor 'mother'	mora	mødrer	mødrene
ei tann 'tooth'	tanna	tenner	tennene
ei tå 'toe'	tåa	tær	tærne
ei ku 'cow'	kua	kyr	kyrne
eit auga 'eye'	auga	augo	augo
eit hjarta 'heart'	hjarta	hjarto	hjarto
eit øyra 'ear'	øyra	øyro	øyro

2. Some Modal Auxiliaries

The verbs *å ha*, *å vera*, and *å verta* or *å bli* are used as helping verbs to form compound tenses or to express the passive voice. In addition to these verbs, there are a number of *modal auxiliaries*. The modal auxiliaries tell us something about the way an utterance is being presented, i.e., whether it is a command, a recommendation, a possibility, etc. A list of the most common modal auxiliaries is presented below.

Notice that after a modal auxiliary, the main verb is always in the infinitive, but it is not preceded by the infinitive marker å: Han skal reisa til Noreg. Kan du koma?

Modal auxiliaries:

Infinitive	Present tense	Past tense	Part participle
å skulla 'to be going to'	skal 'shall'	skulle 'should'	skulla
å vilja 'to wish, to want'	vil 'will'	ville 'would'	vilja
å kunna 'to be able to'	kan 'can'	kunne 'could'	kunna
å byrja 'ought to'	bør 'ought to'	burde 'ought to'	burt
å måtta 'to have to'	må 'must, have to'	måtte 'had to'	måtta
å ljota 'to have to'	lyt 'must, have to'	laut 'had to'	lote
å tora 'dare to'	torer 'dare'	torde 'dared'	tort
å lata 'to let'	lèt 'let'	lét 'allowed'	late
å få 'to get'	får 'get'	fekk 'got'	fått

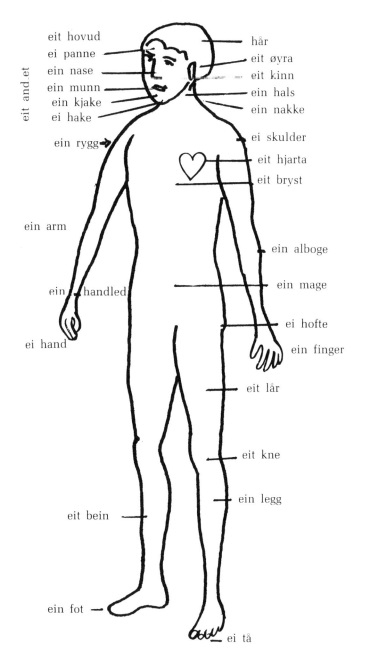

eit hovud
ei panne
ein nase
ein munn
ein kjake
ei hake

eit and et

ein rygg

ein arm

ein handled

ei hand

hår
eit øyra
eit kinn
ein hals
ein nakke

ei skulder
eit hjarta
eit bryst

ein alboge
ein mage
ei hofte
ein finger

eit lår

eit kne

ein legg

eit bein

ein fot

ei tå

Fig. 10.2 Kroppen vår.

103

After a modal auxiliary the main verb may be left out if it denotes motion: Han skal (reisa) til Noreg. Eg må (gå) heim no. The verb 'to do' is sometimes also understood: Det kan eg. 'I can do that.'

Observe carefully the following examples:

1) *Skal and skulle*

Han skal til byen.	He is supposed to go to town.
Han skulle til byen.	He was supposed to go to town.
Han seier at han skal koma.	He says he is coming (intends to, is going to come).
Han sa at han skulle koma.	He said he was coming.

2) *Vil and ville*

Han vil ikkje gå.	He doesn't want to go.
Han ville ikkje gå.	He didn't want to go.
Eg veit ikkje kva eg vil.	I don't know what I want (to do).
Eg visste ikkje kva eg ville.	I didn't know what I wanted (to do).

3) *Må and måtte*

Han må til byen.	He has to go to town.
Han måtte til byen.	He had to go to town.
Eg må kjøpa mjølk.	I have to buy milk.
Eg måtte kjøpa mjølk.	I had to buy milk.

4) *Bør and burde*

No bør du gå heim.	Now you should go home.
No burde du gå heim.	Now you ought to (or should) go home.
Eg burde ha gått heim før.	I ought to have gone home earlier.

Oppgåver

1. List the sentences in 10A in which a modal auxiliary has been used.
2. Fill in the blanks with the correct form of the noun:
   a) Læraren fann . . . . .i oppgåva. (ein feil)
   b) Jenta hadde kvite . . . . (ein sko)
   c) Begge . . . . .var ute. (ein bror)
   d) To . . . . .stod i døra. (ein mann)
   e) Han hadde vondt i begge . . . . .sine. (ein fot)
   f) Lars hadde fem . . . . (ein son)

g) Alle . . . . likte seg godt. (ein bonde)
h) Læraren har kjøpt mange . . . . (ei bok)
i) Dei budde der i to . . . . (ei natt)
j) Begge . . . . var heime. (ei bestemor)
k) Alle . . . . var ute. (ei ku)
l) . . . . hennar var heilt kvite. (ei tann)
m) Han hadde vondt i begge . . . . (eit auga)

3. Translate the following sentences into nynorsk: a) I can go now.
   b) I could go. c) I must go now. d) I had to go. e) I ought to go now.
   f) I ought to have gone home at twelve.

10C Pronunciation/Spelling

The Fricative Consonants /f v s j h/

The fricative consonants (spirants) /kj/ and /sj/ have been discussed
in 6C, and the remaining fricatives /f v s j h/ do not cause many
difficulties. The consonant /j/, however, is pronounced like the
opening sound in *yes* and *yawn* and should not be confused with
the pronunciation of the letter *j* in English.

The sound /j/ is spelled in different ways: 1) *j*: ja, jul 'Christmas',
jamn 'even', jente; 2) *gj*: gjerne, gjest 'guest', gjera; 3) *hj*: hjarta,
hjerne 'brain', hjelp; 4) *lj*: ljom 'ringing sound, echo', ljore 'smoke
vent', ljå 'scythe'; 5) g before *i, y, ei* and *øy* in stressed syllables: gift
'married; poison', gyta 'spawn', geit 'goat', gøyma 'hide'.

Oppgåve
Try to find other examples of the four different ways of spelling the
consonant /j/ in the previous texts.

10D Folketrygda

Den viktigaste sosiale reforma som har vore innført i Noreg, er lova
om folketrygda, som tok til å gjelda frå 1. januar 1967.

Folketrygda er ei felles og obligatorisk trygd og pensjonsordning
for alle som bur i Noreg eller arbeider på norske skip.

Føremålet med folketrygda er å gje stønad ved sjukdom, uførleik,
arbeidsløyse, dødsfall, tap av forsytar og alderdom. Hovudtanken
bak folketrygda er såleis at alle menneske som bur i Noreg eller

arbeider på norske skip, skal ha ein rimeleg levestandard, jamvel om dei misser inntekta si.

Dersom ein person vert sjuk eller ufør til dømes, vil han få ein viss stønad frå staten slik at han kan greia seg. Dersom han vert arbeidslaus, vil han få nok pengar til å dekkja dei faste utgiftene sine. Når han vert gammal, vil han få ein fast alderspensjon.

Det folk flest tenkjer på i samband med folketrygda, er fri lækjarhjelp, fritt sjukehusopphald, trygd ved arbeidsløyse og alderspensjon.

Utgiftene til folketrygda vert dekte ved ei medlemsavgift frå den einskilde personen, ei avgift frå arbeidsgjevaren og tilskot frå staten og kommunen. Medlemsavgifta vert fastsett i prosent av inntekta og er ein del av skatten ein betaler.

ei folketrygd /''fålketrygd/ – national insurance
ei trygd – insurance
ei reform /re'fårm/ – reform
å innføra /'innfø:ra/ – to introduce
å taka til å gjelda – to become effective, to take effect
felles /'felles/ – common
ei pensjonsordning /'pen-'sjo:nsårdning/ – pension system
å bu (bur, budde, butt) – to live
å arbeida (arbeider, arbeidde, arbeidt) – to work
eit skip /sji:p/ – ship
eit føremål /'fø:remå:l/ – purpose
å gje (gjev, gav, gjeve) /je:/ – to give
ein stønad /''stø:na/ – support, relief
ein sjukdom – disease
uførleik /''u:fø:rlæik/ m. – disability
ufør /''u:fø:r/ – disabled
arbeidsløyse f. – unemployment

arbeidslaus – unemployed
eit dødsfall /'døtsfall/ – death
eit tap – loss
ein forsytar /får'sy:tar/ – breadwinner, provider
ein alderdom /'alderdom/ – old age
ein hovudtanke – basic idea
såleis – thus
bak – behind
ein levestandard /''le:vestandar/ – standard of living
å missa (misser, miste, mist) – to lose
ein person /pær'so:n/ – person
viss – certain
staten – the State
nok /nåkk/ – enough
ein alderspensjon – old age pension
folk flest – people in general
i samband med – in connection with
fri – free, gratis
ei lækjarhjelp – medical treatment
eit sjukehusopphald – hospitalization

106

vert dekte – are covered
ei medlemsavgift /"me:dlems-
a:vjift/ – membership fee
einskild /"æinsjild/ – individual
ei avgift – fee
ein arbeidsgjevar – employer

eit tilskot /"tillskå:t/ – support,
subsidy
vert fastsett – is determined
i prosent av – in percentage of
ei inntekt – income
ein skatt – tax, income tax

11A I reisebyrået

Roy Eisel skal til Volda for å byrja på distriktshøgskulen og går inn
på eit reisebyrå for å kjøpa billett.

EKSPEDITØREN	Ver så god.
ROY	Eg skulle ha ein billett til Volda.
EKSPEDITØREN	Kva måte vil du reisa på?
ROY	Eg vil reisa på den måten som er enklast og billegast.
EKSPEDITØREN	Ja, du må ta toget til Bergen. Frå Bergen kan du ta fly, snøggbåt eller vanleg båt. Med fly er reisetida berre ein halv time. Snøggbåten bruker fem og ein halv time til Nordfjordeid, og derifrå går det buss. «Hurtigruta» bruker om lag fjorten timar til Ålesund, og frå Ålesund til Volda må du ta buss og ferje.
ROY	Eg tek «hurtigruta», for eg liker å reisa med båt. Dessutan får eg sjå meir av kysten då. Norske-kysten er så vakker, synest eg.
EKSPEDITØREN	Dersom du tek snøggbåten, får du sjå mykje av fjordane, men du kan vel ta den attende.
ROY	Ja, det var ein god idé. Eg skal attende til Voss ein tur seinare.
EKSPEDITØREN	Ver så god. Her er billettane. – Vil du ha lugar?
ROY	Ja, takk, det vil eg gjerne. Det vert for lenge å sitja oppe heile natta.
EKSPEDITØREN	Ja vel. Eg skal tinga til deg med det same.
ROY	Er det vanskeleg å finna fram i Bergen? Eg er ikkje kjend der.
EKSPEDITØREN	Nei, det er lett, men lettast av alt er å ta drosje frå jarnvegsstasjonen og ut til kaien der båten går frå.
ROY	Ja, då gjer eg det. – Ha det.
EKSPEDITØREN	Ha det, og god tur!

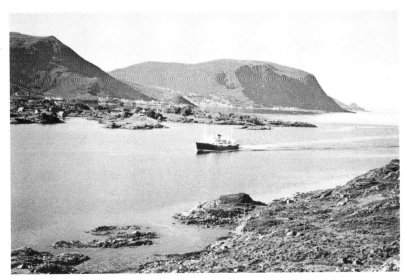

Fig. 11 Frå Herøy, Sunnmøre.
«Hurtigruta» på veg nordover frå Bergen til Ålesund.

eit reisebyrå – travel agency
å byrja (byrjar, byrja, byrja) – to begin
å gå inn på – to go into, to enter
å kjøpa (kjøper, kjøpte, kjøpt) – to buy
ein billett /bi'lett/ – ticket
eg skulle ha – I would like to have
kva måte . . . på – In constructions such as this, prepositions are placed at the end of the clause in questions and subordinate clauses.
å reisa (reiser, reiste, reist) – to travel
eit tog /to:g/ – train
eit fly – (air)plane, aircraft
å ta fly – to go by air, to fly
ein båt – boat
ein snøggbåt – fast ship
å ta båt – to go by boat

ei reisetid – traveling time
å bruka (bruker, brukte, brukt) – to use, to take
halv – half
derifrå – from there
ein buss – bus
«hurtigruta» – the coastal express
ei ferje – ferryboat
å lika (liker, likte, likt) – to like
å reisa med båt – to travel by boat
dessutan /'dessu:tan/ – in addition, besides
ein idé /i'de:/ – idea
ein tur – trip
ein lugar /lu·ga:r/ – cabin
å sitja oppe – to sit up
ja vel – okay
å tinga – to book, to make reservations
med det same – immediately

109

å finna fram – to find one's way
eg er ikkje kjend der – I don't
 know the city well; I'm not
 acquainted there
ein drosje /"dråsje/ – taxi

ein jarnvegsstasjon – railway
 station
ein kai – pier, quay
god tur! – have a nice trip!

Spørsmål

1. Kvar skal Roy Eisel reisa? 2. Kvar tingar han billett? 3. Tek han toget til Volda? 4. Kor lang tid bruker «hurtigruta» frå Bergen til Ålesund? 5. Må han ta buss også? 6. Kvifor liker han å reisa med båt? 7. Kvifor vil han ta snøggbåten attende? 8. Kva skal han gjera i Volda? 9. Er han kjend i Bergen? 10. Tingar han lugar på båten?

11B Grammar

1. The Future

Future time is expressed in different ways in *nynorsk*:

1) By means of the present tense, particularly in connection with adverbial time phrases referring to the future: Eg kjem snart. Han byrjar i morgon. Ho reiser om ei veke 'in a week'. Eg trur eg tek rommet. 'I think I'll take the room.'

2) By means of the present tense of the modal auxiliary *å skulla*, i.e., *skal* 'shall', plus the infinitive of the main verb: Eg skal reisa til Noreg neste år. Kor lenge skal du vera der? Vi skal vera heime dette året, men sonen vår skal reisa til Afrika. Grannane våre skal reisa til utlandet også. Skal de reisa eit anna år, kanskje?

 As can be seen from the examples above, *skal* is used when something *is going to* take place or is predetermined to take place.

3) By means of the present tense of the modal helping verb *å vilja*, i.e., *vil* 'will' plus the infinitive of the main verb: Vil du prøva kjolen? Når vil han koma? Vil far din koma også? Vil han hjelpa oss? Vil de vera med oss? Dei andre vil ikkje reisa.

The distinction between *skal* and *vil* is not very clear. As a general rule we may say that *vil* expresses *volition* in connection with a future action. This is particularly the case with *vil* when the subject is a person, and *vil* is, therefore, mostly used as a helping verb for the future with impersonal subjects: Eg trur det vil ta lang tid. Eg trur det vil bli regn. Ho seier det vil verta vanskeleg. Notice

110

also that *vil* is often used after a conditional clause: Dersom han reiser til Noreg, vil han fort læra norsk. Dersom ho har nok pengar, vil det gå fint med henne.

4) Very often by means of the present tense of *å koma til å*, i.e., *kjem til å*, plus the infinitive of the main verb: Vi kjem til å reisa til Noreg i sommar. Ingen veit kva som kjem til å henda.

5) By means of the present tense of the verb *å få* 'to get', i.e., *får*, plus the infinitive without the infinitive marker *å*: Eg får prøva. Eg får gjera det.

If we want to express that an action is to take place before another one in the future (the future perfect), we use *skal ha* or *vil ha* plus the past participle of the main verb: Brit skal (vil) ha skrive eit brev før ho legg seg. 'Brit will have written a letter before she goes to bed.' Quite often *får* plus the past participle of the main verb is also used about an action completed in the future: Eg skal skriva til deg så snart eg får gjort det. 'I will write to you as soon as I get it done.' Han skal reisa så snart han får selt huset. 'He will leave as soon as he gets the house sold.'

2. The Relative Pronoun **som** and the Relative Adverb **der**

The relative pronoun which is most frequently used is *som*. It renders who, whom, which, that, and as in English.

Som has only one form, and that form refers to persons, things, ideas, etc., in the singular as well as in the plural. It has three main functions:

1) It is used as the *subject* of the relative clause. Han har ei kone som talar nynorsk. Han har ein bror som bur på Voss.
2) It is used as the *object* of the relative clause: Eg har den boka (som) du nemnde 'mentioned'. Astrid hadde ei klokke, som ho hadde fått av far sin.
3) It is used when governed by a preposition at the end of the clause: Det er den mannen (som) eg tala om. Der ser du huset (som) eg bur i.

As in English, a relative pronoun can be omitted when it is not the subject of the clause: Eg har den boka du nemnde. Det er den mannen eg tala om. Notice that the prepositions governing the relative pronoun *som* are always placed at the end of the clause: mannen eg tala om; huset eg bur i.

In sentences like: Den staden *der* han bur, heiter Voss. Vegen *der* ho går, er smal 'narrow', the word der 'where' is called a *relative adverb*.

A relative clause has the same function as an adjective or a prepositional phrase that modifies a noun: Han har ei brun bok. Han har ei bok med brun farge. Han har ei bok som er brun.

Oppgåver
1. Translate the following sentences into *nynorsk*:
    a) Will she write to us?
    b) I will not go there.
    c) He will be here tomorrow.
    d) How long will you stay there?
    e) I think it's going to rain.
2. Combine each pair of sentences below into one sentence using relative pronouns/adverbs.
    a) Mannen er rik. Han bur i det huset.
    b) Ho kjenner ein mann. Han talar nynorsk.
    c) Han har to systrer. Dei bur på Voss.
    d) Eg har den bilen. Du nemnde bilen.
    e) Brit hadde ei fin bok. Ho hadde fått henne av læraren sin.
    f) Bygda heiter Voss. Dei bur der.
    g) Kontoret er fint. Dei arbeider der.

11C Pronunciation/Spelling

The Nasal Consonants /m/ and /n/

The nasal consonants /m/ and /n/ are pronounced as in English, and need no further discussion. The sequence /ng/ is pronounced like ng in English *finger* or *linger* in the western regions of the country, but like that of *sing* and *singer* in the eastern regions. In the sequences /kn/ and /gn/ both sounds are pronounced in *nynorsk*: Knut /knu:t/ (name), gnag /gna:g/ 'gnawing'.

Notice that the letter m is never doubled at the end of a word, e.g., kom, kam 'comb', lam 'lamb', nor is a final n doubled in modal auxiliaries or pronouns, e.g., kan, han, sin.

Oppgåve
Find words containing the nasals /m/ and /n/ in 11A. Practice pronouncing them.

11D Nordmannen

Millom bakkar og berg utmed havet
hovo nordmannen fengo sin heim,
der han sjølv heve tuftene grave
og sett sjølv sine hus oppå deim.

Han såg ut på dei steinute strender;
det var ingen som der hadde bygt.
«Lat oss rydja og byggja oss grender,
og so eiga me rudningen trygt.»

Han såg ut på det bårute havet;
der var ruskut å leggja utpå;
men der leikade fisk nedi kavet,
og den leiken den ville han sjå.

Frampå vetteren stundom han tenkte:
Gjev eg var i eit varmare land!
Men når vårsol i bakkane blenkte,
fekk han hug til si heimlege strand.

Og når liene grønka som hagar,
når det laver av blomar på strå,
og når netter er ljose som dagar,
kan han ingenstad venare sjå.

Av Ivar Aasen

Ivar Aasen (1813–96) var fødd i Ørsta på Sunnmøre. Faren var
bonde, men Ivar synte tidleg at han var meir interessert i bøker enn i
gardsarbeid. Då han vart eldre, voks det fram hjå han eit ønske om å
gjera noko for bondeklassen, og han makta å gjennomføra det som få
hadde tenkt seg: *å skapa eit skriftmål som bygde på målføra i Noreg
og som hadde samanheng med gammalnorsken.*
    Ivar Aasen har også skrive mange vakre dikt, og «Millom bakkar
og berg» er eitt av dei mest kjende. Det er ofte sunge ved festlege
samkomer og er godt likt av alle.

millom /"millom/ – between
  (old form)
ein bakke /"bakke/ – hill
eit berg – mountain
utmed /"u:tme/ – along, near

heve /"he:ve/ – has (old form)
fenge /"fenge/ – past participle
  of å *få* (old form)
ein heim – home
ei tuft – (building) site

å grava (grev, grov, grave) – to dig
å setja (set, sette, sett) – to set, to put
oppå /"oppå/ – upon
deim – them (old form)
å byggja (byggjer, bygde, bygt) – to build
å rydja (ryd, rudde, rudt) – to clear (land of trees, bushes, and stones)
so /so:/ – so, then (old form)
eiga – present tense pl. of å eiga (old form)
me = vi (optional form)
ein rudning – clearing, piece of new land
trygt – safely
bårut – wavy, billowy
ruskut – rough, stormy
å leggja utpå – to set out on
leikade – played (old form)
nedi /"ne:di/ – down in
eit kav – deep, the depths of the sea
ein leik – play, playing
frampå /"frampå/ vetteren – late in the winter
stundom – now and then
gjev eg var – I wish I were
ei vårsol /"vå:rso:l/ – spring sun
å blenkja (blenkjer, blenkte, blenkt) – to shine, to gleam
å få hug til – to get a mind to, to like
heimleg – home, homelike
ei li – hillside
å grønka – to grow (or become) green
å lava – to hang down in rich clusters

ein blom – flower
eit strå – stem or stalk of tall grass
ljos /jo:s/ – light
ingenstad – nowhere
ven – pretty, beautiful
var fødd – was born
å syna (syner, synte, synt) – to show
tidleg /"ti:leg/ – early
interessert /intre'se:rt/ – interested
eit gardsarbeid /'ga:rsarbæi/ – work on a farm
å veksa (veks, voks, vakse) – to grow
å veksa fram – to develop
fram – ahead, forward
eit ønske – wish
ein bondeklasse – the farmers
å makta (maktar, makta, makta) – to manage
å gjennomføra – to carry out, to accomplish
få – few
å skapa (skaper, skapte, skapt) – to create
eit skriftmål – written language
eit målføre – dialect
ein samanheng – connection
gammalnorsk m. – Old Norwegian, also used for Old Norse
å skriva (skriv, skreiv, skrive) – to write
mest – most
kjend – well known
å syngja (syng, song, sunge) – to sing
festleg – festive
ei samkome /"samkå:me/ – meeting, gathering

114

12A Snakk dialekt – skriv nynorsk!

Roy har byrja å studera nynorsk i Volda, og ein dag talar han med Liv, som er aktiv i målrørsla.

ROY   Hei!
LIV   Hei!
ROY   Snakkar du alltid dialekt, Liv?
LIV   Ja, det gjer eg. Eg veit at somme målfolk meiner at ein skal normera talemålet også, men det er eg usamd i. Det første språket du lærer, er dialekten. Dialekten din bruker du i leik og arbeid, han vert ein del av deg sjølv. Du kastar han ikkje av deg med fritidskleda.
ROY   Kva meiner du med dialekt?
LIV   Dialekt eller målføre er det språket folk snakkar i ei grend, ein by eller delar av ein by. Dialektane har utvikla seg noko ulikt i dei ulike landsdelane, men alle dialektar her i landet har viktige drag felles. Somme er opplærte til å snakka bokmål. Også dei har som regel innslag av dialektformer, men skriftspråket har vore mønster for talemålet deira.
ROY   Korleis ser du på bydialektane?
LIV   Bydialektane er ikkje mindreverdige variantar av bokmål, men norske dialektar, i slekt med dei andre dialektane her i landet.
ROY   Kvifor skal vi gå over til nynorsk når bokmål dominerer slik det gjer i samfunnet i dag?
LIV   Det som skil nynorsk frå bokmål, er at det nynorske skriftmålet byggjer på målføra, medan bokmålet samsvarar dårleg med dialektane. Når du skriv nynorsk, byggjer du på dialekten din. Skal folket få eit skriftmål som byggjer på dialektane, må nynorsken verta teken i bruk.
ROY   Ville det ikkje vera lettare for meg å snakka ein normert nynorsk?

115

LIV Jau, for ein utlending ville vel det vera enklast, men du fortalde i går at mor di snakka Vosse-mål. Etter mitt syn er det ein menneskerett å få snakka slik ein vil, men vi må ha nokolunde faste reglar for skriftspråket. Og det må byggja på talemålet til folk flest, ikkje talemålet til ein kulturell og økonomisk elite.

å snakka (snakkar, snakka, snakka) – to speak

å tala (talar, tala, tala) – to speak, to talk

aktiv /'akti:v/ – active

målrørsla f. – the New Norwegian language movement

ein dialekt /dia'lekt/ – dialect

å vita (veit, visste, visst) – to know

somme – some

målfolk n.pl. – adherents of New Norwegian

å meina (meiner, meinte, meint) – to think, to be of the opinion that

å normera (normerer, normerte, normert) – to standardize, to normalize

eit språk – language

eit talemål – spoken language, speech

å vera usamd i – to disagree about

å læra (lærer, lærte, lært) – to learn

ein del – part

å kasta (kastar, kasta, kasta) – to throw

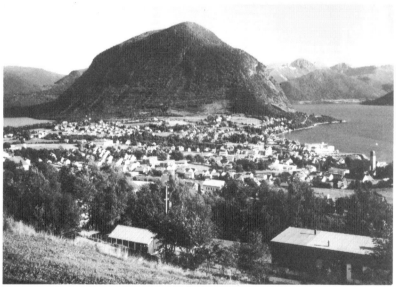

Fig. 12.1 *I Volda er det mange skular.*

116

å kasta av – to take off
fritidsklede /'fri:ti:skle:e/ n.pl. –
casual clothes
å utvikla (utviklar, utvikla, utvikla) /'u:tvikla/ – to develop
ein landsdel /'lansde:l/ – region
her i landet – in this country
er opplærte til – have been
trained to
eit innslag – element
eit mønster /'mønster/ – model,
pattern, norm
ein bydialekt – urban dialect
deira – their
å sjå på – to consider, to think
of
mindreverdig /'mindreværdi/ –
inferior
ein variant /vari'ant/ – variant
i slekt med – related to
å gå over til – to go over to, to
change to
å dominera (dominerer, domi-
nerte, dominert) /domi'ne:ra/
– to dominate

eit samfunn – society
å skilja (skil, skilde, skilt) – to
distinguish
medan /"me:an/ – while
å samsvara med (samsvarar,
samsvara, samsvara) – to correspond to
dårleg – poorly
i bruk – into use
ein utlending – foreigner
å fortelja (fortel, fortalde,
fortalt) /får'telja/ – to tell
Vosse-mål – the dialect of Voss
etter mitt syn – in my opinion
eit syn – view, opinion
ein menneskerett – human
right
nokolunde – somewhat, to a
certain degree
ein regel /'re:gel/ – rule
kulturell /kultur'ell/ – cultural
økonomisk /øko'no:misk/ – financial, economic
ein elite /e'li:te/ – elite

Spørsmål
1. Kva gjer Roy i Volda? 2. Kva heiter jenta som han snakka med? 3.
Talar ho alltid dialekt? 4. Kva er ein dialekt? 5. Kva er ein bydialekt?
6. Kvifor bør ein skriva nynorsk? 7. Kva for mål byggjer nynorsken
på? 8. Kvifor bør alle få snakka slik dei vil? 9. Kva for talemål bør
skriftspråket byggja på? 10. Kva er ditt syn?

12B Grammar

1. Eg veit (at), eg kjenner (han), eg meiner (at)
The English verb *to know* is translated by two different words in
nynorsk: *å vita* and *å kjenna*. *Å vita* means to know a fact, or that
something is true, whereas *å kjenna* means to be acquainted with or
familiar with someone or something: Eg veit at Roy er frå USA. Eg

117

kjenner han godt. The phrase *å kjenna til at* is synonymous with *å vita at*: Eg kjenner til at Roy er frå USA. The phrase *å kjenna att* means 'to recognize': Eg kjende han att med det same.

The nynorsk verb *å meina* means 'to think, to be of the opinion that', and in some cases 'to mean': Eg meiner at ein skal tala dialekt. 'I think that people should speak their dialects.' Kva meiner du med dialekt? 'What do you mean by dialect?' The English verb *to mean* in the sense of 'to signify' is translated by *å tyda* in most cases: Kva tyder det ordet? 'What does that word mean?'

2. The Conjugation of Verbs

We have already briefly discussed the infinitive (3B3), the present tense (1B3, 7B3), the past tense (5B3), the present perfect tense (9B1), and the future tense (11B1). We have also stated that a verb is usually listed with four forms in a dictionary: the infinitive, the present tense, the past tense, and the past participle.

As we mentioned in 5B3, the verbs in nynorsk are grouped into two classes according to the way the past tense is formed. Those verbs that have a grammatical ending in the past tense (usually a dental suffix) are called *weak verbs*, while those without any ending but usually having a change of the vowel of the stem are called *strong verbs*. In addition to these two classes, there is a relatively large group of irregular verbs. Below the basic patterns for the conjugation of weak and strong verbs are listed according to verb class. The past participle is listed with its neuter form only.

The conjugation of weak verbs:

Infinitive	Present tense	Past tense	Past participle
1. å kasta 'to throw'	kastar -ar	kasta -a	kasta -a
2. å dømma 'to judge, sentence'	dømmer	dømde	dømt
å tenkja 'to think'	tenkjer -er	tenkte -de, -te	tenkt -t
3. å tru 'to believe'	trur -r	trudde -dde	trutt or trudd -tt or -dd
4. å telja 'to count'	tel -	talde -de	talt -t

The conjugation of strong verbs:

Infinitive	Present tense	Past tense	Past participle
1. å bita 'to bite'	bit -i-	beit -ei-	bite -i-
2. å bryta 'to break'	bryt -y-	braut -au-	brote -o-
3. å finna 'to find'	finn -i-	fann -a-	funne -u-
4. å bera 'to carry'	ber -e-	bar -a-	bore -o-
5. å lesa 'to read'	les -e-	las -a-	lese -e-
6. å fara 'to go'	fer -a(e)-	fór -o-	fare -a-
7. å blåsa 'to blow'	blæs -å(æ)-	bles -e-	blåse -å-

3. The Numerals. Cardinal Numbers (continued)

Review all the numbers given so far (see 4B3 and 6B2). The remaining cardinal numbers are: ein million /milli'o:n/, pl. millionar; ein milliard /milli'ard/, pl. milliardar (American: billion), ein billion /billi'o:n/, pl. billionar (trillion; British: billion).

In compound numbers ein is usually not inflected, e.g., tjueein poeng, trettiein bilete, even though both poeng and bilete are neuter nouns. The same is the case with year numbers: nittentrettiein (1931).

In writing, the only difference between the cardinal number ein (ei, eitt) and the indefinite article ein (ei, eit) is, as you can see, the double -t in the neuter form of the cardinal number. In speech, however, the difference is clear, since the cardinal number is stressed, whereas the indefinite article is unstressed.

As you probably already have noticed, compound numbers are formed in the same way as in English, i.e., with the decimal first: tjueein (21), tjuefem (25), førtifire (44).

As will be seen from 4B3, all cardinal numbers from 13 to 19 end in -ten. A teenager is, therefore, called ein tenåring in nynorsk.

Year numbers from the year 1100 to 1999 can be read in two ways, e.g., 1979: nittensyttini or nittenhundreogsyttini. Notice that if you read nitten hundre, the conjunction og must always be added.

For the years before and after the period 1100–1999, both the word *hundre,* resp. *tusen,* and the conjunction *og* must be read, e.g., 850: åttehundreogfemti; 2010: totusenogti.

A comma is used for the decimal point.

Numbers like *11,5 prosent* are read as *elleve komma fem prosent.*

Oppgåver

1. Put these sentences into the past tense:
   a) Lækjaren kastar jakka si.
   b) Roy tenkjer på far sin.
   c) Liv trur at det skal gå bra.
   d) Guten fortel ein stubb.
   e) Dei finn lett vegen heim.
   f) Liv les lekser.
   g) Roy fer til byen.

2. Translate into *nynorsk:*
   a) I know that he has been here before.
   b) I recognized my old teacher at once.
   c) I'm going to meet him at five o'clock.
   d) I know that family very well.
   e) I think that students should respect their teachers.
   f) What do you mean by that?
   g) What does 'lærar' mean?
   h) Do you mean me?
   i) Do you think we'll meet any of our students there?

12C Pronunciation/Spelling

One or Two Consonants?

In writing, a double consonant is reduced to a single one before a grammatical ending that starts with a consonant: trygg – trygt; vill 'wild' – vilt; å byggja – bygde, bygt; å spenna 'kick, stretch' – spente, spent.

The double consonant is kept, however, in compounds and before the genitive *-s:* fjelltopp, tryggleik 'safety', til fjells, manns mot 'a man's courage'.

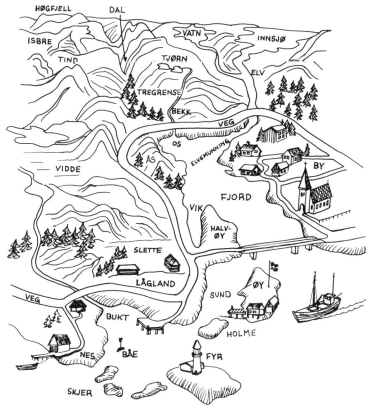

Fig. 12.2 Norsk natur er ulik frå stad til stad.
Viktige ord: ein bekk, ei bukt, ein by, ein båe, ein dal, ei elv, ein elvemunning, ein fjord, ein fyr, ei halvøy, ein holme, eit høgfjell, ein innsjø, ein isbre, eit lågland, eit nes, ein os, eit skjer, ei slette, eit sund, ein tind, ei tjørn, ei tregrense, eit vatn, ein veg, ei vidde, ei vik, ei øy, ein ås.

Oppgåver
1. Find words in 12A and 12D where a double consonant has been reduced to a single one.
2. Find words in the same texts that have kept the double consonant.

12D Norsk målreising

Då unionen med Danmark vart oppløyst i 1814, stod det danske skriftspråket sterkt i Noreg. Først ikring 1830 tok det til å koma til

121

orde eit nytt syn på dansken, og den leiande talsmannen for det nye synet var *Henrik Wergeland* (1808–45). Han ville fornorska det danske skriftspråket ved å gje rom for norske ord og norske bøyingsformer. Både nasjonale, stilistiske og demokratiske omsyn burde tilseia at skriftspråket kom nærare det talemålet folket hadde, meinte han.

Den mest aktive representanten for *fornorsking* av dansken etter Wergelands tid var *Knud Knudsen* (1812–95), og litt etter litt fekk denne politikken tilslutning. Det tok til å utvikla seg eit skriftspråk i Noreg som inneheldt så mange norske former at det ikkje lenger kunne kallast dansk. Vi kallar det derfor *norsk-dansk*, og det er dette språket som er grunnlaget for moderne bokmål.

Norsk talemål vart ikkje borte i dansketida. Til dagleg brukte mange byborgarar eit talemål som var prega av dansk, men også av dialekten på staden. Bønder og arbeidsfolk snakka dialekt.

Dei norske dialektane var utvikla av gammalnorsk og utgjorde eit levande og ekte talemål. Livsverket til *Ivar Aasen* (1813–96) vart å samla inn opplysningar om desse dialektane og å leggja dei til grunn for eit ekte norsk skriftspråk. Aasen kalla dette språket for *landsmål* (1929: nynorsk).

Eit viktig spørsmål er om bokmål og nynorsk før eller sidan kan gå saman til eitt språk, og dette har ført til ein langvarig språkstrid. Striden mellom bokmål og nynorsk var særleg kvass ikring 1900. Det vart derfor skipa organisasjonar på begge sider. Hovudorganisasjonen til målrørsla – *Noregs Mållag* – vart skipa i 1906 er ein landssamskipnad for lokallaga og fylkeslaga.

målreising f. – New Norwegian language movement
ein union /uni'o:n/ – union
vart oppløyst – was dissolved
å stå (står, stod, stått) – to stand, to be
det stod sterkt – it had a strong position
først ikring – not until around
å koma til orde – to appear, to be expressed
leiande /"læiande/ – leading
å fornorska /får'nårska/ – to Norwegianize

å gje rom for – to give room for, to allow
ei bøyingsform – grammatical form
nasjonal /nasjo'na:l/ – national
stilistisk /sti'listisk/ – stylistic
demokratisk /demo'kra:tisk/ – democratic
eit omsyn – consideration
å tilseia (tilseier, tilsa, tilsagt) /'tillsæia/ – to indicate
nær – close
ein representant /represen-'tant/ – representative

122

ei fornorsking /får'nårsking/ – Norwegianization
litt etter litt – little by little
ein politikk /puli'tikk/ – policy
ei tilslutning /'tillslutning/ – approval, support
å innehalda (inneheld, inneheldt, innehalde) – to contain
å kallast – to be called
å kalla (kallar, kalla, kalla) – to call
derfor /'dærfår/ – therefore
eit grunnlag – basis
å verta borte – disappear
dansketida f. – the Danish period (1380–1814)
til dagleg – ordinarily, every day
ein byborgar /'by:bårgar/ – city-dweller
var prega av – was marked by, was characterized by
arbeidsfolk n.pl. – working people
å utgjera /'u:tje:ra/ – to constitute, to make up
levande – living, vital
ekte – genuine
eit livsverk /'lifsværk/ – life-work

å samla inn – to gather
ei opplysning /opp'ly:sning/ – piece of information
desse – these
å leggja (legg, la, lagt) – to lay
å leggja til grunn – to use as a basis
å gå saman – to merge
å føra til – to lead to
langvarig – long-lasting
ein språkstrid – language conflict
ein strid /stri:/ – conflict, controversy
særleg – particularly
kvass – sharp, acute
å skipa /"sji:pa/ (skipar, skipa, skipa) – to establish
ein organisasjon /årganisa'sjo:n/ – organization
hovud- – main-
ein landssamskipnad /'lansamsji:pna/ – national organization
eit lokallag /lo'ka:l-la:g/ – local organization
eit fylkeslag – county organization
eit fylke – county. There are 19 counties in Norway.

13A På fest i ungdomslaget

Liv og Roy har vorte gode vener og går på fest i ungdomslaget.

LIV   Gjekk du på fest i ungdomslaget på Voss?
ROY   Nei, eg var berre med på festane og samkomene på folkehøgskulen, og det likte eg godt.
LIV   Det var vel mykje folkedans der?
ROY   Ja, det var ein del, og det var mange som kunne spela hardingfele. Men det var størst interesse for folkeviseleik, for då kunne vi dansa saman i ein ring, og alle kunne vera med.
LIV   Gjekk ungdomen i bunad der slik som her?
ROY   Ja, jentene hadde ofte bunad, men berre nokre få av gutane gjekk i bunad.
LIV   Synest du Vosse-bunaden er vakrare enn Sunnmørs-bunaden?
ROY   Nei, det veit eg ikkje. Eg tykkjer dei er så vakre begge to, og eg har lyst å skaffa meg ein mannsbunad, men dei er så dyre.
LIV   Veit du kvar min bunad er frå?
ROY   Eg er ikkje heilt sikker, men eg trur han er frå Austlandet ein stad.
LIV   Ja, han er frå Gudbrandsdalen.
ROY   Skal det vera mykje program her i kveld?
LIV   Ja, det skal det, men det er alltid gildt her. Først skal dei syna eit spelstykke, så skal vi ha mat, og til slutt skal det vera leik og gammaldans. Dei har eige spelemannslag her, så det skal verta mykje moro.
ROY   Eg kan ikkje nokon av desse dansane, eg kan berre litt folkeviseleik – slik som «Per spelemann» og eit par andre.

124

LIV   Eg skal læra deg. Du kan ikkje reisa attende til USA utan å kunna gammaldans og folkeviseleik. Så kan du læra venene dine der borte norske dansar.

RØY   Ja, det ville vera fint.

ein fest – party, celebration
på fest – at a party
eit ungdomslag – youth association, youth organization
fest i ungdomslaget – entertainment and dance in the Young People's Society
ein ven, pl. vener – friend
folkedans m. – folk dancing
ei interesse /inter'esse/ – interest
folkeviseleik m. – dance accompanying singing of folksongs
ei folkevise – folk song, popular ballad
å dansa (dansar, dansa, dansa) – to dance

ein ring – ring, circle
å vera med – to join in
ein ungdom – youth, young people
ein bunad /"bu:na/ – national (regional) costume
å gå i – to wear
nokre få – a few
Vosse-bunad – bunad from Voss
Sunnmørs-bunad – bunad from Sunnmøre
å skaffa seg – to get hold of
Gudbrandsdalen – valley in Eastern Norway
gildt /jilt/ – fun
å syna (syner, synte, synt) – to show

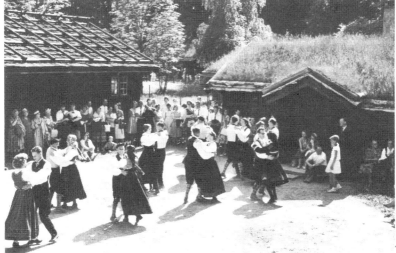

Fig. 13 På fest i ungdomslaget.

125

eit spelstykke – play
leik m. = folkeviseleik
gammaldans m. – oldfash-
  ioned dancing
eit spelemannslag – band

moro – fun
nokon – any(one)
ein dans – dance
å reisa attende – to go back
utan å – without. . .ing

Spørsmål

1. Kvar går Liv og Roy på fest? 2. Har Roy vore på fest i eit ungdomslag før? 3. Var det folkedans på folkehøgskulen? 4. Kva var det størst interesse for på folkehøgskulen? 5. Gjekk både jentene og gutane i bunad? 6. Tykkjer Roy at Vosse-bunaden er vakrast av alle? 7. Har han bunad sjølv? 8. Har Liv bunad? 9. Kvar er hennar bunad frå? 10. Har Roy hug til å læra gammaldans og folkeviseleik?

13B Grammar

1. Att, å læra

The word *att (igjen)* has four different meanings: 'back', 'left', '(left) behind', and 'again'. Examples:

a) *'Back'*: Når læraren kjem *att*, skal vi seia det.
   This meaning of *att* is usually found with verbs like *å få, å ha, å koma*. Both the words *attende* and *tilbake* are used with the same meaning.

b) *'Left, remaining'*: Det var berre ein billett *att* (igjen).
   Har du ingenting *att* (igjen)?
   This meaning of *att* is usually found with verbs like *å vera* and *å ha*.

c) *'(Left) behind'*: Kor mykje plar ein leggja *att* i drikkepengar 'tip'?
   Det er synd at bilen min står *att* på kaien.
   This meaning of *att* is usually found with verbs like *å leggja, å liggja, å sitja, å stå, å verta, å bli*.

d) *'Again'*: Det var hyggeleg å møta deg *att*. Remember that *å kjenna att* means 'to recognize'. Another expression with similar meaning that can often be used in place of *att* in this sense is *ein gong til*: Vil du seia det ein gong til?

   The verb *å læra* translates both *to teach* and *to learn* in English. Notice, for example, that *a teacher* is called *ein lærar* in nynorsk.

126

2. The Numerals. Ordinal Numbers

Each of the cardinal numbers has a corresponding ordinal number, and we have had some of them in the titles of the lessons. The general rule for the formation of ordinal numbers from cardinal numbers is to add -ande to all numbers except 1–6, 11, 12, 100, 1000, and 1,000,000.

All the ordinal numbers from 1 to 1000 are:

første	first	syttande	seventeenth
andre	second	attande	eighteenth
tredje	third	nittande	nineteenth
fjerde	fourth	tjuande	twentieth
femte	fifth	tjueførste	twentyfirst
sjette	sixth	tjueandre	twentysecond
sjuande	seventh	trettiande	thirtieth
åttande	eighth	førtiande	fortieth
niande	ninth	femtiande	fiftieth
tiande	tenth	sekstiande	sixtieth
ellevte	eleventh	syttiande	seventieth
tolvte	twelfth	åttiande	eightieth
trettande	thirteenth	nittiande	ninetieth
fjortande	fourteenth	hundrede	hundredth
femtande	fifteenth	tusende	thousandth
sekstande	sixteenth	millionte	millionth

Notice *den hundrede, den tusende,* and *den millionte.*

When written as numerals, the ordinals are written as cardinals with a period after them, e.g., 1., 2., 3., etc. Dates can be written with or without *den: den 17. mai* or *17. mai.*

Notice that *nynorsk* has no equivalent to *on* before dates, or *of* before the name of the month. The number in dates cannot be placed after the name of the month. *May 17,* for example, must be written *den 17. mai* or *17. mai.*

The term *1300-talet* instead of *det 14. hundreåret* (14th century) is preferred today, since it will never cause misunderstanding: På slutten av 1800-talet kom elektrisiteten i bruk.

3. Fractions

In fractions both the numerator (*teljaren*) and the denominator (*nemnaren*) are cardinal numbers, but with the ending *-del,* pl. *delar,* in the denominator: *ein tredel* ($\frac{1}{3}$), *to femdelar* ($\frac{2}{5}$), *fire femtendelar* ($\frac{4}{15}$).

127

If the denominator is a number between 1 and 12, however, one is allowed to use ordinal numbers in the denominator: ein tredel = ein tredjedel (1/3); to femdelar = to femtedelar (2/5), ein tolvdel = ein tolvtedel (1/12); but: ein trettendel (1/13); fire femtendelar (4/15).

The fraction 1/1 is called ein heil, 1/2 ein halv, 1/4 ein kvart or ein firedel (fjerdedel). Ein halv is declined like an adjective: ein halv kopp, ei halv flaske, eit halvt glas, to halve flasker.

In mixed numbers where the numerator is 1, the following noun is in the singular: to og ein halv kopp, to og ei halv flaske, to og eit halvt glas.

4. The Indefinite Pronouns and Adjectives

The indefinite pronouns and adjectives are inflected in gender and number. The most common of them are listed in the chart.

The indefinite pronoun ein cannot be used as an adjective. It is the equivalent of en or man in the other Scandinavian languages: Ein trur. 'It is believed.'

The indefinite pronoun det is used to form impersonal constructions, which is so characteristic of all the Scandinavian languages: Det kjem post. 'Mail is arriving.' Det kom to gutar. 'Two boys came along.'

Masculine	Feminine	Neuter	Plural, all genders
all 'all'	all	alt	alle 'every(one)'
annan 'other'	anna	anna	andre
(no form)	(no form)	det 'it, there'	dei 'they'
ein 'one, you, they'	(no form)	(no form)	(no form)
einkvan 'some, somebody'	eikor	eitkvart	(no form)
ingen 'no, nobody'	inga	inkje	ingen
kvar 'every, everybody, each'	kvar	kvart	(no form)
mang ein 'many a'	mang ei	mangt eit	mange
nokon 'some, somebody, any, anybody'	noka	noko	nokre, nokon
(no form)	(no form)	somt 'something'	somme 'some'

Except for *ein* and *det*, all the indefinite forms listed in the chart above, can be used both as pronouns and adjectives. The pronoun *einkvan*, for example, stands for *some, somebody, someone,* and *someone or other.* Examples: Einkvan hadde vore der. Han venta på einkvan. Han bur einkvan stad her. Eikor jente sa det.

The pronoun *nokon* not only covers *some* and *somebody,* but also *any* and *anybody.* Notice that *noko* can be used before words of all three genders in the singular and in the plural: Han kjøpte noko smør 'some butter'. Han kjøpte noko bær 'some berries'. The plural form *nokon* is mostly used in questions and negations: Ser du nokon bilar på vegen? Det var ikkje nokon studentar der. But: Nokre studentar stod utanfor døra.

Instead of the pronoun *ingen, ikkje nokon,* and instead of the neuter form *inkje, ingenting* or *ikkje noko* are usual.

Oppgåver

1. Identify the indefinite pronoun *det* in the dialogue as opposed to the personal pronoun *det.*
2. Make up 5 sentences with the indefinite pronoun *det.*
3. Translate into *nynorsk:*
   a) I have only two days left in this country.
   b) Then I have to go back to America.
   c) Did you meet her again?
   d) Yes, I met her only once more.
   e) Here is my new car.
   f) I got it back yesterday.

13C Pronunciation/Spelling

Vowel Quantity (Length)

We have mentioned earlier (Sounds and Letters) that difference in vowel quantity (length) may distinguish between words in *nynorsk,* cf. the minimal pair *gul* /gu:l/ adj. and *gull* /gull/ n.

Uttaleøving

Drill on long and short vowels by saying these pairs aloud several times: vis 'wise', viss 'certain'; pen 'pretty', penn 'pen'; været 'the fishing station', verre 'worse'; hat 'hatred', hatt 'hat'; våt 'wet', vått 'wet' (neuter form); rot 'root', rott 'rowed'; brun 'brown', brunn 'well'; syn 'view; sight', synd 'sin'; søt 'sweet', søtt 'sweet' (neuter form).

129

As can be seen from the pairs mentioned above, vowel length is indirectly shown in writing: A long vowel is followed by one consonant, whereas a short vowel is followed by two consonants. American students tend to pronounce a long vowel too short.

13D Noregs Ungdomslag

Noregs Ungdomslag er ein landssamskipnad for dei frilyndte ungdomslaga i Noreg. Han vart skipa i Trondheim i 1896, men har hovudkontoret i Oslo. I åra 1913–56 hadde Noregs Ungdomslag og Noregs Mållag sams sekretariat, som vart kalla Skrivarstova.

Noregs Ungdomslag har eit vidt arbeidsområde. Alt som kan tena til å gjera ungdomslivet lettare og lysare, vert rekna som godt arbeid. Lagsarbeidet som har vore drive, har vore ein viktig samlings- og kulturfaktor både i bygdene og mellom bygdeungdomen i byane. Norsk bygdekultur har nemleg alltid vore i framgrunnen i lagsarbeidet.

I ei særstode står *folkedansen*, som har vorte vekt til nytt liv i ungdomslaga rundt om i landet. Noregs Ungdomslag vert rekna som den einaste folkedansorganisasjonen i Noreg, og kvart år vert det halde ei mengd folkedanskurs. Saman med arbeidet for folkedansen har ein også arbeidd med å få i bruk att *bygdebunadene*, som i dag har vunne seg ein trygg plass. Lokale spelemannslag syter for musikk til folkedansen, og norsk *folkemusikk* har ein sentral plass i lagsarbeidet.

Somme ungdomslag har synt ei særleg stor interesse for *amatørteater*, og mange spelstykke vert innøvde med jamne mellomrom. *Studiearbeidet* har også vore ei viktig arbeidsgrein, og arbeidet for målsak, skogsak, helse og edruskap har hatt stort rom i programmet.

Noregs Ungdomslag har frå første stund vore aktivt med i alt norsk reisingsarbeid. I all verksemd vert nytta nynorsk, og både einskildlag, fylkeslag og landslaget har vore i fremste rekkja med å gje nynorsken ein rettkomen plass i samfunnsliv og kulturliv. Ei viktig arbeidsoppgåve har derfor vore spreiing av nynorsk litteratur.

Mange møtehus, kaffistover og bondeheimar har vorte reiste, og rørsla har samarbeidt med andre ungdomsorganisasjoner og med folkehøgskulane.

frilyndt /"fri:lynt/ – liberal, broad-minded
eit frilyndt ungdomslag – a liberal association of youth (without religious or political affiliation)

eit kontor /kon'to:r/ – office
sams – common
eit sekretariat /sekreta:ri'a:t/ – sekretariat
vid /vi:/ – broad
eit arbeidsområde – field of activity
å tena til (tener, tente, tent) – to serve to, to help to
eit ungdomsliv – life of a youth
lys – light, bright
vert rekna som – is considered
eit lagsarbeid – work carried out by (ungdoms)laget
ein samlingsfaktor – uniting factor
ein kulturfaktor – cultural factor
ein bygdeungdom – young person from a rural district
ein bygdekultur – rural (peasant) culture
nemleg – namely; the fact is
ein framgrunn – foreground
ei særstode /"sæ:rstå:e/ – exceptional position
å vekkja til nytt liv (vekkjer, vekte, vekt) – to revive, to start again
rundt om i landet – throughout the country
den einaste – the only (one)
å halda eit kurs – to give (arrange) a course
ei mengd – a lot of
å vinna (vinn, vann, vunne) – to win
å vinna seg ein trygg plass – to acquire a solid position
å syta for (syter, sytte, sytt) – to provide

folkemusikk m. – folk music
amatørteater /ama'tø:rtea:ter/ n. – amateur theater
å øva inn (øver, øvde, øvt) – to rehearse
med jamne mellomrom – at regular intervals
eit studium – study
eit studiearbeid – studying activity, studies
ei arbeidsgrein – branch of work
målsak f. – language movement
skogsak f. – protection and preservation of forest
edruskap m. – promotion of temperance
reisingsarbeid n. – restoration of the essentially Norwegian in language and culture
ei stund – while, time, moment
frå første stund – right from the start
ei verksemd – activity
å nytta (nyttar, nytta, nytta) – to use
i fremste rekkja – at the front of the line
rettkomen – just, legitimate
ei arbeidsoppgåve – task
ei spreiing – spread, diffusion
eit møtehus – assembly hall
ei kaffistove – coffee house, cafeteria
ein bondeheim – farmers' inn, hotel
å reisa – to build, to erect
ei rørsle – movement
å samarbeida med – to cooperate with, to collaborate with

131

14A Nynorsk dikting

Liv og Roy har vore på ei førelesning om skodespelet *Tusen fjordar, tusen fjell* av Edvard Hoem (f. 1950).

LIV   Har du lese noko nynorsk litteratur før du kom hit?

ROY   Ja, eg har lese nokre bøker av dei nynorske klassikarane, og så hadde vi eit kurs om nynorske diktarar på folkehøgskulen på Voss.

LIV   Kva for bøker har du lese då?

ROY   Eg har lese heile *Symra* av Ivar Aasen, så har eg lese utdrag frå *Ferdaminne* av A. O. Vinje, og *Fred* og nokre dikt frå *Haugtussa* av Arne Garborg. I fjor las eg fleire dikt av Tor Jonsson og Olav Aukrust, og i år held eg på med *Fuglane* av Tarjei Vesaas og *I eventyre* av Olav Duun. Duun er litt vanskeleg for meg, for han bruker så mange ord og former frå dialekten i Namdalen.

LIV   Kva forfattar liker du best?

ROY   Det er ikkje lett å svara på, men eg trur det må vera Garborg.

LIV   Har du oppdaga noko felles drag hjå desse diktarane?

ROY   Ja, eg trur det. – Dersom du ser på dei under eitt, ser det ut til at kvar landsdel har sin eigen diktar, og at det er *bygda* som utgjer miljøet i bøkene.

LIV   Meiner du at bøkene er altfor lokale?

ROY   Nei, på ingen måte. Jamvel om dei bruker mange ord og former frå dialektane og handlinga går føre seg i ei lita bygd, er problema dei skildrar universelle.

LIV   Kjenner du andre enn Edvard Hoem som skriv på nynorsk i dag?

ROY   Eg veit iallfall om ein – Kjartan Fløgstad, for han har eg lese om i *Ny Verd*, som er eit målblad som kjem ut i USA. I 1978 fekk han Nordisk Råds litteraturpris for romanen *Dalen Portland*. Prisen var på 75 000 kroner, men han gav heile

	prisen til Noregs Mållag. Det var same prisen Vesaas fekk i 1962 for romanen *Is-slottet*.
LIV	Ja, du veit meir enn eg. – Har de verkeleg mållag i USA?
ROY	Ja, det har vi. Det heiter *Vinlands Mållag* og gjev ut bladet *Ny Verd* tre eller fire gonger i året.
LIV	Kjenner du andre unge forfattarar som bruker nynorsk?
ROY	Nei, eg veit berre namnet på eit par stykke: Tor Obrestad, Einar Økland og Paal-Helge Haugen.

dikting f. – fiction, poetry
ei førelesning om – lecture about
eit skodespel av – play by
ein klassikar – classic
ein diktar – writer, poet, author
å lesa (les, las, lese) – to read
Symra – *Anemone*
eit utdrag – extract
Ferdaminne – *Travel Memoirs*
Fred – *Peace*
Haugtussa – collection of poems
i fjor – last year
å halda på med – to be doing something
eg held på med – I'm reading
I eventyre – *In Fairyland*
Namdalen – valley in North Trøndelag
ein forfattar – author
å svara på – to answer
å oppdaga (oppdagar, oppdaga, oppdaga) – to discover
eg trur *det* – I think *so*
under eitt – as a whole

altfor /'altfår/ – too
på ingen måte – not at all
ei handling – action
å gå føre seg – to take place
å skildra /'sjildra/ (skildrar, skildra, skildra) – to describe
universell /univær'sell/ – universal, general
iallfall – at any rate
å lesa om – to read about
eit målblad – *nynorsk* newspaper
kjem ut – is published
Nordisk Råd – the Nordic Council
ein pris – a prize
ein roman /ro'ma:n/ – novel
Is-slottet – *The Ice Palace*
å gje (gjev, gav, gjeve) – to give, to donate
verkeleg – really
eit mållag – *nynorsk* language society
å gje ut – to publish
eit blad – newspaper

NY VERD
(NEW WORLD)

35 cents

Vinlands Mållag
Nr. 2, 1978   Blad for norsk fedra-arv i Nord-Amerika / Norwegian heritage newspaper for North America   6. argang 6th year

Fig. 14.1 *Eit amerikansk målblad.*

133

Spørsmål

1. Kven har skrive skodespelet dei høyrer om? 2. Hadde Roy lese nynorsk litteratur før han kom til Volda? 3. Kva for bøker hadde han lese? 4. Kva forfattar liker han best? 5. Kva er det som gjer Duun så vanskeleg å forstå for han? 6. Kva for felles drag hadde han oppdaga hjå desse diktarane? 7. Tykkjer han bøkene deira er for lokale? 8. Kva er *Noregs Mållag*? 9. Kva er *Vinlands Mållag*? 10. Kva er *Ny Verd*?

14B Grammar

1. The Past Perfect Tense

The past perfect tense is formed, as in English, by using the past tense of the verb å ha, i.e., hadde, plus the past participle of the main verb: Dei hadde sett eit skodespel. Han hadde lese ei bok.

The past tense of the helping verb å vera, i.e., var, can be used instead of hadde when the main verb is å bli, å verta, or a verb denoting motion: Han hadde vorte bleik 'pale'. Han var vorten bleik. Han var blitt bleik. Ho hadde reist til Noreg. Ho var reist til Noreg.

2. The Interrogative Pronouns, Adjectives and Adverbs

In 1B4 we mentioned some of the most frequent interrogatives. Below we will discuss both the interrogative pronouns and the interrogative adverbs in some detail.

The *interrogative pronouns* are kven, kva, and kva for ein (ei, eit).

Examples:

Kven tok bilen?	Who took the car?
Kven talar du om?	Who are you talking about?
Kven sin bil er dette?	Whose car is this?
Kven si bok er dette?	Whose book is this?
Kven sitt hus er dette?	Whose house is this?
Kven sine bilar er dette?	Whose cars are these?
Kva sa du?	What did you say?
Kva bok las du?	What book did you read?
Kva mann var det?	What man was that?
Kva talar du om?	What are you talking about?
Kva tenkjer du på?	What are you thinking of?

Kva for ein var det?	'Which one was it?
Kva for (ein) mann var det?	Which man was that?
Kva for (ei) bok var det?	Which book was that?
Kva for (eit) hus bur han i?	Which house does he live in?
Kva for (nokre) bøker er dette?	Which books are these?

As can be seen from the examples above, only the interrogative pronoun *kva for ein (ei, eit)* is inflected in gender and number, whereas *kven* and *kva* have only one form. *Kven* is used both as a pronoun and an adjective (modifying a noun); it can refer both to persons and things. *Kva for ein (ei, eit)* usually modifies a noun, and in those cases *ein, ei, eit* may be left out, but it can also be used as a pronoun in some cases.

When an interrogative pronoun is governed by a preposition, the preposition is placed at the end of the clause: Kven talar du om? Eg spurde kven han hadde tala med.

Instead of expressing possession by means of *kven sin (si, sitt, sine)*, it is quite common to use a prepositional or verbal construction: Kven sin son er han? – Kven er han son til? 'Whose son is he?' Kven sitt hus er det? – Kven eig det huset? 'Who owns that house?'

The English expression *which of* about persons is rendered by *kven av*: Kven av studentane har du skrive til? 'Which of the students have you written to?'

The interrogative pronouns and adjectives:

kven	who
kven . . . . om, på, etc.	about whom
kven sin (si, sitt, sine)	whose
kva	what
kva + noun	what
kva . . . . om, på, etc.	about what
kva for ein (masculine)	which one
kva for ei (feminine)	which one
kva for eit (neuter)	which one
kva for nokre (plural, all genders)	which ones

The most frequent *interrogative adverbs* are *kor* 'how', *korleis* 'how', *kvar* 'where', *kvar helst* 'where', *kvifor* 'why', and *når* 'when'.

Examples:

Kor mange var der?	How many were present?
Korleis veit du det?	How do you know that?
Kvar kom dei frå?	Where did they come from?
Kvar helst kom dei frå?	Where did they come from?
Kvifor kom dei?	Why did they come?
Når kom dei?	When did they come?

3. The Months of the Year

The names of the months are: januar /janu'aːr/, februar /feːbru'aːr/, mars, april /a'priːl/, mai /'maːi/, juni /'juːni/, juli /'juːli/, august /æu'gust/, september /sep'tember/, oktober /ok'toːber/, november /no'vember/, desember /de'sember/.
Notice that the names of the months are not capitalized.

Oppgåver

1. Make up 10 questions using both interrogative pronouns and interrogative adverbs.
2. Write a short letter to a friend.

14C Pronunciation/Spelling

Word Stress

Difference in word stress does not distinguish between words as it does in English, cf. the noun 'transport, which has the main stress on the first syllable, and the verb to trans'port, which has the main stress on the last syllable. In nynorsk the main stress is normally on the root syllable of the word, which in most cases is the first syllable: 'frimerke, "grønsaker, "menneske, 'vinter. This stress pattern is typical of the Germanic languages. Loanwords from non-Germanic languages usually keep the stress pattern of the language they are borrowed from, e.g., tek'nikk, ek'samen, an'nonse 'advertisement', medi'sin, favor'itt, kata'log, sensa'sjon, interes-'sant.
The word stress can be realized as sentence stress. The words which are felt to be the most important ones in the sentence are said with stronger stress than others: Eg "kjenner "ikkje 'mannen.
By putting extra strong stress on one particular word in a

136

sentence, we can express different shades of meaning (contrastive stress): Eg kjenner ikkje *'mannen* (men eg kjenner "kona). 'Eg kjenner ikkje mannen (kanskje *'du* kjenner han?).

Oppgåve

Identify all words of more than one syllable in the dialogue which have the stress on a syllable other than the first one.

14D Duskeluva

Immatrikuleringsdagen kom.

Daniel Braut drog på seg sine svarte klede og sette høgtidsamt duskeluva på hovudet sitt. No var han student. Med bankande hjarta gjekk han framfor spegelen. No hadde han nått sitt store mål; no ville han sjå seg sjølv. Han venta å få sjå eit hamskifte.

Duskeluva sat ikkje rett; han drog ho meir ned mot det eine øyra. Men endå sat ho ikkje rett. Han drog ho ned mot det andre øyra.

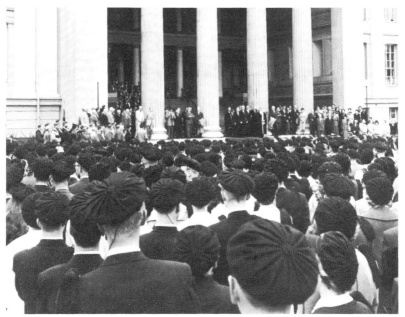

Fig. 14.2 *Immatrikulering ved Universitetet i Oslo.*

137

Men det hjelpte ikkje heller. Så sette han ho midt på skolten; – like nære. Han freista på alle vis, sette ho lenger bak, eller lenger fram, litt meir på skakke, litt mindre på skakke; det nytta ikkje. Det var som duskeluva ikkje ville høva åt hans hovud.

Daniel kolna der han stod. Han freista på nytt; lagde dusken bak; lagde dusken fram; lagde dusken midt på aksla; nei. Det vart ikkje den rette svingen. Og frakken, – frakken sat, som alle frakkar hadde sete. Han såg ikkje ut som student. Han var ikkje student. Han var ein forkledd bonde.

Bleik og modfallen stod han og glodde på seg sjølv i spegelen. Han tykte han vart seg sjølv så framand. Det breie godslege andletet hadde vorte så langt og magert. Munnen såg styven ut; og augo, som ein gong hadde vore så blanke, hadde krympa i hop og vorte sundsprengde og dauvvorne. Men akslene var gruve; han såg liksom nedtyngd ut; laut retta seg opp når han ville nå si høgd; annleis hadde han sett ut i sine studentdraumar. Nå; det laga seg vel. Men kald om hjarta rusla han til universitetet etter det akademiske borgarbrevet, som han no skjøna ikkje heller kunne gjera underverk.

Og då han kom der opp, og såg på alle dei unge bystudentane, som kom strykande fine og lette som fuglar i sol og bar duskeluva så flott og fjongt som ho skulle vera støypt til dei, då kjende han seg framand i dette laget. Han hadde berre ei trøyst, og den var skral: dei andre bondestudentane tok seg for det meste ikkje stort betre ut enn han med duskeluva.

Frå *Bondestudentar* (1883)
Av *Arne Garborg*

Eit stykke sør for Stavanger ligg Jæren, som er eitt av dei mest produktive jordbruksområda i heile landet. Diktaren og språkpolitikaren *Arne Garborg* (1851–1924) var fødd her, og mange av bøkene hans er inspirerte av Jæren. Meir enn nokon annan var han med på å utvikla det nynorske skriftmålet. Han skreiv politiske artiklar, romanar, dikt og skodespel. På mange måtar er han ein av dei mest særprega personane innanfor norsk litteratur. Han er klartenkt, kjenslevar og grublande, og alltid på leiting etter sanninga.

ei duskeluve – tasseled cap, esp. a black cap worn by those who have passed the matriculation examination

ein immatrikuleringsdag – day of university matriculation
å dra(ga) på seg (dreg, drog, drege) – to put on

138

høgtidsamt – solemnly
å banka (bankar, banka, banka) – to beat, throb
framfor – in front of
ein spegel – mirror
eit mål – goal
å venta (ventar, venta, venta) – to expect
eit hamskifte – changing of the outer appearance; trans-figuration
å sitja rett – to sit straight or right; to fit well
endå – still
ein skolt – head
like nære – just the same
å freista (freistar, freista, freista) – to try
ei vis – way
på skakke – on one side
det nytta ikkje – it was useless
å høva (høver, høvde, høvt) – to fit
åt – to
å kolna (kolnar, kolna, kolna) – to run cold, to shudder
ein dusk – tassel
ei aksel (aksla, aksler, akslene) – shoulder
den rette svingen – the right style, elegance
ein frakk – overcoat
forkledd – disguised
bleik – pale
modfallen – discouraged, down-cast
å glo (glor, glodde, glott) (på) – to stare (at)
framand – strange
brei – broad
godsleg – friendly, pleasant
eit andlet – face

mager – thin
styven – stupid
blank – bright
å krympa i hop   to shrink
sundsprengd – put at a variance
dauvvoren – indifferent
gruv – bent forward, stooping
liksom – kind of, as
nedtyngd – weighed down
å retta seg opp – to straighten one's back
ei høgd – height
annleis – different
ein draum – dream
det lagar seg vel – things will be all right, I guess
å rusla (ruslar, rusla, rusla) – to walk slowly
eit akademisk borgarbrev – cer-tificate of matriculation
å skjøna (skjønar, skjøna, skjø-na) – to understand, to real-ize
eit underverk – miracle
ein bystudent – student from a city
dei kom strykande – they came walking elegantly
flott – elegantly, smartly
fjong /fjång/ adj. – elegant, smart
som – as if
å støypa (støyper, støypte, støypt) – to cast
eit lag – company
å kjenna seg framand – to feel a stranger
ei trøyst – comfort
skral – poor
ein bondestudent – student from the country

å ta(ka) seg ut – to look, to appear
for det meste – for the most part
eit stykke sør for – a little ways south of
å liggja (ligg, låg, lege) – to lie, to be situated
produktiv /'proddukti:v/ – productive
eit jordbruksområde – farming district
ein språkpolitikar – politician involved in the language conflict

er inspirerte av – are inspired by
meir enn nokon annan – more than anybody else
ein artikkel – article
på mange måtar – in many ways
særprega – distinctive
innanfor – within
klartenkt – clear thinking
kjenslevar – sensitive
grublande – brooding
på leiting etter – in search of
ei sanning – truth

15A Påske på fjellet

Foreldra til Liv har gard i Gudbrandsdalen og seter på fjellet. Liv har invitert Roy og to andre studentar med seg på setra i påskehelga.

ROY Eg hadde aldri trutt det kunne vera så fagert nokon stad. – Djup snø og fin sol. – Det er godt forståeleg at nordmenn liker å feira påske på fjellet.

LIV Ja, har du først vore her ein gong, lengtar du attende til stilla og freden. Dette gamle selet set oss også i ei romantisk stemning.

ROY Har de buskapen på setra om sommaren framleis?

LIV Nei, no bruker vi setra berre til feriestad. Vi har lagt om jordbruket til korndyrking.

LEIF Skal eg kløyva litt småved så vi kan få fyr i omnen?

LIV Ja, takk, det er mykje ved i fjøset, og han er tørr og fin.

AUD Ver så god! No er det mat å få! Eg har laga til litt god norsk mat.

– – –   (Litt seinare)

LEIF Vi må gå tidleg til sengs i kveld, for i morgon skal vi ta oss ein lang skitur innover vidda.

LIV Har du gått på ski før, Roy?

ROY Eg har prøvt så vidt å køyra slalåm, men det gjekk ikkje så bra.

LIV Det er lettare med turski, og Leif er ein god læremeister. Han veit alt om både skitypar, skismurning og skiløyper. I fjor vann han til og med eit lokalt hopprenn.

LEIF Ja, men du vart nummer to i eit langrenn. – Forresten, kvar skal Roy og eg liggja?

LIV De får liggja i koven, og så får Aud og eg liggja her.

ROY God natt, og takk for i dag.

LIV God natt, og sov godt.

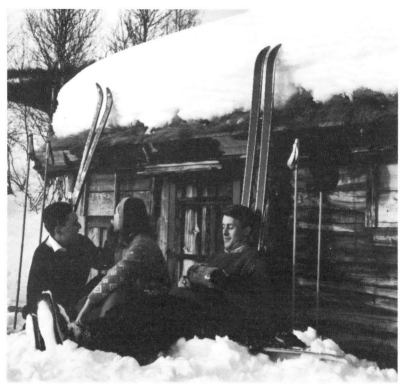

Fig. 15 *Påske på fjellet.*

Fjellreglane

1. Dra ikkje ut på langtur utan trening.
2. Meld frå om kvar du går.
3. Vis respekt for fjellet og vêrmeldingane.
4. Høyr på røynde fjellfolk.
5. Ver utrusta mot uvêr jamvel på korte turar.
6. Hugs kart og kompass.
7. Gå aldri åleine.
8. Snu i tide, det er inga skam å snu.
9. Spar på kreftene og grav deg ned i snøen om det er naudsynt.

ei påske – Easter
påske på fjellet – Easter holidays in the mountains

ei seter (setra, setrar, setrane)
  /'se:ter/ – summer dairy (usually in the mountains)

142

å invitera /invi'te:ra/ – to invite
ei påskehelg – Easter holidays
fager /'fa:ger/ – beautiful
djup /ju:p/ – deep
ein snø – snow
forståeleg /får'stå:eleg/ – understandable
å feira (feirar, feira, feira) – to celebrate
å lengta etter (lengtar, lengta, lengta) – to long for
ei stille – silence
ein fred – calmness, peace
eit sel – living-house of a seter
romantisk /ro'mantisk/ – romantic
ei stemning – mood
ein buskap – cattle, livestock on a farm
om sommaren – in the summer
framleis – still
ein feriestad /'fe:riesta:/ – vacation place
å leggja om – to change, to reorganize
jordbruk n. – farming
korndyrking f. – grain cultivation
å kløyva ved – to cut up firewood
småved m. – kindling
ein omn /åmn/ – stove; furnace
å få fyr i omnen – to light the fire
tørr – dry
å gå til sengs – to go to bed
i morgon – tomorrow
å ta(ka) seg ein lang skitur – to go on a long ski trip, to go out some distance skiing
innover vidda – across the plateau

å gå på ski – to go skiing
det gjekk ikkje så bra – it didn't turn out so well
å prøva (prøver, prøvde, prøvd) – to try
å køyra slalåm – to ski slalom, to go downhill skiing
slalåmski /'sla:låmsji:/ f. – slalom ski
turski /'tu:rsji:/ f. – cross-country ski
ein læremeister – teacher
ein skitype /'sji:ty:pe/ – type of ski
ein skismurning /'sji:smurning/ – ski wax
ei skiløype /'sji:løype/ – ski track, ski trail
til og med – even
lokal /lo'ka:l/ – local
eit hopprenn /'håpprenn/ – jumping competition
hoppski /'håppsji:/ f. – jumping ski
eit langrenn – cross-country race
eit nummer /'nommer/ – number
kvar skal eg liggja? – where am I supposed to sleep?
ein kove /''kå:ve/ – alcove, small room
å sova (søv, sov, sove) – to sleep
ein fjellregel – guideline for hiking (or skiing) in the mountains
ein langtur – long trip
å dra ut på – to go on
ei trening – training
å melda frå om – to report, to tell

143

å visa respekt for – to show respect for
ei vêrmelding – weather forecast
å høyra på – to listen to
røynde fjellfolk – experienced mountain people
å vera utrusta – to be equipped, fitted out
eit uvêr – storm
eit kart – map

ein kompass /kom'pass/ – compass
åleine /å"læine/ – alone
å snu i tide – to turn in time
ei skam /skamm/ – shame
å spara på kreftene – save one's energy
å grava seg ned – to dig oneself a hole in the snow to stay in
om naudsynt – if necessary

Oppgåve

1. Memorize *Fjellreglane*.
2. In *Fjellreglane* a number of verbs are used in the imperative. List the infinitives of the verbs and the imperative forms.

15B Grammar

1. The Demonstrative Pronouns and Adjectives

The most important demonstrative pronouns and adjectives are *den* (that, that one), *denne* (this, this one), and *hin* (the other, the second of two). Others are: *slik* (such, of that kind), *sjølv* (self, -self, -selves), *same* (the same), and *begge* or *båe* (both).

Same, *begge*, and *båe* are indeclinable, whereas *den*, *denne*, *hin*, and *slik* are inflected in gender and number; *sjølv* has only one form in the singular and one form in the plural.

The demonstrative pronouns and adjectives:

	Singular		Plural
Masculine	Feminine	Neuter	All genders
den 'that'	den 'that'	det 'that'	dei 'those'
denne 'this'	denne 'this'	dette 'this'	desse 'these'
hin 'the other'	hi 'the other'	hitt 'the other'	hine 'the others'
slik 'such'	slik 'such'	slikt 'such'	slike 'such'
sjølv 'self'	sjølv 'self'	sjølv 'self'	sjølve 'selves'

The demonstrative pronouns and adjectives are stressed in connected speech since they have the function of pointing out particular objects or persons: *Den* bilen var god. *Den* boka var

144

interessant. *Det* huset er fint. *Dei* epla er sure. 'Those apples are sour.'

Notice that the demonstrative pronoun/adjective *den* (*det, dei*) is identical in form with the definite article of the adjective (see 6B1), and that the forms *det* and *dei* are identical with the personal pronouns *det* and *dei* (see 6B3). They differ, however, in stress and function.

The demonstrative pronoun/adjective *den* (*det, dei*), which is always stressed, is used to refer to somebody or something remote from the person speaking. To emphasize this function, the adverb *der* 'there' is often placed after the noun or after the form of *den*: Den guten *der* er sterk. Det huset *der* er fint. Den *der* guten er sterk. Det *der* huset er fint.

The demonstrative pronoun/adjective *denne* (*dette, desse*) is used to refer to persons or objects which are close to the speaker. This function is often emphasized by placing the adverb *her* 'here' after the noun or the form of *denne*: Denne guten *her* er sterk. Denne bilen *her* var god. Dette huset *her* er fint.

her 'here' this	der 'there' that
Denne guten (her) er sterk.	Den guten (der) er sterk.
Denne boka (her) er god.	Den boka (der) er god.
Dette huset (her) er fint.	Det huset (der) er fint.
Desse husa (her) er fine.	Dei husa (der) er fine.

A noun which is modified by a demonstrative adjective always takes the definite form. A demonstrative pronoun can be used alone as a pronoun, i.e., without adding *one*: Vil du selja 'sell' bilen din? Nei, *den* vil eg ha så lenge eg kan.

Even though both *det* and *dette* are neuter singular forms, they are used to refer to persons and objects both in the masculine, the feminine, the neuter, singular and plural, in connection with the verb *å vera*:

Dette er bilen min.   This is my car.
Det er ei dårleg bok.   That is a poor book.
Dette er bøkene mine.   These are my books.
Det der er gode bøker.   Those are good books.

Oppgåver
1. Make up 10 sentences which use the demonstratives listed in the chart above.

145

2. Discuss the use of *den* *(det, dei)* in the following sentences: Den gamle bilen var dårleg. Den som eg no har, er god. Den kjøpte eg i fjor. Det nye huset der borte er vakkert. Det har eg ikkje sett før.
3. Fill in the correct form of the demonstrative pronoun:
   a) . . . . . . guten der kastar stein på bilen.
   b) . . . . . . guten her er flink 'clever'.
   c) Ser du . . . . . . huset der?
   d) Kven bur i . . . . . . huset der?
   e) Kva gjer . . . . . . gutane her?
   f) . . . . . . bilane her er amerikanske.
4. Translate into *nynorsk*:
   a) How long are you going to stay in that community?
   b) How long have you been in this city?
   c) Sit on that table!
   d) I bought these skis two years ago.
   e) This house is very large.
   f) Those mountains are very large.
   g) That mountain is larger than this mountain.
   h) Take this chair!
   i) Take this book!

15C Pronunciation/Spelling

Tonemes (Word Tone)

Unlike English and other Germanic languages except Swedish, difference in word tone may distinguish meanings in Norwegian in words of two or more syllables. There are only two contrastive tone patterns, referred to as *Toneme 1* and *Toneme 2*. If the sequence /so:la/, for example, is pronounced with Toneme 1, it means 'the sun', whereas it means the place name *Sola* near Stavanger if it is said with Toneme 2.

Toneme 1 is shown by placing *the sign* ' before the stressed syllable, and Toneme 2 by placing *the sign* " before the stressed syllable.
Examples:

Toneme 1	Toneme 2
(eit) 'brukar 'bridge pile or pier'	(ein) "brukar 'user'
(den) 'gjelda 'the debt'	(å) "gjelda 'to concern'
(to) 'hender 'two hands'	(det) "hender 'it happens'
(den) 'tanken 'the tank'	(den) "tanken 'the thought'
(to) 'tenner 'two teeth'	(han) "tenner 'he lights'

146

Even though there is no tonemic contrast between monosyllabic words, it is usual to say that they are pronounced with Toneme 1.

Some Norwegian dialects do not have any tonemic contrast at all, particularly in Northern Norway – the main part of Finnmark, large parts of Troms, and some parts of Nordland. There is also a region north of Bergen that does not have this contrast, whereas the city of Bergen itself has it. In very few cases, however, will this lack of tonemic contrast cause any trouble for the dialect speakers from these regions, since the context will indicate the meaning of the word.

A very interesting thing to notice is the fact that in Eastern Norway, in the midland regions, and in the county of Trøndelag, the stressed syllable is said on a low note and the unstressed syllable on a higher note, whereas northern and western dialects have a high note on the stressed syllable and a falling tone on the unstressed one.

The tonemes are not shown in writing.

Oppgåve
Drill on Toneme 1 and Toneme 2 by reading aloud the examples mentioned above.

15D Dei tre bukkane Bruse

Det var ein gong tre bukkar som skulle gå til setra og gjera seg feite. På vegen var det ei bru over ein foss, som dei skulle over, og under den brua budde det eit stort fælt troll med augo som tinntallerkar og nase så lang som eit riveskaft. Først kom den yngste bukken Bruse og skulle over brua. Tripp, trapp, tripp, trapp, sa det i brua. – «Kven er det som trippar på mi bru?» skreik trollet. – «Å, det er den minste bukken Bruse; eg skal på setra og gjera meg feit,» sa bukken; han var så fin i målet. – «No kjem eg og tek deg!» sa trollet. – «Å nei, ta ikkje meg, for eg er så liten; bi berre litt, så kjem den mellomste bukken Bruse; han er mykje større.» – «Eg får vel det,» sa trollet.

Om ei lita stund kom den mellomste bukken Bruse og skulle over brua. Tripp, trapp, tripp, trapp, tripp, trapp, sa det i brua. – «Kven er det som trippar på mi bru?» skreik trollet. – «Å, det er den mellomste bukken Bruse, som skal på setra og gjera seg feit,» sa bukken; han var ikkje så fin i målet, han. – «No kjem eg og tek deg!» sa trollet. – «Å nei, ta ikkje meg, men bi litt, så kjem den store bukken Bruse; han er mykje, mykje større.» – «Eg får vel det då!» sa trollet.

Rett som det var, så kom den store bukken Bruse: tripp, trapp, tripp, trapp, tripp, trapp, sa det i brua; han var så tung at brua både knaka og braka under han. – «Kven er det som trampar på mi bru?» skreik trollet. – «Det er den store bukken Bruse!» sa bukken; han var fælt grov i målet. – «No kjem eg og tek deg!» skreik trollet. – «Ja, kom du!» sa bukken, og dermed rauk han på trollet og stakk augo ut på det, knasa både merg og bein og stanga det ut i fossen, og så gjekk han til setra. Der vart bukkane så feite, så feite at dei mest ikkje orka å gå heim att; og er ikkje feittet gått av dei, så er dei der enno. Og snipp, snapp, snute, her er eventyret ute.

Norsk eventyr

feit – fat
å gjera seg feit – to get fat
ei bru – bridge
fæl – terrible
eit troll /tråll/ – monster
ein tinntallerk – pewter plate
så ... som – as ... as
eit riveskaft – rake handle
tripp, trapp – sound of short steps on bridge
å trippa (trippar, trippa, trippa) – to trip, to toddle
var fin i målet – had a nice voice
å bia (biar, bia, bia) – to wait
å skrika (skrik, skreik, skrike) – to shout
den mellomste – the middle one
eg får vel det – I guess I may as well
rett som det var – in a little while, then all at once

tung – heavy
å knaka (knakar, knaka, knaka) – to creak, to crack
å braka (brakar, braka, braka) – to bang, to crack
å trampa (trampar, trampa, trampa) – to tramp
var grov i målet – had a coarse voice
å ryka på (ryk, rauk, roke) – to attack
å stikka ut (stikk, stakk, stukke) – to poke out
å knasa (knasar, knasa, knasa) – to smash
ein merg – marrow
eit bein – bone
å stanga (stangar, stanga, stanga) – to push (with horns), to butt
å orka /"årka/ (orkar, orka, orka) – to manage
eit feitt – fat

16A Husmann og bonde

Ein kveld det er styggevêr på setra, fortel Liv om den gamle
husmannsskipnaden i Noreg.

ROY Var det dei fattige bøndene på små og dårlege gardar som
     hadde det verst før i tida?
LIV Nei, det var det ikkje. Dei brukte ofte det gamle ordtaket:
     «Det er alltid ei trøyst at einkvan har det verre». Og
     husmennene på storgardane hadde det iallfall verre enn dei.
ROY Ja, eg veit at mange husmannssøner drog over til USA utover
     på 1800-talet. – Var det ikkje plass til dei i Noreg?
LIV På 1700-talet auka folketalet mykje i landet, og det var jorda
     som måtte skaffa leveveg til dei fleste. Derfor vart det dyrka
     opp mykje jord i denne tida. Det byrja gjerne slik at ein mann
     fekk lov til å dyrka opp ubrukt jord hjå ein bonde som hadde
     ein stor gard. Der fekk mannen byggja seg eit lite hus for seg
     og familien sin. Huset var gjerne endå mindre enn hjå dei
     fattigaste av dei sjølveigande bøndene. Den jorda husman-
     nen fekk lov til å dyrka, låg ofte i utkanten av garden, og
     jorda var ofte mager og skrinn. Som leige for plassen måtte
     husmannen arbeida hjå den bonden som åtte jorda. Dersom
     husmannen og huslyden hans ikkje gjorde det arbeidet som
     vart pålagt dei, måtte dei utan vederlag fara frå plassen.
ROY Korleis var tilhøvet mellom bonden og husmannen?
LIV Dei ættestolte odelsbøndene såg ned på husmannen og
     huslyden hans, og det vart snart gløymt at dei første
     husmennene var bondesøner som ikkje hadde nokon gard å
     overta. For mange barn sveid det hardt å verta kalla
     «husmannsunge». USA vart derfor draumen og vona for dei.
ROY Finst det husmenn og husmannsplassar i dag?

149

LIV   Nei, i dag utgjer ikkje husmenn noka eiga sosial gruppe. Industrialisering, omlegging av jordbruket, flytting innanfor landet og utvandring til USA førte til at husmannsskipnaden vart oppløyst. Mange husmannsplassar vart slegne saman med garden eller nedlagde. Andre vart kjøpte, og jordlova frå 1928 gav husmannen rett til å løysa inn plassen.

ROY   Kvifor er det så mange som vil kjøpa husmannsplassar i dag?

LIV   Dei vil ha dei til feriestad.

eit styggevêr – nasty weather
ein husmannsskipnad – system of tenant farmers
fattig – poor
før i tida – formerly, in the old days
å ha det vondt (verre, verst) – to be miserable, unhappy
utover /'u:tå:ver/ på 1800-talet – throughout the 19th century
på 1700-talet – in the 18th century
å auka (aukar, auka, auka) – to increase
eit folketal – population
ein leveveg – way to make a living, employment
til dei fleste – for the majority
å dyrka (dyrkar, dyrka, dyrka) – to cultivate
i denne tida – in this period
å få lov til – to be permitted to
ubrukt jord – land not in use
ein sjølveigande bonde – free-holding farmer
i utkanten av – on the outskirts of
mager jord – lean (or poor) soil
skrinn jord – barren (or poor) soil
ein (husmanns)plass – cottager's farm
å eiga (eig, åtte, ått) – to own

ein huslyd – family
å påleggja nokon – to impose on smb.
eit vederlag – compensation
å fara frå plassen – to leave the farm
eit tilhøve – relationship
ættestolt – proud of one's family
ein odelsbonde /'o:delsbonde/ – allodial owner
å sjå ned på – to look down on
å overta – to take over
å svida (svid, sveid, svide) – to hurt, to burn
ei von – hope
å finnast (finst, fanst, funnest) – to be, to exist
ei gruppe – group, class
ei industrialisering – industrialization
ei omlegging /'omlegging/ – change, rearrangement
ei flytting – moving, change of residence
ei utvandring /'u:tvandring/ – emigration
å løysa opp (løyser, løyste, løyst) – to dissolve
å slå saman (slår, slo, slege or slått) – to combine
vart slegne saman – were combined

å leggja ned (legg, la, lagt) – to desert

ein nedlagd gard – deserted farm

ei jordlov /ˈjoːrlɑːv/ – law relating to land problems

å løysa inn – to buy

Spørsmål

1. Kva er ein husmann? 2. Kva er ein odelsbonde? 3. Kva er ei seter? 4. Kvifor drog mange husmannssøner over til USA? 5. Kva var viktigaste levevegen i Noreg på 1700-talet? 6. Kva er viktigaste levevegen i Noreg i dag? 7. Kvar helst på garden låg oftast den jorda husmannen fekk lov å dyrka? 8. Var denne jorda god? 9. Korleis var tilhøvet mellom bonden og husmannen? 10. Kva rett fekk husmennene i 1928?

16B Grammar

1. The Different Functions of det 'it, there'

As was seen in 1B2 and 6B3, *det* is used to refer to a noun of the neuter gender, i.e., it is used as a personal pronoun: Barnet skrik. Det skrik. Biletet er fint. Det er fint. *Det* sometimes refers to a whole idea and is then translated into English as 'so': Eg trur det. Eg vonar det.

Another function, which is very common, is the use of *det* as an indefinite pronoun in impersonal expressions. This construction corresponds to English *it* used as a formal subject: Det regnar. 'It is raining.' Det snøar. 'It is snowing.' Det er langt å gå. 'It is a long way to walk.' Det er lett å kritisera andre. 'It is easy to criticize others.' Det vart fortalt at han var uærleg. 'It was told that he was dishonest.'

Det is also used in expressions corresponding to English *there is/are*: Langt inne i skogen låg det ei hytte. 'Far away in the middle of the woods, there was a cabin.' Det var ein gong ein konge som hadde ei dotter. 'Once upon a time there was a king who had a daughter.'

This construction is also found with verbs with the same meaning as *å vera*, e.g., *å finnast* and *å eksistera*: Det finst mange parkar i denne byen. 'There are many parks in this city.' Det eksisterer ingen med det namnet her. 'There is nobody by that name here.'

The neuter form singular of the definite article of the adjective and of the demonstrative pronoun or adjective *den* is also *det*: Det vakre landet; Det huset er fint. However, when used as a

151

demonstrative pronoun with the verb å vera, det refers to all genders: Det er ei dårleg bok. 'That is a poor book.' Det der er gode bøker. 'Those are good books' (see 15B1).

In many cases det has no equivalent in English. Det often begins a sentence in which the actual subject, which follows the verb, is a noun in the indefinite form with the indefinite article or modified by an indefinite adjective like nokon, mange, ingen: Det kom ein mann gåande nedover gata. 'A man came walking down the street.' Det har butt mange nordmenn i Madison. 'Many Norwegians have lived in Madison.' Det kjem ingen studentar i kveld. 'No students are coming tonight.'

Det can also be used in a construction which emphasizes a particular element in the sentence. Instead of: Eg gjorde det, one can emphasize the subject: Det var eg som gjorde det. 'I'm the one who did it', or the object: Det var det (som) eg gjorde. 'That is what I did.'

With the verb å vera, det is often used to refer to persons or things mentioned immediately before, whereas English uses he, she, or they in such cases: Kven er den guten der? Det er son min. 'Who is that boy? He is my son.' Her er to vakre jenter. Det er Brit og Kari. 'Here are two pretty girls. They are Brit and Kari.'

The use of det:

1. Biletet er fint. Det er fint. Eg trur det. The picture is nice. It is nice. I believe so.	Personal pronoun it (sometimes 'so')
2. Det regnar. Det er langt å gå. It is raining. It is a long way to walk.	Indefinite pronoun it
3. Det var ein gong ein konge som hadde ei dotter. Once upon a time there was a king who had a daughter.	Indefinite pronoun there
4. det vakre landet the pretty country	Definite article of the adjective the
5. Det er ei dårleg bok. That is a poor book.	Demonstrative pronoun that, those
6. Det kom ein mann gåande nedover gata. A man came walking down the street.	Indefinite pronoun No equivalent
7. Det var eg som gjorde det. I'm the one who did it.	Indefinite pronoun No equivalent
8. Kven er den guten? Det er son min. Who is that boy? He is my son.	Demonstrative pronoun he, she, they

152

2. The Passive Voice

When a sentence is changed from active to passive, the object of the verb in the active sentence becomes the grammatical subject of the new sentence. The person performing the action – the logical subject – may be mentioned in a prepositional phrase. Example:

The active voice:

Subject	Verb	Object
Vaktmeisteren The janitor	stengjer closes	porten the gate

The passive voice:

Grammatical subject	Verb	Logical subject
Porten The gate	vert stengd is closed	av vaktmeisteren by the janitor

In nynorsk the passive is usually formed by means of the helping verb å verta or å bli plus the past participle of the main verb (see 9B2). To each tense in the active voice, there is a corresponding tense in the passive voice. Only the helping verb changes to form different tenses: å verta, vert, vart, har vorte, hadde vorte, skal/vil verta, skulle/ville verta.

Examples:

The present: stengjer: Porten vert stengd.
           The gate is closed.

The past: stengde: Porten vart stengd.
           The gate was closed.

The present perfect: har stengt: Porten har vorte stengd.
           The gate has been closed.

The past perfect: hadde stengt: Porten hadde vorte stengd.
           The gate had been closed.

The future: skal/vil stengja: Porten vil verta stengd.
           The gate will be closed.

153

In the present perfect it is quite common to write *Porten er vorten stengd* or only *Porten er stengd*, and in past perfect *Porten var vorten stengd* or only *Porten var stengd*, i.e., the helping verb *å vera* can be used in these cases.

The corresponding tenses of the helping verb *å bli* are: blir, blei, har blitt, skal/vil bli, skulle/ville bli.

In addition to this way of forming the passive voice, some verbs have a particular passive form ending in *-st*, e.g., *å stengjast* 'to be closed', *å seljast* 'to be sold'. However, the passive in *-st* is normally used with modal auxiliaries only: Porten skal stengjast klokka 23. 'The gate is to be closed at 11 o'clock.' Klippfisken skulle seljast i Bergen. 'The dried cod was to be sold in Bergen.' Porten kan stengjast klokka 23. Klippfisken måtte seljast i Bergen.

Oppgåver

1. Put the following sentences into the passive voice:
   a) Han kastar steinen.
   b) Ho sende boka i går.
   c) Han sender brevet i dag.
   d) Ho kjøpte hytta på auksjon.
   e) Hunden beit mannen.
   f) Han har lese artikkelen to gonger.
2. Translate into *nynorsk*:
   a) Do you think you'll get the job? – Yes, I hope so.
   b) It was told in the city that he had sold his farm.
   c) Once upon a time there was a king who had three sons.
   d) In the middle of the farm there was a very big tree.
   e) There are many small lakes in this area.
   f) Many Americans have lived in Stavanger.
   g) Who is that girl? – She is my daughter.
   h) I'm the one who did it.

16C Pronunciation/Spelling

Intonation

By intonation we mean the inflection of voice in a sentence. There are recurrent tone patterns which occur and make a syntactical or emotional distinction, for example, between a declarative sentence and a question.

Intonation differs from tonemes in several ways:

1. It is connected to the whole utterance, not to the different syllables or words like the tonemes are.
2. Intonation does not only distinguish between words, like the tonemes do, but rather has a meaning by itself.
3. The meaning which is associated with intonation patterns is not a lexical or grammatical meaning as is the case with tonemes, but tells us something about the speaker's *attitude*, i.e., whether he is confident or doubtful, enthusiastic or sceptical, indifferent or surprised, servile or commanding, friendly or rough, etc.

Each language or dialect has its own characteristic intonation patterns, and these patterns are probably the most difficult aspect of any language for the foreigner to learn. In many languages, however, a rising intonation is associated with a question, whereas a falling intonation is associated with a complete statement.

In 17C and 18C we will briefly discuss falling and rising intonation in *nynorsk*.

16D Kvardagshelten

Verda treng heltar ho kan dyrka og beda til. Det må vera ei lysande bragd kring dei av dåd og djervskap. – Men vi har andre heltar òg. Desse som bøyer ryggen i hard trass mot gråstein og ulende og som vier livet sitt til seigt slit, for å leggja eit mål jord til fedrelandet. Mannen som vert krøkt i ryggen og grå i håra, lenge før han er gammal av alder. Eller kona som går og steller på garden, frå tidleg til seint, dag ut og dag inn, år etter år, utan å tenkja på noko som heiter ferie. Ho lever for arbeidet, og gjer si plikt i kjærleik.

Men det lyser ikkje nokon helteglorie over desse. Einaste bautaen som vert reist, er store steinrøysar ein kan sjå, som vitnar om ein beisk strid for tilværet og ein seig vilje til å leva.

Eller vi ser det bløma på barnekinn. Det vitnar om ei kjærleg morshand som gjer alt for sine. Det vert ikkje spørsmål om å sjå til med seg sjølv først. Her er alt for borna.

Slike kvardagsheltar finn vi rundt om.

Det er mange av dei.

Det er dei som byggjer landet!

Frå *Nesler. Ny samling* (1952)
Av *Tor Jonsson*

155

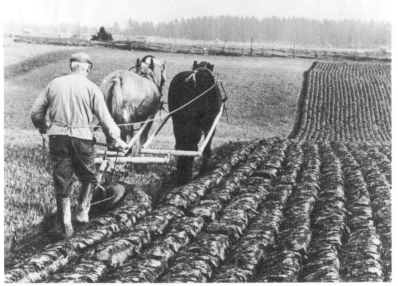

Fig. 16 *På storgarden måtte husmannen og familien hans arbeida hardt.*

Tor Jonsson (1916–51) vart født i Lom i Gudbrandsdalen. Han var son til ein husmann og opplevde på kroppen sosial utnytting og fattigdom. Mange av dikta og artiklane han skreiv, er fulle av sosialt opprør, men han har også skrive om andre emne, som t.d. i diktet *Norsk kjærleikssong.*

Norsk kjærleikssong

Eg er grana, mørk og stur.
Du er bjørka. Du er brur
under fager himmel.
Båe er vi norsk natur.

Eg er molda, djup og svart.
Du er såkorn, blankt og bjart.
Du ber alle voner.
Båe er vi det vi vart.

Eg er berg og naken li.
Du er tjørn med himmel i.
Båe er vi landet.
Evig, evig er du mi.

ein helt – hero
ein kvardagshelt – everyday
  hero

ei verd /væ:r/ – world
å trenga (treng, trong, trunge) –
  to need

156

å dyrka (dyrkar, dyrka, dyrka) –
to adore, to worship
å be(da) til (bed, bad, bede) – to
worship
ei bragd – deed, exploit
ei lysande bragd – a brilliant
exploit
ein dåd /då:d/ – deed; achievement
ein djervskap – daring, boldness
å bøya (bøyer, bøygde, bøygd) –
to bend
ein trass – defiance; obstinacy
ein gråstein – gray rock
eit ulende /"u:lende/ – rugged
ground
å via (vier, vigde, vigt) – to
dedicate
seig – heavy, hard
eit slit – hard work, toil
eit mål – 1 000 square meters
eit fedreland – fatherland, native
country
krøkt – bent, stooped
grå – gray
ein alder /'alder/ – age
å stella (steller, stelte, stelt) – to
work
frå tidleg til seint – early and
late
dag ut og dag inn – day after
day
å leva for (lever, levde, levt) – to
live for
ei plikt – duty
ein kjærleik – love
å lysa (lyser, lyste, lyst) – to
shine
ein helteglorie – heroic halo

ein bauta /'bæuta/ – monolith
ei steinrøys – heap of stones,
cairn
å vitna om (vitnar, vitna, vitna)
– to bear witness to
beisk – bitter
eit tilvære – life
ein vilje – will
å bløma (blømer, blømde,
blømt) – to flourish, to
blossom
eit barnekinn /"ba:rnekjinn/ –
child's cheek, face
kjærleg – loving
å sjå til med seg sjølv – to think
of oneself
eit barn, pl. barn or born – child
å oppleva – to experience
ei utnytting /'u:tnytting/ – exploitation
fattigdom m. – poverty
eit opprør – protest, rebellion
eit emne – subject
ein kjærleikssong – love song
ei gran – spruce
mørk – dark
stur – solemn
ei bjørk – birch tree
ei brur – bride
båe – both
ein natur /na'tu:r/ – nature
ci mold /måld/ – soil, earth
eit såkorn /"så:korn/ – seed
bjart – bright
å bera (ber, bar, bore) – to carry
eit berg – rock
naken – bare
ei tjørn /kjø:rn/ – pond, small
lake
evig – forever

17A Norsk næringsliv

Roy er interessert i norsk næringsliv, og Liv svarar på spørsmåla hans.

ROY   Når du talar om næringsvegane i Noreg, vil du då seia at Noreg er eit jordbruksland eller industriland?

LIV   Noreg er i dag eit moderne industriland, men grunnlaget for Noregs økonomi er jordbruk, skogbruk, fiske, skipsfart, vasskraft og dei norske oljefelta i Nordsjøen. Handelen med utlandet er sjølvsagt vesentleg.

ROY   Har talet på gardsbruk gått mykje ned i dei siste åra?

LIV   Ja, det skal vera visst. I året 1900 t.d. var 40 prosent av alle arbeidsplassane i landet i primærnæringane jordbruk, skogbruk og fiske, og i 1973 var talet kome ned i litt over 10 prosent. Samstundes har talet på personar som arbeider i industrien og i ulike tenesteyrke auka tilsvarande. I 1973 var heile 55 prosent sysselsette i tenesteyrke, undervisning og administrasjon.

ROY   Flyttar folk inn til byar og sentrale strok her som andre stader?

LIV   Ja, det ser ut til å vera uråd å stogga den tendensen. I 1930 t.d. budde litt over halvparten av folket i grisgrendte strok og resten i tettstader eller i byar. I 1970 var tala etter tur ein tredel og to tredelar.

ROY   Korleis ser du på oljeindustrien i denne samanhengen?

LIV   Eg ser det slik at oljeleitinga i Nordsjøen, og oljeindustrien i det heile, vil forsterka denne tendensen, særleg i visse område i landet. Men det er visst god forretning for landet. – All sentralisering inneber ein fare for nynorsken og målføra, og no får vi presset frå engelsk i tillegg, t.d. med lånord som 'blow-out', 'off-shore' osv.

eit næringsliv – economic life of a nation, esp. commercial and industrial life, trade, industry

ein næringsveg – (branch of) trade (or industry); livelihood

interessert i – interested in

eit industriland /indu'stri:land/ – industrial country

eit grunnlag – basis, foundation

ein økonomi /økono'mi:/ – economy

skogbruk /"sko:gbru:k/ n. – forestry, lumbering

fiske n. – fishing

skipsfart /'sjipsfa:rt/ m. – shipping industry

vasskraft f. – water power

eit oljefelt – oil field

handel /'handel/ m. – commerce, trade

utlandet /"u:tlande/ – the outside world, foreign countries

sjølvsagt – of course

vesentleg /'ve:sentleg/ – essential

eit gardsbruk /'ga:rsbru:k/ – farm

å gå ned – decrease

det skal vera visst – to be sure, decidedly so

ein arbeidsplass – job

ei primærnæring /pri'mæ:r-næ:ring/ – primary industry

ein industri /indu'stri:/ – industry

eit tenesteyrke – service industry

tilsvarande /'tillsva:rande/ – proportionally

å sysselsetja (set, sette, sett) – to employ

undervisning /under'vi:sning/ f. – education

administrasjon /administra-'sjo:n/ m. – administration

å flytta (flyttar, flytta, flytta) – to move

eit strok /strå:k/ – area

det ser ut til – it looks as if

det er uråd /"u:rå:/ – it is impossible

å stogga (stoggar, stogga, stogga) – to stop

ein tendens /ten'dens/ – tendency, trend

eit grisgrendt strok – sparsely populated area

etter tur – respectively

ein samanhang – connection

oljeleiting f. – oil exploration

Nordsjøen – the North Sea

i det heile – on the whole

å forsterka (forsterkar, forsterka, forsterka) /får'stærka/ – to strengthen

det er visst – I suppose it is

forretning /få'retning/ f. – business

ei sentralisering – /sentrali-'se:ring/ – centralization

å innebera /"innebe:ra/ – to imply

ein fare – danger

eit press – pressure

i tillegg – in addition

eit lånord – loanword

osv. = og så vidare – and so forth

Spørsmål

1. Er Noreg eit jordbruksland eller industriland? 2. Kva er grunnlaget for Noregs økonomi? 3. Har talet på gardsbruk auka dei siste åra? 4. Kvar finn ein dei fleste arbeidsplassane i dag? 5. Kva for strok flyttar folk til? 6. Kva kan oljeindustrien føra til? 7. Kvifor kan sentralisering vera ein fare for nynorsken og målføra i landet? 8. Kvifor er presset frå engelsk så sterkt i dag?

17B Grammar

1. The Inflection of the Past Participle

As can be seen from 9B1 and 12B2, the past participle may have different forms depending on the verb class to which it belongs: kasta 'thrown', kjøpt 'bought', trutt 'believed', talt 'counted', svike 'betrayed', lese 'read', etc. All the above mentioned participles are listed with their *neuter form*, which is always used with the helping verb å *ha* to form the present perfect and the past perfect: Han har kasta ballen. Ho hadde kjøpt bilen hans. Dei hadde talt epla. Han hadde svike kona si. Ho har lese boka om Ibsen.

However, when the past participle is used together with the various forms of the helping verbs å *vera*, å *verta*, and å *bli* to form the passive, and when it is used as an adjective to modify a noun, it has inflectional forms. Just like an adjective, it agrees in gender and number with the noun or pronoun it refers to or modifies.

The past participle of weak verbs. Basic pattern:

	Masculine	Feminine	Neuter	Plural, all genders
1	Steinen er kasta. ein kasta stein -a	Boka er kasta. ei kasta bok -a	Brevet er kasta. eit kasta brev -a	Dei er kasta. kasta steinar -a
2	Mannen vert dømd. ein dømd mann -d	Kona vert dømd. ei dømd kone -d	Barnet vert dømt. eit dømt barn -t	Dei vert dømde. dømde folk -de
3	Mannen vert trudd. ein trudd mann -dd	Kona vert trudd. ei trudd kone -dd	Barnet vert trutt. eit trutt barn -tt	Dei vert trudde. trudde folk -dde
4	Bilen vert kjøpt. ein kjøpt bil -t	Hytta vert kjøpt. ei kjøpt hytte -t	Huset vert kjøpt: eit kjøpt hus -t	Bilane, hyttene, husa vert kjøpte. kjøpte bilar, hytter, hus -te

In the two charts, these two different functions and the different endings of the past participle are shown. As you can see, only weak verbs of Class 1 have one form of the past participle (kasta), whereas all the other verb classes have two or three forms.

The past participle of strong verbs. Pattern:

Masculine	Feminine	Neuter	Plural, all genders
Mannen vart sviken. 'betrayed' ein sviken mann -en	Kona vart sviken. ei sviken kone -en	Barnet vart svike. eit svike barn -e	Dei vart svikne. svikne folk -ne
Artikkelen vart lesen. ein lesen artikkel -en	Boka vart lesen. ei lesen bok -en	Brevet vart lese. eit lese brev -e	Artiklane, bøkene, breva vart lesne. lesne artiklar, bøker, brev -ne

Notice that the inflection of the past participle of all strong verbs is the same (-en, -en, -e, -ne).

2. The Conditional

The conditional is formed with *skulle* or *ville* (should or would) in the same way as the future tense is formed with *skal* or *vil* (shall or will):

Eg skal (vil) koma.   I shall (will) come.
Eg skulle (ville) koma.   I should (would) come.

Notice that *skal, skulle* also renders English *am (are, is) to*: Hurtigruta skal gå innom Ålesund. 'The Coastal Express is to call at Ålesund', and *be about to*: Vi skal nettopp eta frukost. 'We are just about to have breakfast.'

The conditional:

The Past Future Tense	The Past Future Perfect Tense
Intention: Han skulle koma i dag. He was supposed to come today.	Han skulle ha kome i dag. He was supposed to have come today.
Volition: Han ville koma i dag. He wanted to come today.	Han ville ha kome i dag. He would have come today.

161

3. The Conjunction **dersom**

Dersom det vert fint vêr i morgon, vil vi reisa til Bergen. = Vert det fint vêr i morgon, vil vi reisa til Bergen. 'If the weather is fine tomorrow, we will go to Bergen.'

Dersom han skulle reisa til Bergen, ville han ta paraply med. = Skulle han reisa til Bergen, ville han ta paraply med. 'If he were to go to Bergen, he would take along an umbrella.'

Oppgåver

1. Fill in the correct form of the past participle:
   a) Læraren er .... (å dømma)
   b) Ein .... mann (å dømma)
   c) Mennene vart .... (å dømma)
   d) Båten vart .... (å kjøpa)
   e) Båtane vart .... (å kjøpa)
   f) .... bilar (å kjøpa)
   g) Boka er .... (å skriva)
   h) Eit .... brev (å skriva)
   i) Breva er .... (å skriva)

2. Translate the following sentences into nynorsk:
   a) Mother said she was going to town.
   b) She wanted to buy some milk.
   c) Where are you going?
   d) He said that he was coming.
   e) I wanted to be the teacher.
   f) What did you want?
   g) Did you have to go?
   h) He had to go home without food.

17C Pronunciation/Spelling

Falling Intonation

We know rather little about the intonation of nynorsk, partly because it is very complex, and partly because very few linguists have tried to analyze it. There is a complicated interplay of intonation and the tonemes. As words of one or more syllables are combined into sentences, Toneme 1 and Toneme 2 are extended to include entire utterances. They thus characterize the intonation patterns. In addition, certain rhythmic patterns are combined with the intonation patterns.

It is very difficult to give general rules for the intonation of nynorsk, but one basic rule can be given: *Statements are finished with a falling intonation.*
Examples:
Han heiter Per Nes.
Ho kjem i morgon.
Klokka er fem.
Noreg er eit land i Skandinavia.
Roy Eisel bur på Voss.

In writing, falling intonation is normally indicated by means of a period. In fact, the intonation alone can distinguish between a statement and a question in the following utterances: Han kjem i morgon. – Han kjem i morgon?

17D Oljeeventyret

Etter folketalet er Stavanger nummer fire i rekkja av norske byar etter Oslo, Bergen og Trondheim. Viktige byar er også Kristiansand, Haugesund, Ålesund, Molde, Narvik, Bodø og Tromsø.

Stavanger er eit aktivt senter for Rogaland fylke. Her ligg fylkesadministrasjonen, Rogaland distriktshøgskule og andre høgskular, og byen er eit gammalt bispesete med ei vakker domkyrkje frå mellomalderen.

Stavanger er ein travel handels- og industriby, og han er sentrum for oljeleitinga i Nordsjøen. Dette har ført med seg at talet på utlendingar, særleg ekspertar frå USA, har auka sterkt.

Oljeindustrien er ei ny næringsgrein i Noreg, men industrien er frå før hovudnæringsvegen i landet. Av ulike grunnar knyter det seg størst interesse til oljeindustrien i dag, kanskje først og fremst fordi ein trur at denne industrien vil få svært mykje å seia for norsk økonomi i framtida. Dessutan er det spanande å driva stort! For å gje eit inntrykk av storleiken kan vi nemna at kontraktprisen på *Statfjord B-plattforma* var på om lag 600 millionar kroner (1978). Den nye bustadplattforma til Phillips Petroleum Company, Noreg, har 212 sengeplassar fordelte på 106 tomanns-lugarar. Alle lugarane har dusj og toalett, slik at det nærmar seg hotellstandard. Byggjekostnaden var på om lag 2,8 mill. kr. for kvar sengeeining.

163

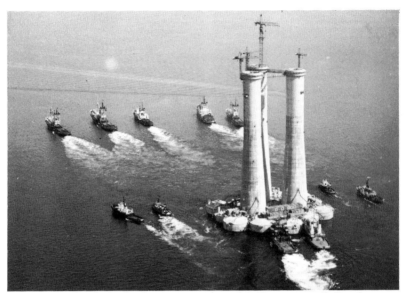

Fig. 17 *Statfjord A-plattforma vert slept frå Stavanger til Stord.*

I bustadblokka er det ein stor kinosal som tek 115 personar, scene, mosjonsrom, badstove, spelerom, musikk- og leserom, stor kantine, hyggeleg salong, konferanserom, sjukestove og kapell. Det er også lagt vinn på tryggingstiltak. Bustadblokka ligg godt unna produksjonseiningane, og ho er utstyrt med helikopterdekk, livbåtar og flåtar.

oljeeventyret – the oil adventure
etter folketalet – according to (or: with respect to) population
ei rekkje – row
eit bispesete – episcopal residence, cathedral city
ei domkyrkje /'dommkyrkje/ – cathedral
mellomalderen – the Middle Ages
travel – busy
å føra med seg – to lead to
ein ekspert /ek'spært/ – expert

ei næringsgrein – branch of industry
å knyta seg til (knyter, knytte, knytt) – to be attached to
først og fremst – above all, first and foremost, primarily
å få mykje å seia for – to become important for
ei framtid – future
spanande – exciting
å driva stort (driv, dreiv, drive) – to do big business
eit inntrykk /'inntrykk/ – impression
ein storleik – size

å nemna (nemner, nemnde, nemnt) – to mention
ein kontrakt /kon'trakt/ – contract
ein kontraktpris – contract price
ei plattform /'plattfårm/ – platform
bustadplattform /'bu:staplattfårm/ – platform containing living quarters, cabins
ein sengeplass – bed
ei seng – bed
å fordela (fordeler, fordelte, fordelt) /får'de:la/ – to distribute
ein tomanns-lugar – cabin for two, double room
ein dusj – shower
eit toalett /toa'lett/ – toilet
å nærma seg (nærmar, nærma, nærma) – to get close to, to approach
ein standard /'standar/ – standard, quality
ein byggjekostnad – construction cost
ei eining – unit
ei sengeeining – bed unit
ei bustadblokk = ei bustadplattform

ein kinosal /'kji:nosa:l/ – movie theater
eit mosjonsrom /mo'sjo:nsromm/ – room for physical exercise
ei badstove /'ba:dstå:ve/ – room for hot steam baths, sauna
eit spelerom – game room
eit musikkrom /mu'sikkromm/ – music room
ei kantine /kan''ti:ne/ – canteen, snack bar
ein salong /sa'lång/ – lounge
eit konferanserom /konfe'ranseromm/ – conference room
ei sjukestove – nurse's office, infirmary
eit kapell /ka'pell/ – chapel
å leggja vinn på – to stress
eit tryggingstiltak – security measure
godt unna – far away from
ein produksjon /produk'sjo:n/ – production
eit helikopterdekk – helicopter pad
ein livbåt – lifeboat
ein flåte – raft, float

18A Fiske og fiskarar

Liv og Roy samtalar om fisket langs Norskekysten.

ROY Korleis ser fiskarane i Noreg på oljeboringa i Nordsjøen?

LIV Eg trur at mange oppfattar oljeindustrien som eit trugsmål mot fiskerinæringa. Dei er redde for at dei gode fiskefelta skal verta øydelagde av oljesøl og oljeavfall.

ROY Eksporterer Noreg mykje sild og fisk?

LIV Ja, det gjer vi. Det var dei store sesongfiskeria som gav slike fiskemengder at fisket kunne løna seg som eigen næringsveg både for den einskilde fiskar, for oppkjøparar og fabrikkeigarar. Storparten av dei silde- og torskemengdene som vert oppfiska, vert eksportert til framande land, og sildemjøl er også ein god eksportartikkel.

ROY Er ikkje fiskarane redde for at all silda og fisken skal verta oppfiska?

LIV Jau, det er mykje snakk om den faren i dag. Det store omskiftet kom med nota. Med nota kunne ein stengja av små vikar og fjordarmar, og så var det berre å ausa silda opp or sjøen. Så lenge ein brukte garn som fiskereiskap, var det ingen fare. Det var mange som var imot notbruk, fordi dei meinte at all fisk kom til å verta utrydda, og stundom vart det forbode å bruka not. Same redsla har mange fiskarar i dag når det gjeld bruk av trål, som er ein endå meir effektiv fiskereiskap enn nota.

ROY Er dei norske fiskebåtane moderne og lettdrivne?

LIV Ja, utviklinga av nye båttypar og fiskereiskapar har gått så fort at det er heilt uråd å følgja med. Dei nye havgåande kraftblokkbåtane, som bruker snurpenot, og fabrikktrålarane, som bruker moderne trål, er så effektive at styremaktene har sett seg nøydde til å innføra restriksjonar, t.d. faste kvotar for sild og makrell, for å hindra at fiskeressursane i havet vert øydelagde.

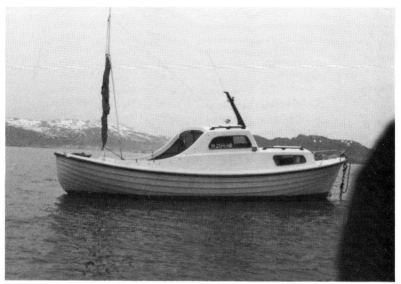

Fig. 18.1 *Ein moderne plastsjark.*

ein fiskar – fisherman
å sjå på – to think of
ei oljeboring – drilling for oil
å oppfatta (oppfattar, oppfatta,
   oppfatta) – regard, conceive
eit trugsmål /'trugsmå:l/ – threat
ei fiskerinæring – fishing industry
å vera redd for – to fear
eit fiskefelt – fishing ground(s)
å øydeleggja (øydelegg, øydela,
   øydelagt) – to ruin
eit oljesøl – oil slick
eit oljeavfall – oil residue
å eksportera /ekspor'te:ra/ (eksporterer, eksporterte, eksportert) – to export
ei sild – herring
ein fisk – fish
eit sesongfiskeri /se'sångfiskeri/
   – seasonal fishing
ei fiskemengd – quantity of fish

ein oppkjøpar – buyer
ein fabrikkeigar /fa'brikkæigar/
   – factory owner
storparten av – the greater part
   of, the majority of
ein torsk /tårsk/ – cod
å fiska opp (fiskar, fiska, fiska)
   – to catch
sildemjøl n. – herring meal
eit snakk – talk
eit omskifte /"omsjifte/ –
   change
ei not, pl. nøter – trawl net,
   seine
ei vik (vika, vikar, vikane) – bay
ein fjordarm – arm of a larger
   fjord
å ausa opp (auser, auste, aust) –
   to scoop
or – out of
ein fiskereiskap – fishing gear
   or tackle

167

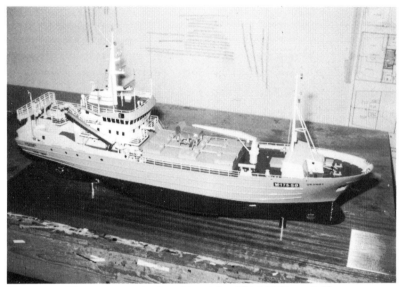

Fig. 18.2 «*Uksnøy*» *er ein kombinert kraftblokkbåt og trålar.*

eit notbruk – the use of trawl nets

å rydda ut (ryddar, rydda, rydda) – to kill off, to exterminate

ei redsle – fear

forbode – illegal, forbidden

når det gjeld – as for . . ., as far as . . . is concerned

ein trål – trawl net

ein fiskebåt – fishing boat

lettdriven – easily operated or run

å følgja med (følgjer, følgde, følgt) – to keep up with

havgåande – seafaring, seagoing

ein kraftblokkbåt /'kraftblåkkbå:t/ – fishing boat equipped with a purse net, seine

ei snurpenot – purse net, purse seine

ein fabrikktrålar /fa'brikktrå:lar/ – big trawler (factory trawler)

styremaktene f.pl. – the authorities

å sjå seg nøydd til – to feel forced to

å innføra /'innfø:ra/ – to introduce

ein restriksjon /restrik'sjo:n/ – restriction

ein kvote – quota

ein makrell /ma'krell/ – mackerel

å hindra (hindrar, hindra, hindra) – to prevent

ein fiskeressurs – fishing resource

Spørsmål

1. Kva slags fiskereiskapar vert brukte i dag? 2. Kva slags fisk fiskar dei i dag? 3. Kvifor var nota ein effektiv fiskereiskap? 4. Korleis kan oljeindustrien vera eit trugsmål mot fisket? 5. Kva gjer ein med all fisken ein får? 6. Kvifor var mange fiskarar lenge imot notbruk? 7. Kva vert gjort for å verna 'protect' om fiskeressursane i havet? 8. Kva trur du mange fiskarar seier om fabrikktrålarane?

18B Grammar

1. Frequent Words and Forms

Below is a list of 100 words and forms which have a very high frequency in nynorsk. They are listed in order of frequency and should be memorized by the student.

i	in	om	about
og	and	frå	from
det	it (the)	han	he
er	is (are, am)	men	but
som	who (whom, which, that)	var	was (were)
		vi	we
til	to	seg	himself (herself, etc.)
ein	one; a (an)	kan	can
av	of	vil	will
på	on	så	then
for	for	ved	by
å	to	vart	became
at	that	også	too
med	with	dette	this
dei	they, them (the)	skal	shall
den	that (the)	eg	I
har	has (have)	vera	be
ikkje	not	eller	or
eit	a (an)	år	year
alle	all, everybody	få	get
mot	against, toward	slik	thus
nokon	somebody	mykje	much
andre	others	desse	these
bli	become	sine	his, her, its, their
opp	up	dag	day

169

to	two	første	first
enn	than	ville	would
kunne	could	skulle	should
etter	after	kva	what
vore	been	heile	whole
ha	have	mellom	between
mange	many	oss	us
der	there	nye	new
inn	into	store	great, big
hans	his	før	before
sjølv	myself (himself, etc.)	sitt	his, her, its, their
meir	more	si	his, her, its, their
kvar	where (each)	tid	time
under	under	går	goes (go)
her	here	sidan	since
denne	this	får	gets (get)
blir	becomes (become)	no	now
sin	his, her, its, their	siste	last
då	then	kjem	comes (come)
må	must	seier	says (say)
over	over	alt	everything
hadde	had	kom	came
ut	out	ta	take
berre	only	blitt	become
når	when	vorte	become
noko	something		

2. Compound Verbs and Verbs + Adverb/Preposition

One way of making new verbs in nynorsk is to attach a stressed adverb or a stressed preposition to a verb. The most frequent adverbs and prepositions thus prefixed to verbs are: av, etter, fram, frå, inn, om, opp, over, på, til, ut, ved. Examples:

å avfolka 'to depopulate' – avfolkar – avfolka – har avfolka
å avtala 'to agree upon' – avtalar – avtala – har avtala
å etterlikna 'to imitate' – etterliknar – etterlikna – har etterlikna
å oppdaga 'to discover' – oppdagar – oppdaga – har oppdaga
å oppmoda 'to encourage' – oppmodar – oppmoda – har oppmoda
å tilby 'to offer' – tilbyd – tilbaud – har tilbode
å undervise 'to teach' – underviser – underviste – har undervist

170

In compound verbs of this category, the two parts of the verb (the particle and the verb) are inseparable in all tenses and forms, and are, therefore, easy to use correctly. However, a more common way of making new verbs in nynorsk is to combine an adverb or a preposition with a verb. Examples: å fiska opp 'to catch'; å gje ut 'to publish'; å kasta bort 'to throw away'; å koma ut 'to be published'.

When this type of verb is used together with the verb å ha to form compound tenses, the verb and the particle are always separated: Dei har gjeve ut boka. Ho hadde kasta bort brevet. But the particle is prefixed to the participle if one of the helping verbs å vera, å verta, or å bli is used to form the passive: Boka vart utgjeven. Brevet var bortkasta. Compare: Han gjev ut boka. Han gav ut boka. Han har gjeve ut boka. Han vil gje ut boka. – Boka vert utgjeven. Boka vart utgjeven. Boka vil verta utgjeven.

Today the distinction between the two categories of verbs mentioned above is not so clear as it used to be. In some cases, however, there is a difference of meaning between a compound verb and a verb + an adverb/preposition. Usually the compound verb has a more figurative meaning whereas the verb + adverb/preposition conveys a more literal meaning of the elements. Examples:

å innsjå	to understand	å sjå inn	to look in
å innvenda	to object	å venda inn	to turn inwards
å oppleva	to experience	å leva opp	to grow up
å oversjå	to overlook	å sjå over	to look over
å utføra	to do	å føra ut	to export

3. Derivational Verbs

A large number of verbs have been formed by means of derivation, i.e., a prefix or a suffix has been added to some other word. In contrast to adverbs and prepositions, prefixes and suffixes cannot be used by themselves, even though they may have a more or less definite meaning. Examples: å betala 'to pay', å forstå 'to understand', å ekspedera 'to send, to wait on', å låsa 'to lock' (from eit lås 'lock').

Oppgåver

1. Analyze the formation of the verbs used in 18A.
2. Translate into nynorsk:
   a) Some parts of the country have been depopulated.
   b) She was good at imitating her teacher.

171

c) Who discovered America?
d) They said that they wanted to publish his book.
e) He had experienced many things.

18C Pronunciation/Spelling

Rising Intonation
Unlike English, both questions starting with an interrogative word
and yes/no questions are said with rising intonation in *nynorsk*.

Examples:
Kva heiter han?
Kven bur på Voss?
Kvar skal Brit reisa?
Kvifor kjem dei hit?
Korleis er tilhøva i Noreg?
Bur han på Voss?
Liker du nynorsk?

A subordinate clause is also said with a rising tune when it is
placed first in a sentence. Examples:
Dersom han kjem, går eg.
Då ho hadde gjort arbeidet, gjekk ho heim.
Sidan dei ikkje ville arbeida, gjekk det dårleg.

In writing, rising intonation is usually indicated by means of a
question mark. A comma may also indicate rising intonation, but
the usual function of a comma is to indicate a pause.

18D Til fiskeskjer

Dersom ein samanliknar moderne fiske med fisket etter havtorsk
(skrei) på Lofothavet i eldre tid, ser ein kor fort utviklinga har gått.
Revolusjonen kom med båtmotoren. Nordlandsbåtane hadde råsegl,
slik dei gamle vikingskipa hadde, og dei var også utan dekk.
Frå sør og nord langs kysten drog fiskarane til Lofoten i januar.
Dei rekna med å vera heimanfrå i tre månader. Mat hadde dei med
seg i kister og tønner. Det var smør og mjøl, kjøt og flatbrød og anna

172

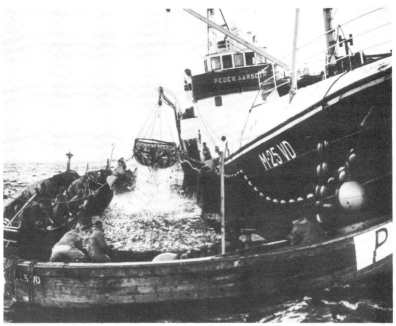

Fig. 18.3 Snurpebåten «Peder Aarseth» har fått full nota av sild.

som dei kunne trenga. Dei som var att heime, gav gladeleg frå seg mest alt for at lofotkarane skulle få kraftig kost til det harde arbeidet vinterstid.

I ei god hamn nær fiskefeltet hadde fiskarane små hus som vart kalla rorbuer, og i Lofoten var det mange slike. Mannen som åtte staden, vart kalla væreigar, og dei betalte væreigaren leige for rorbua. Dei betalte med fisk, og væreigarane vart ofte rike folk.

Rorbua hadde jordgolv og open eldstad. Langs veggene var det briskar til å liggja på. I rorbua åt og sov fiskarane. Her stelte dei fiskereiskapane sine, og her vart det fortalt segner og soger når det var storm og landlege. Ingen stad i Noreg har den sterke og humørfylte forteljekunsten stått så høgt som mellom fiskarane nordpå.

På dei moderne fiskebåtane er lugarane så fine og maten så god at det minner om hotell, men så har også fiskaryrket vorte heilårsyrke. Mange ligg på opne havet i lange bolkar både utanfor Norskekysten og i framande farvatn, t.d. utanfor Afrika-kysten, i Barentshavet osv.

173

Til fiskeskjer

Ro, ro til fiskeskjer.
Kor mange fiskar fekk du der?
Ein til far, og ein til mor,
ein til syster, ein til bror,
og ein til den som fisken fekk,
og det var vesle Olav.

Voggesong

eit skjer /sje:r/ – skerry, rock
eit fiskeskjer – fishing ground
near a skerry
ein havtorsk = ein skrei –
spawning cod that gather on
the banks offshore in winter
Lofothavet /"loffo:tha:ve/ – the
Lofoten Sea
i eldre tid – in former times
ein revolusjon /revolu'sjo:n/ –
revolution
ein båtmotor /"bå:tmoto:r/ – boat
engine
ein Nordlands-båt – special
type of boat from the county
of Nordland
eit råsegl /"rå:segl/ – square sail
eit vikingskip /"vi:kingsji:p/ –
viking ship
eit dekk – deck
heimanfrå – away from home
ein månad (månaden, månader,
månadene) – month
ei kiste /"kjiste/ – trunk, chest
ei tønne – barrel, cask
smør n. – butter
mjøl n. – flour
gladeleg – gladly
kraftig – substantial
ein kost /kåst/ – food
vinterstid – in winter

ei hamn – port
ei rorbu – fisherman's shanty
eit vær – place where men
gather to form fishing expe-
ditions, fishing station
ein væreigar – owner of a vær
eit jordgolv – dirt floor
langs – along
ein eldstad – fireplace
ein brisk – bunk
å eta (et, åt, ete) – to eat
ei segn – legend
ei soge /"så:ge/ – story, yarn
ein storm /stårm/ – storm
ei landlege – time ashore because of bad weather
humørfylt /hu'mø:rfylt/ – humorous
ein forteljekunst – art of telling
a story
nordpå /'no:rpå/ – in the north
å minna om (minner, minte,
mint) – to remind one of
eit fiskaryrke – fisherman's
trade
ein bolk /bålk/ – period
eit farvatn – waters
utanfor kysten – off the coast
å ro (ror, rodde, rott) – to row
ein voggesong /"våggesång/ –
lullaby

19A Det går alltid eit tog

Roy skal attende til USA for å studera vidare, og han skal byrja ved Universitetet i Wisconsin, som har ei stor norskavdeling. Før han reiser, vil han stogga i Oslo eit par dagar. Han tek toget frå Åndalsnes, og Liv er med han.

ROY	Har du kjøpt billettar til oss begge?
LIV	Ja, det har eg. – Når ein skal reisa langt med tog her i landet, bør ein helst kjøpa billettar nokre dagar før ein skal dra av stad.
ROY	Eg kan gå i kiosken og kjøpa noko lesestoff for turen, medan vi ventar på at toget skal gå. – Kva vil du ha?
LIV	Du kan kjøpa eit par aviser og eit vekeblad.
ROY	Ja vel. Eg har så mykje bagasje at eg må ekspedera han som reisegods.
– – –	(Litt seinare)
LIV	Kva for aviser har du kjøpt?
ROY	Eg har kjøpt «Sunnmørsposten» og «Dagbladet».
LIV	Eg ville no helst hatt ei nynorskavis, t.d. «Dag og Tid» eller ei lokalavis.
– – –	(Litt seinare)
JARNBANE-FUNKSJONÆREN	Ta plass! Ta plass! Steng dørene!
ROY	Er du svolten? Skal vi gå inn i restaurantvogna og få oss litt mat?
LIV	Ja, det ville vera koseleg. Det er alltid så hyggeleg å reisa med dagtoget, for då får ein sjå mykje, og så kan ein kosa seg i matvogna. (Dei sit og røykjer.)
ROY	Sist reiste eg med nattoget. – Det var bra det òg.

175

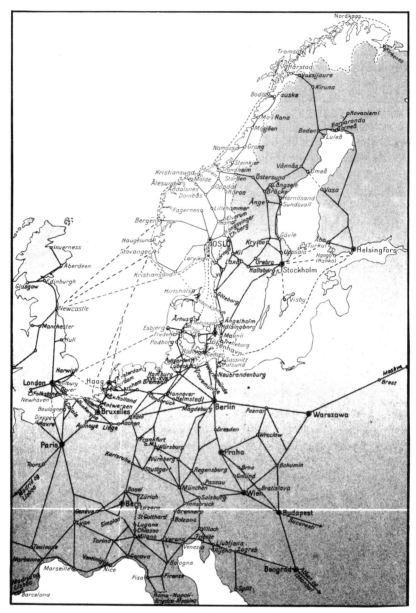

Fig. 19.1 Jarnbaneruter og båtruter i Skandinavia.

176

KONDUKTØREN	Billettane, takk! – De kan ikkje røykja her, for dette er ein kupé for ikkje-røykjarar. Dersom de skal røykja, må de gå inn i røykjekupéen ved sida av.
– – –	(Litt seinare)
ROY	Det er veldig interessant med alle stadnamna ein kan sjå langs jarnbanelina.
LIV	Ja, stadnamn er dikting på ein måte, og syner kor stor fantasi eller skapingsevne folk hadde. Dei er eigentleg stutte skildringar av korleis det ser ut på staden, eller av noko som peikar han ut frå andre stader.

å studera vidare – to continue with one's study

ei avdeling /av'de:ling/ – section, department

å dra av stad – to leave

ein kiosk /kjåsk/ – kiosk, newsstand

eit lesestoff /"le:seståff/ – reading material

eit vekeblad /"ve:kebla:/ – weekly magazine

ein bagasje /ba'ga:sje/ – baggage, luggage

reisegods n. – baggage

eg ville no helst hatt – I would prefer (The helping verb ha is usually dropped in constructions like this in conversation: ville (ha) hatt.)

ein jarnbanefunksjonær – railroad official

ta plass – sit down, take your seats

svolten /"svålten/ – hungry

ei vogn /vågn/ – coach, car; wagon

koseleg /"ko:seleg/ – nice

eit dagtog /"da:gto:g/ – morning (day) train

å kosa seg (kosar, kosa, kosa) – to enjoy oneself

sist – last time

eit nattog – night train

ei matvogn /"ma:tvågn/ = restaurantvogn – dining-car

ein kupé /ku'pe:/ – compartment

å røykja (røykjer, røykte, røykt) – to smoke

ein røykjekupé – smoking compartment

ved sida av – next door

eit stadnamn /"sta:namn/ – place name

ei jarnbaneline – railway line

på ein måte – in a way

ein fantasi /fanta'si:/ – imagination

ei skapingsevne – creative ability

eigentleg – actually, in reality

stutt – short

ei skildring /"sjildring/ – description

å peika ut (peikar, peika, peika) – to point out, to distinguish

Spørsmål

1. Kva skal Roy gjera når han kjem attende til USA? 2. Kvifor vil han studera vidare i Wisconsin? 3. Korleis reiser han til Oslo? 4. Reiser han åleine? 5. Reiser dei med dagtoget eller nattoget? 6. Kva gjer Roy med all bagasjen sin? 7. Kva for aviser les dei på vegen? 8. Har dei med seg mat? 9. Kva seier konduktøren til dei? 10. Korleis kan stadnamna vera dikting?

19B Grammar

1. The Formation of Nouns

The majority of the nouns of *nynorsk* are *derivatives* and *compounds*; new nouns are also formed in this way. A derivative is formed by adding a prefix or a suffix, or both, to some other word. Examples: *mistake* 'mistak', *samtale* 'conversation'; *bunad* 'costume', *fisking* 'fishing'; *betaling* 'payment'; *førebuing* 'preparation'.

A prefix or a suffix may have a more or less definite meaning, but it cannot be used by itself. The most common prefixes are: an-, be-, for-, fore-, føre-, er-, ge-, and the most common suffixes are: -ar, -er, -an(ar), -(n)ing, -semd, -dom, -døme, -leik, -skap, -nad, -sel, -sle, and -eri.

Compound nouns in *nynorsk* are usually written as one word, whereas the corresponding English compound words are often written as two words or hyphenated. In *nynorsk* a compound has only one primary stress, which usually falls on the first part of the compound. If the last part of the compound is an *ein-, ei-,* or *eit*-noun, the entire compound belongs to the same gender. Examples:

ein vårdag	a spring day	(cf. ein dag)
ei matvogn	a dining-car	(cf. ei vogn, but: ein mat)
eit lesestoff	reading material	(cf. eit stoff)

If three identical consonants follow each other in a compound, e.g., fjell-land, natt-tog, the compound can be written in two ways: either as *fjelland* and *nattog* with two consonants, or as *fjell-land* and *natt-tog* with a hyphen. Some other long compounds are also hyphenated now and then, e.g. norsk-avdeling, engelsk-kurs, etc.

Adjectives, nouns, and verbs may all enter into compounds. In some cases an -e- or an -s- is inserted between the two parts.

178

Examples:

Noun + noun:	dagtog, nattog, bygdekultur, vekeblad, skapingsevne, årstid.
Adjective + noun:	flathrød, gammaldans, storby.
Verb + noun:	byggjemåte, leveregel, spekemat.

Oppgåver

1. Analyze the formation of the nouns used in 19A.
2. Translate into *nynorsk*:
   a) They met in a dining-car on a lovely spring day.
   b) They had both taken the morning train to get back early.
   c) When they had eaten, they went back to their own compartment.
   d) Last time they had taken a night train.
   e) They were both interested in the place names they saw along the railway line.

19C Pronunciation/Spelling

The Spelling of Consonants

In 12C and 13C we gave the basic rule for the spelling of vowels and consonants in nynorsk: A long vowel (always stressed) is followed by one consonant, whereas a short stressed vowel is followed by two or more consonants. Examples: gul, gull; tak, takk; vis, viss.

Below we will discuss the spelling of consonants in some detail:

1. A double consonant is reduced to a single one before a grammatical ending that starts with a consonant. This will apply to:
   a) the neuter form of adjectives (with -*t* added): trygg – trygt, vill – vilt,
   b) the past and past participle of verbs before the endings -*de*, -*d*, -*te*, *and* -*t*: å byggja – byggjer – bygde – bygt; å spenna – spenner – spente – spent,
   c) contracted forms of adjectives and nouns: lubben – den lubne 'fat', vakker – den vakre; ein gaffel – gaflar; ein sommar – somrar.

2. A double consonant is reduced to a single one before the following derivational endings (suffixes): -na, -ning, -sel, -sle, -ling, and -sk. Examples: tjukk 'thick' – å tjukna 'to become thick'; å byggja – ein bygning 'building'; redd – ei redsle 'fear'; ei ætt – ein ætling 'relative'; eit troll – trolsk 'troll-like'.

3. The letter m is never doubled at the end of a word: kom, eit lam 'lamb', and final l and n are not doubled in modals or pronouns: skal, vil, kan; but: ein hall, ein kall 'fellow', ein mann, sann 'true'.

4. A number of very common short words end in a single consonant even though the vowel may be short and stressed: at, for, men, nok, når, til.

A double consonant is kept in the following cases:

1. Before the following derivational endings: -dom, -leg, -leik, -laus, -løyse, -sam, -semd, -skap.
Examples: ein mann – ein manndom 'manhood'; lett – lettleg 'handy'; stutt – ein stuttleik 'shortness'; eit vett 'intelligence' – vettlaus 'foolish'; rett – ei rettløyse 'unlawfulness'; ein takk – takksam 'grateful'; ein takk – ei takksemd 'gratitude'; eit troll – ein trollskap 'witchcraft'.

2. In compounds (see 19B1): ein fjelltopp, ein tannverk, eit nattog, eit fjelland.

3. Before the genitive -s: til fjells, i manns minne.

4. In some words to avoid confusion with other words: full – fullt (cf. ful – fult 'sly'), viss – visst (cf. vis – vist), å søkkja 'to sink' – søkkte (cf. å søkja 'to search' – søkte), å sleppa 'to drop' – sleppte (cf. å slepa 'to drag, to tow' – slepte).

5. In verbs which are derived from nouns ending in a double consonant: ein lakk 'varnish' – å lakkera 'to varnish', ein plass – å plassera 'to place', ein trafikk – å trafikkera.

Oppgåver

1. List words spelled with a single or double consonant in 19A.
2. Put the following nouns in the definite form plural:
ein artikkel, ein sommar, ein sykkel 'bike', ein spegel.
3. Put the following adjectives in the neuter form singular: kvass, stygg, skakk.
4. Put the following verbs in the past tense: å kjenna, å skjenna 'to scold', å kneppa 'to press'.

180

19D Førenamn og etternamn i Noreg

Alle nordmenn har både førenamn og etternamn. Når ein skal velja førenamn, har den gamle skikken med å «kalla opp» foreldre eller avlidne skyldfolk framleis mykje å seia. Same førenamnet går ofte att i fleire ættleder i same ætta, t.d. Gunnar, Olav osv.

I vikingtida var mest alle førenamn av nordisk opphav, t.d. Torbjørn, Tordis, Åshild, men då kristendomen vart innført omkring år 1000, kom mange kyrkjelege namn av latinsk opphav inn, t.d. Jon (av Johannes), Nils (av Nikolaus), Lars (av Laurentius), Pål (av Paulus), Maria og Cecilia. Litt seinare i mellomalderen kjem Peter, Andreas, Simon, Tomas, Benedikt, Stefan, Katarina, Margareta o.fl.

I slutten av mellomalderen, då sambandet med Nord-Tyskland var særleg sterkt, fekk vi inn mange tyske namn: Henrik, Engelbrekt, Konrad, Hermann, Kristian, Ludvig, Otto, Gjertrud, Kristina o.fl.

Dei nordiske namna heldt seg likevel forholdsvis godt ved sida av dei kyrkjelege og dei tyske. Særleg var namnet Olav godt likt. Det var både eit gammalt nordisk namn og eit kyrkjeleg namn.

Men etter reformasjonen (1537) tok prestane til å arbeida for å få bort dei gamle nordiske namna, fordi dei minte om heidenskapen, og dei greidde å trengja ut mange nordiske namn.

Frå midten av 1800-talet kjem det ei endring. Det heng saman med den aukande interessa for nordisk kultur og historie (nasjonalromantikken). Frå den tid til i dag har dei gamle nordiske namna

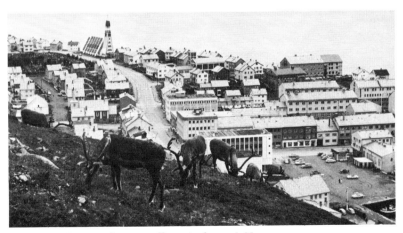

Fig. 19.2 *Hammerfest, nordlegaste byen i Noreg.*

181

vore populære, jamvel om ei heil rekkje utanlandske namn, særleg frå engelsk, også vert nytta.

Når det gjeld *etternamn*, er stoda i dag den at dei fleste nordmenn anten har eit *gardsnamn* eller eit *-sen-namn* til etternamn. Heilt frå 1200-talet har det vore vanleg i norske bygder å bruka gardsnamnet til etternamn, av og til med farsnamnet som mellomnamn: Aasmund Olavsson Vinje. Dei som flytta til byane, tok gjerne etternamnet med seg. Derfor har så stor del av byfolket i Noreg eit gardsnamn til etternamn.

I viktingtida og mellomalderen var det oftast farsnamnet som vart nytta til å laga etternamn: Olav Tryggvason, Håkon Håkonsson. Med dansken (1400–1800) kom former som *-søn* og *-sen* inn i staden for *-son*: Jens Nilssøn, Christen Jenssøn, og etter ei tid sigra *-sen* heilt. Namn som Hansen, Jensen, Larsen, Olsen vart vanlege, særleg i byane, og desse namna gjekk over til å verta faste familienamn som kunne brukast om kvinner også. Dersom Olav Hansen t.d. hadde ein son som heitte Gunnar, ville han kalla seg Gunnar Hansen (ikkje Gunnar Olavsen).

eit førenamn /'fø:renamn/ – given name
eit etternamn /'etternamn/ – family name, surname
å velja (vel, valde, valt) – to choose
ein skikk /sjikk/ – custom
å kalla opp (kallar, kalla, kalla) – to name after
avliden, pl. avlidne /'a:vli:den/ – deceased, dead
skyldfolk /'sjyldfålk/ n.pl. – relatives, kinsmen
å gå att – to recur
ein ættled /'ættle:/, pl. ættleder – generation
vikingtida f. – the viking period
eit opphav – origin
kristendomen m. – Christianity
kyrkjeleg /'kjyrkjeleg/ – religious, biblical
latinsk /la'ti:nsk/ – Latin

o.fl. = og fleire
i slutten av – at the end of
eit samband – contact, communication
Tyskland – Germany
tysk – German
nordisk /'nordisk/ – Nordic, Scandinavian
å halda seg godt – to hold their own
forholdsvis – relatively
reformasjonen /refårma'sjo:nen/ – the Reformation
ein prest – minister, clergyman
å få bort – to get rid of, to abolish
heidenskapen m. – paganism
å greia (greier, greidde, greitt) – to manage
å trengja ut (trengjer, trengde, trengt) – to force out, to replace

ei endring – change
å hanga (heng, hang, hange) – to hang
det heng saman med – it is related to
aukande – increasing
historie /hi'sto:rie/ f. – history
nasjonalromantikk m. – national romanticism, national feeling
ei stode /"stå:e/ – situation
eit gardsnamn /'ga:rsnamn/ – farm name

heilt frå – all the way from
eit farsnamn /'fa:rsnamn/ – father's name
eit mellomnamn – middle name
byfolk /'by:fålk/ – townspeople
dansk – Danish
i staden for – instead of
etter ei tid – after some time
å sigra (sigrar, sigra, sigra) – to win, to prevail

ESSON 20

20A Har De ledige rom?

Liv og Roy er komne til Oslo og prøver å finna ein stad å bu. Dei går
først på Bondeheimen og spør der.

ROY	Orsak, har De ledige rom?
PORTIEREN	Nei, dessverre, alle romma er opptekne i dag. Det er så mange turistar i byen no.
ROY	Veit De om ein annan stad, kanskje?
PORTIEREN	Eg er lei for at det er så fullt hjå oss, men eg veit om ein stad der dei leiger ut rom. Romma er enkle, men reine og fine, og det er svært billeg der.
LIV	Ja, det ville høva godt for oss. Kunne De gje oss namnet og telefonnummeret?
PORTIEREN	Ja, med glede. Eg kan ringja bort dit for Dykk, om De vil. Her er adressa. Det er eit stykke herifrå.
LIV	Det var veldig snilt av Dykk. Tusen takk.
ROY (TIL LIV)	Kom så tek vi ein bil.
— — —	(Litt seinare)
ROY	God kveld. Har De eit par rom som er ledige?
MANNEN	Ja, vi har to små rom. Det er varmt vatn på begge romma, og det er dusj og toalett på gangen.
ROY	Ja, det er godt nok for meg. – Kva seier du, Liv?
LIV	Er det godt nok for deg, er det godt nok for meg også.
	– Kva kostar romma?
MANNEN	Dei kostar to hundre kroner til saman for ei natt.
ROY	Då tek vi dei. – Veit De om det er vanskeleg å få billett til Det Norske Teatret no?
MANNEN	Så vidt eg veit, er det god plass midt i veka.
ROY	Kunne vi låna telefonen og tinga herifrå?
MANNEN	Ver så god.

6 *trafikkreglar*
1. Køyr til høgre!
2. Sjå deg om før du går over gata!
3. Ta meir omsyn til andre i trafikken!
4. Gå på venstre sida av vegen!
5. Køyr varsamt!
6. Vent på grønt lys før du kryssar køyrebanen!

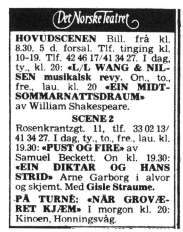

(Det Norske Teatret)

HOVUDSCENEN Bill. frå kl. 8.30, 5 d. forsal. Tlf. tinging kl. 10-19. Tlf. 42 46 17/41 34 27. I dag, ty., kl. 20: «L/L **WANG & NILSEN** musikalsk revy. On., to., fre., lau. kl. 20 «**EIN MIDT-SOMMARNATTSDRAUM**» av William Shakespeare.

SCENE 2
Rosenkrantzgt. 11, tlf. 33 02 13/41 34 27. I dag, ty., to., fre., lau. kl. 19.30: «**PUST OG FIRE**» av Samuel Beckett. On kl. 19.30: «**EIN DIKTAR OG HANS STRID**» Arne Garborg i alvor og skjemt. Med **Gisle Straume.**

PÅ TURNÉ: «NÅR GROVÆRET KJÆM» I morgon kl. 20: Kinoen, Honningsvåg.

Fig. 20 *Det Norske Teatret er eitt av dei leiande teatra i landet.*

ledig /"le:di/ – vacant
ein portier /porti'e:/ – doorman
oppteken, pl. opptekne /"opp-te:ken/ – occupied, taken
ein turist /tu'rist/ – tourist
eg er lei for at – I'm sorry that
å leiga ut (leiger, leigde, leigt) – to let, to have rooms for rent
å høva (høver, høvde, høvt) – to suit
ein telefon /tele'fo:n/ – telephone
eit telefonnummer /tele'fo:-nommer/ – telephone number
med glede – gladly

å ringja (ringjer, ringde, ringt) – to call
om De vil – if you want me to
ei adresse /a'dresse/ – address
eit stykke herifrå – some distance from here
det var veldig snilt av Dykk – that's very kind of you
kom så tek vi ein bil – let's take a cab
ein bil – cab; car
varm – hot, warm
ein gang – hallway, corridor
på gangen – in the hallway
til saman – all together
så vidt eg veit – as far as I know

185

å låna (låner, lånte, lånt) – to borrow
ein trafikkregel /tra'fikkre:gel/ – traffic law, regulation
å køyra (køyrer, køyrde, køyrt) /"kjøyra/ – to drive
ta omsyn til andre – have consideration for others, respect others
varsamt – carefully
å kryssa (kryssar, kryssa, kryssa) – to cross
ein køyrebane – traffic lane

Spørsmål

1. Kvar er Liv og Roy no? 2. Kvar helst prøver dei å få rom? 3. Kvifor var det så vanskeleg å finna rom i Oslo på denne tida? 4. Kor mange senger måtte dei ha? 5. Korleis kom dei seg frå Bondeheimen til den andre staden? 6. Korleis var romma? 7. Var det dyrt å bu der? 8. Kor mykje kosta romma til saman? 9. Kva spør dei om? 10. Kva seier trafikkreglane?

20B Grammar

1. Expressions of Time

Some types of time expressions have already occurred now and then, and it will be helpful to summarize the most frequent ones:

1. Expressions used to refer to an event that happened (or will happen) within a specific period of time.

i:

i dag	today
i dag tidleg	this morning, early today
i morgon	tomorrow
i morgon tidleg	tomorrow morning
i overmorgon	the day after tomorrow
i går	yesterday
i går kveld	yesterday evening
i natt	last night, or tonight, depending on the context: I natt sov eg dårleg. 'Last night I slept poorly.' I natt dreg vi på fisketur. 'Tonight we are going fishing.'
i føremiddag	this forenoon
i ettermiddag	this afternoon
i år	this year

i sommar	this summer, or last summer, depending on the context
i vinter	this winter, or last winter, depending on the context
i vår	this spring, or last spring, depending on the context
i haust	this fall, or last fall, depending on the context
i fjor sommar	last summer
i fjor vinter	last winter

2. Expressions used to state that something happens repeatedly or regularly within or during a certain period of time.

om:

om morgonen	in the morning
om ettermiddagen	in the afternoon
om kvelden	in the evening
om fredag (på fredag)	on Friday
om våren	in (the) spring
om sommaren	in (the) summer
om hausten	in (the) fall
om vinteren	in (the) winter
om natta	at (during the) night
om dagen	during the day, or per day, depending on the context

3. Expressions used to state how soon something will take place, reckoning from the present moment.

om:

om ei veke	in a week
om tre månader	in three months
om eit år	in a year
om fem timar	in five hours
om ti minutt	in ten minutes

4. Expressions used to state the period of time since something happened.

for – sidan:

| for ei veke sidan | a week ago |
| for tre månader sidan | three months ago |

for eit år sidan	a year ago
for femti år sidan	fifty years ago
for lenge sidan	long ago

5. Expressions used to state the length or duration of an activity.
i:

i ei veke	for a week
i tre månader	for three months
i femti år	for fifty years
i fem dagar	for five days
i ti minutt	for ten minutes
i mange år	for many years

When the statement is negated, the preposition *på* is used, e.g., Eg har ikkje sett henne på fem år. 'I haven't seen her for five years.'

6. Expressions to state the hour, day, month or season of the occurrence of an event.

The preposition *i* or *ved* is used for approximations to the hour, *på* is used with the days of the week, *i* is used with months, *til* is used with approaching seasons, and the article *den* (without a preposition) is used for the days of the month.

i (ved) fem-tida	about 5 o'clock
i (ved) halv åtte-tida	about 7:30
på måndag	on Monday
på laurdag	on Saturday
i mars	in March
til våren (i vår)	next spring
til sommaren (i sommar)	next summer
den niande april	on the 9th of April

2. Courtesy Phrases
Most of the courtesy phrases of nynorsk have occurred in the lessons, and they are listed below, along with some more phrases that are relatively common.

1. Greeting		Reply
Hei! (Informal. Very Common)	Hi!	Hei!

188

188

God dag. (More formal)	How do you do?	God dag.
God morgon.	Good morning.	God morgon.
God kveld.	Good evening.	God kveld.
Hallo! (Esp. as a telephone greeting)	Hello! Hey! Hey there!	Hallo!

2. How are you?

		Reply
Korleis står det til? (Correct and formal)	How are you?	Berre bra, takk.
Korleis har du det? (More personal)	How's life at the moment?	Takk, berre bra.
Korleis går det? (Often used by adults talking to young people)	How's it going?	

3. Farewell

		Reply
Ha det. (Very common)	Bye-bye. So long.	Ha det.
Ha det bra (godt, hyggeleg).	So long.	Ha det (bra).
Ha det bra så lenge.	So long.	Ha det.
Adjø. (Formal)	Good-bye.	Adjø.
Far vel. (Formal)	Good-bye.	Far vel.
God middag.	'Have a nice dinner.'	God middag.
God natt.	Good night.	God natt.

4. Please

Ver så gild (snill, venleg) å ...
Eg skulle gjerne ha ...
Eg skulle ha to kilo, takk.

5. Apologizing

Orsak.	Excuse me.
Eg er lei for at ...	I'm sorry that ...
Dessverre ...	Unfortunately, ...

6. Thanking

		Reply
Takk. (Normal and neutral way of expressing thanks)	Thank you.	Ver så god.

Tusen takk. (Shows more appreciation)	Ver så god. Or: Ikkje noko å takka for.	
Mange takk. (A little more formal than *tusen takk*)		
Takk skal du (De) ha. (Warm and personal)		
Takk for det. (No particular feeling of warmth)		
Takk for hjelpa.	'Thanks for your help.'	
Takk for lånet.	'Thanks for the loan.'	

Takk for maten.	'Thanks for the food.'	Ver så god.
Takk for meg (oss).	(Said by the guests to their host as they leave)	Sjølv takk.
Takk for i dag.	(Said at the end of a day's work)	Takk, det same.
Takk for i kveld.	(Said after a pleasant evening together)	Takk like eins.
Takk for no.	(Used between people who know each other well)	

Takk for samværet (laget).	Thank you for a very pleasant time.
Takk for samtalen (praten).	It was nice talking to you.
Takk for i går.	'Thank you for yesterday.'
Takk for sist.	'Thank you for last time.'

7. General good wishes		Reply
God jul.	Merry Christmas.	God jul. Or: Takk det same.
Godt nyttår.	Happy New Year.	Godt nyttår.
God påske.	Happy Easter.	God påske.
God pinse.	Happy Pentecost.	God pinse. (Takk like eins.)
God sommar.	Have a good summer.	God sommar.
God helg.	Have a nice weekend.	God helg.
God sundag.	Have a nice Sunday.	God sundag.
Til lukke.	Congratulations.	Takk.
Gratulerer med dagen. Or: Til lukke med dagen.	Happy birthday.	Takk skal du ha.

Lukke til.	Good luck.	Tusen takk.
God betring.	Get well soon.	Mange takk.
God ferie.	Happy holidays.	

As can be seen from the list above, it is not possible to give even a rough translation of a high number of the phrases which is at all satisfactory. In *nynorsk* there is a greater range of courtesy phrases than in English. *Nynorsk* also has a number of courtesy phrases pertaining to situations where in English we say nothing at all, or try to express our pleasure, appreciation, or enjoyment in a rather round-about way. For example, English has no equivalent for *takk for maten* or *takk for sist* other than general comments to the hostess that the meal is good, or similarly, saying something nice about last time we were together instead of saying *takk for sist*.

Oppgåver

Translate the following sentences into *nynorsk*:
1. I was late for school this morning.
2. He usually goes skiing in the evening.
3. It's so cold here in the winter.
4. I didn't sleep well last night.
5. I'm going to the university in three months.
6. I've been in high school for two years.
7. I began to study *nynorsk* one year ago.
8. I haven't seen my professor for two weeks.
9. He said he would be back on Monday.
10. Next spring I'll do a lot of work.

20C Pronunciation/Spelling

The Spelling of Abbreviations

The most important rules for the spelling of abbreviations in *nynorsk* are as follows:
1. Abbreviations for weights and measures have no periods:
   kg (kilogram or kilo), hg (hektogram or hekto), g (gram). 1 kg = 2.2 lbs., 1 lb. = 0,45 kg, 1 hg = 3½ oz., 1 oz. = ¼ hg (28 gram), 1 g = 1/30 oz.
   km (kilometer), m (meter), cm (centimeter); 1 km = ⅝ mile,

1 mile = 1,6 km, 1 m = 39⅜ in., 1 yd. = 91 cm, 1 ft. = 30 cm,
1 cm = ⅜ in., 1 in. = 2½ cm;
l (liter), *dl* (desiliter), *cl* (centiliter); 1 l = 1.1 qt., 1 gal. = 3,8 l,
1 qt. = 0,9 l.

As can be seen from the examples above, the system of
measurement is the *metric* one. Three fundamental units of
measure are used: The *gram* /gramm/ for weight, the *meter* /'me:ter/
for length, and the *liter* /'li:ter/ for volume. Each of these gets a
Greek or Latin prefix to indicate larger or smaller units: milli-
(¹⁄₁₀₀₀), centi- (¹⁄₁₀₀), deci- (¹⁄₁₀), deka- (10), hekto- (100), kilo- (1000).
Notice that instead of decimal points, commas are used.

The fundamental monetary unit *krone*, pl. *kroner*, is abbreviated
as *kr* without a period. When writing large numbers, we use spaces
or periods to separate groups of three numerals, not commas, e.g.,
10 000, 100 000, or 10.000, 100.000.

2. Abbreviations which consist of capital letters are usually written
   without a period between each letter or at the end: NATO,
   UNESCO, USA, NSB (Noregs Statsbanar).

3. The following abbreviations are written with a period at the end:
   dvs. (det vil seia), *etc.* (et cetera = og anna), *jfr.* (jamfør), *osb.*
   (og så bortetter), *osv.* (og så vidare), *vsa.* (ved sida av).

4. Some very common abbreviations have a period after each
   member: *bl.a.* (blant anna, blant andre), *m.a.* (mellom anna),
   m.m. (med meir), *o.a.* (og anna, og andre), *o.fl.* (og fleire), *o.l.* (og
   liknande).

20D Det Norske Teatret

Det Norske Teatret vart skipa i 1912, og oppgåva skulle vera å gje
framsyningar på nynorsk i Oslo og utover landet. Den første
styreformannen var Hulda Garborg, kona til Arne Garborg, og første
teatersjefen var skodespelar Rasmus Rasmussen.

Teatret hadde opningsframsyning 2. januar 1913 i Kristiansand
med *Ervingen* av Ivar Aasen. Den første framsyninga i Oslo var
Jeppe på Berget, omsett til nynorsk av Arne Garborg. Denne
framsyninga vart følgd av ei rekkje pipekonsertar som heldt fram på
spelferda i austlandsbygdene.

Hulda og Arne Garborg arbeidde for at Det Norske Teatret skulle verta eit heilnorsk nasjonalteater, som kunne føra fram det beste i verdsdramatikken i eit mål og ei spelform som var i samsvar med norsk lynne. Dei vona også at teatret skulle verta ein trygg voksterstad for nynorsk talemål.

Første åra la derfor teatret stor vekt på å skapa ei ekte og naturleg framstelling av bønder på scenen. Repertoaret bygde særleg på breie folkekomediar med einskilde alvorlege skodespel som *Læraren* av Arne Garborg. I denne tida drog teatret på mange spelferder rundt i heile landet, og vart ein førelaupar for Riksteatret.

Gjennom sitt ypparlege ensemble og ikkje minst på grunn av Agnes Mowinckels instruksjon utvikla teatret etter kvart sitt kunstnarlege område. Klassiske skodespel og moderne skodespel frå ulike land vart synte, og Det Norske Teatret vart eitt av dei leiande teatra i landet.

Etter at Tormod Skagestad i 1953 vart kunstnarleg leiar og hovudinstruktør, seinare teatersjef, har teatret på ny gjennomgått ei kunstnarleg utvikling. Blant framsyningar som fekk særleg mange lovord, kan nemnast *Kristin Lavransdatter* av Sigrid Undset, *Lang dags ferd mot natt* av Eugene O'Neill, *Den kaukasiske kritringen* av Bertolt Brecht og songspela *Oklahoma, West Side Story* og *Spelemann på taket*.

Skagestad har også sytt for å skaffa fast plass for Ibsen og Strindberg på repertoaret.

ei oppgåve – task; purpose
ei framsyning /'"frammsy:ning/ – performance
ein styreformann /'"sty:refår-mann/ – chair(man) of the board
ein teatersjef /te'a:tersje:f/ – theater manager
ein skodespelar /'"skå:espe:lar/ – actor
ei opningsframsyning – opening performance
Ervingen – The Heir, play by Ivar Aasen
Jeppe på Berget – Jeppe on the Hill, play written in Danish by Ludvig Holberg

å omsetja (omset, omsette, omsett) – translate
ein pipekonsert /'"pi:pekon-sært/ – jeering
å halda fram – to continue
ei spelferd /'"spe:lfæ:r/ – tour
ei austlandsbygd = ei bygd på Austlandet
heilnorsk /'"hæilnårsk/ – wholly Norwegian
å føra fram – to put on, to present
verdsdramatikken m. – the world's dramatic literature
ei spelform /'"spe:lfårm/ – style, form
i samsvar med – in accordance with

193

eit lynne – character, temperament

å vona (vonar, vona, vona) – to hope

ein voksterstad /'våkstersta:/ – place of growth

å leggja vekt på – to emphasize

ei framstelling /'frammstelling/ – presentation

eit repertoar /repærto'a:r/ – repertoire

ein folkekomedie – popular comedy

ein førelaupar /"fø:relæupar/ – forerunner, precursor

ypparleg – excellent

eit ensemble /an'sambel/ – cast

på grunn av – on account of

ein instruksjon /instruk'sjo:n/ – direction, instruction

å utvida (utvidar, utvida, utvida) /'u:tvi:a/ – to expand

kunstnarleg – artistic

etter kvart – little by little, gradually

ein leiar – leader

ein hovudinstruktør – producer

å gjennomgå – to go through

eit lovord /"lå:vo:r/ – word of praise

eit songspel – musical

21A Styreform og politiske tilhøve

Det er første gongen Roy er i Oslo, og han og Liv ser seg om i sentrum av byen.

ROY   Kva heiter denne gata her? – Det ser ut til å vera hovudgata i byen.

LIV   Dette er Karl Johans gate eller Karl Johan, som vi kallar henne til vanleg. Den store bygningen der borte er slottet, og rett bak oss har vi stortingsbygningen. På høgre sida eit stykke nedanfor slottet ligg det gamle universitetet, som vart skipa i 1811, og rett overfor universitetet ligg Nationaltheatret.

ROY   Kan du forklara enkelt for meg kva for styreform Noreg har?

LIV   Eg skal freista. – Noreg er eit konstitusjonelt, arveleg monarki, eller kongedøme, og har vore det sidan 17. mai 1814. Som du veit, er 17. mai den største festdagen vi har. Då feirar vi at vi fekk vår eiga grunnlov, og at unionen med Danmark vart oppløyst.

ROY   Er det Kongen som har makta i Noreg då?

LIV   Nei, den politiske makta ligg hjå nasjonalforsamlinga, eller Stortinget, som det heiter. Stortinget har i dag 155 representantar, som vert valde av folket, og det er val kvart fjerde år.

ROY   Kor gammal må ein vera for å ha lov til å røysta?

LIV   18 år.

ROY   Kva for politiske parti er representerte i Stortinget?

LIV   Hjå oss kan det variera frå periode til periode. I denne valperioden er det følgjande parti: Arbeidarpartiet (76), Høgre (41), Kristeleg Folkeparti (22), Senterpartiet (12), Venstre (2) og Sosialistisk Venstreparti (2).

ROY   Kva kallar de regjeringssjefen?

LIV   Han vert kalla statsminister og tilhøyrer det partiet eller den partigruppa som har regjeringa. Ein regjeringsmedlem vert

195

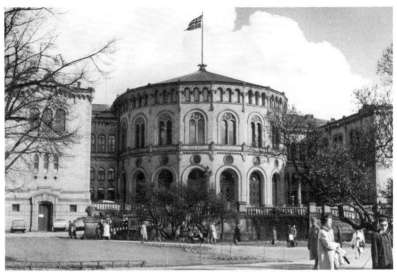

Fig. 21.1 *Stortingsbygningen i Oslo. Her har Stortinget møta sine.*

kalla statsråd eller minister. Kongen styrer møta i statsråd på
slottet.

ROY Kor mange fylke er det i Noreg?

LIV Det er 19 fylke, med unntak av Oslo er kvart fylke delt opp i
kommunar. Eit fylke vert styrt av eit fylkesting, og ein
kommune av eit kommunestyre.

ROY Har Noreg ein offisiell religion?

LIV Ja, det er den evangelisk-lutherske læra, som vart innført ved
reformasjonen i 1537, og Den norske kyrkja er ei statskyrkje
med Kongen som overhovud. Over 90% av alle innbyggjar-
ane i Noreg er medlemer av statskyrkja.

ei styreform /''sty:refårm/ –
 form of government
Stortinget – the Parliament
ein bygning – building
eit slott /slått/ – palace
nedanfor – further down
rett overfor – right across from
å forklara (forklarer, forklarte,
 forklart) /får'kla:ra/ – to explain

konstitusjonell   /kånstitusjo-
 'nell/ – constitutional
arveleg /''arveleg/ – hereditary
eit monarki /monar'ki:/ – monarchy
eit kongedøme – monarchy
ein festdag /'festda:g/ – holiday
ei grunnlov /''grunnlå:v/ – constitution
å løysa opp – to dissolve

196

ein konge /"kånge/ – king
ei makt – power
ei nasjonalforsamling – national assembly, parliament
ein representant /represen'tant/
– representative
eit val – election
å ha lov til – to be allowed to, to
have the right to
å røysta (røystar, røysta, røysta)
– to vote
ein periode /peri'o:de/ – period
ein valperiode /'va:lperio:de/ –
electoral period
Arbeidarpartiet – the Labor
Party
Høgre – the Conservative Party
Kristeleg Folkeparti – the
Christian Democratic Party
Senterpartiet – the Center Party
Venstre – the Liberal Party
Sosialistisk Venstreparti – the
Socialist Left Party
ein regjeringssjef /re'je:ringsje:f/
– head of government
ein statsminister /'sta:tsminis-
ter/ – prime minister

å tilhøyra /'tillhøyra/ – to belong to
ein regjeringsmedlem, pl.
-medlemer – member of the
Cabinet, Cabinet minister
ein statsråd /'sta:tsrå:d/ – Cabinet minister
eit statsråd – Cabinet meeting
eit unntak – exception
eit fylkesting – county council
eit kommunestyre – local
council (city, town or village)
å styra (styrer, styrte, styrt) – to
govern
ein religion /religi'o:n/ – religion
offisiell /åfisi'ell/ – official
evangelisk-luthersk – evangelical Lutheran
ei lære /"læ:re/ – doctrine
Den norske kyrkja – the Norwegian Church
ei statskyrkje – state church
eit overhovud – head
ein innbyggjar /"innbygjgjar/ –
inhabitant
ein medlem /"me:dlem/, pl.
medlemer – member

Spørsmål
1. Kva heiter hovudgata i Oslo? 2. Kvar ligg det gamle universitetet?
3. Når vart Universitetet i Oslo skipa? 4. Kva styreform har Noreg? 5.
Kven styrer møta i statsråd? 6. Kven er statsminister no? 7. Kva
heiter dei største politiske partia? 8. Når fekk Noreg si eiga
grunnlov? 9. Kor mange representantar har Stortinget? 10. Kor
mange fylke er det i Noreg? 11. Korleis vert eit fylke styrt? 12. Kven
styrer ein kommune? 13. Kva meiner ein med *statskyrkje*?

21B Grammar

1. The Co-ordinating Conjunctions

The co-ordinating conjunctions combine together main or independent clauses, parts of a sentence, or words. They do not count in word order. Remember the main rule for word order in main clauses is *verb second* (see 2B1).

The most common co-ordinating conjunctions are:

og	and
både – og	both – and
eller	or
anten – eller	either – or
korkje – eller	neither – nor
men	but
for	for

2. The Subordinating Conjunctions

The subordinating conjunctions introduce subordinate clauses. A subordinate clause is one which cannot stand alone. It is subordinate to another clause and functions as part of the other clause. In the sentence 'When he comes we can go', we have two clauses, i.e., two sets of subject and verb: 1) when he comes, 2) we can go. The clause 'when he comes' cannot stand alone; it functions as an adverbial giving the *time* when 'we can go'. Its function is just like that of the time adverb *now* in 'now we can go'. The clause 'when he comes' is also introduced by a subordinating conjunction (when), which also indicates that it is a subordinate clause.

The most common subordinating conjunctions used in *nynorsk* are:

a) Denoting time: *då* ('when', single past event), *når* ('when', referring to what usually happens or happened or what will happen in the future), *etter (at)* 'after', *før (enn)* 'before, till', *medan* 'while', *så snart (som)* 'as soon as', *så lenge (som)* 'as long as'. Note that *som* is often dropped when a clause follows: Eg kjem så snart eg kan.

b) Denoting cause: *fordi* 'because', *av di* 'because', *sidan* 'since'.

c) Denoting condition: *dersom* 'if', *i fall* 'in case', *utan* 'unless', *med mindre* 'unless', *om* 'if'.

Notice that a condition also can be expressed just by placing the conjugated verb first (see 2B2).

d) Denoting concession: *endå (om)*, *jamvel om* 'even though', *trass i* 'despite', *sjølv om* 'even if'.
e) Denoting purpose: *for at* 'so that', *så* 'so that'.
f) Denoting consequence: *så*, *så at* or *slik at* 'so that',
g) Denoting comparison: *som* or *liksom* 'as', *så – som* 'as – as, so – as', *dess – dess* or *di – di* 'the – the', *enn* 'than', *som om* 'as if'.
h) In front of a noun clause: *at* 'that', *om* 'if, whether'.
i) In front of a relative clause: *som* 'who, whom, that, which'.

Notice that a noun clause can also be introduced by an interrogative pronoun (kven, kva, kva for ein) or an interrogative adverb (kor, korleis, kvar, kvar helst, kvifor, når). See 14B2.

A relative clause is often introduced by the relative adverb *der* instead of *som* (see 11B2). For the word order of subordinate clauses see 2B2.

3. Omission of at and som

The subordinating conjunctions *at* and *som* are often dropped, although one is still dealing with a subordinate clause:
Han sa at han kunne koma. = Han sa han kunne koma.
He said that he could come. = He said he could come.
Mannen som eg tala med, var utlending. = Mannen eg tala med, var utlending.
The man with whom I talked was a foreigner. = The man I talked with was a foreigner.

Notice that the adverb *ikkje* is placed before the conjugated verb in a subordinate clause: Han sa at han *ikkje* kunne koma.
For the omission of *som*, see 11B2.

4. That = det, at, som

There are four types of 'that' in English and three different words in *nynorsk* which correspond to and translate 'that':

that table	*det* bordet (demonstrative)
I saw *that*.	Eg såg *det*. (demonstrative, stressed)
	Det såg eg.
He said *that* he was coming.	Han sa *at* han skulle koma.
The book *that* he was reading, . . .	Boka *som* han las, . . .

199

Oppgåver

1. Analyze the function of the subordinate clauses in 21A.
2. Make up a list of all the conjunctions you can find in the dialogue, and classify them according to function.
3. Translate into *nynorsk*:
   a) Can you tell me where the post office is?
   b) She told me that she had been there before.
   c) I have to shave since I'm going to the theater this evening.
   d) He asked me if I could help him with his homework.
   e) When I was in Norway, I visited an old friend of mine who lives in Bergen.

21C Pronunciation/Spelling

Punctuation

By punctuation we mean the use of standard marks and signs in writing and printing to separate words into sentences, clauses, and phrases in order to clarify meaning. Punctuation also gives an indication of intonation. Basically, the function of punctuation in *nynorsk* and English is the same, i.e., to indicate pauses and intonation in speech. There are some differences, however.

1. The period (punktum)
   Unlike English, a period is used in the following cases:
   a) After ordinal numbers: 1., 5., 101. (første, femte, hundreogførste).
   b) When writing large numbers to separate groups of three numerals (not commas): 10.000, 100.000, 10.000.000 (ti millionar).
   c) To separate hours, minutes, and seconds: kl. 07.12.20.
   Concerning periods after abbreviations see 20C.
2. The comma (komma)
   Commas are used in the following cases:
   a) Between co-ordinated clauses combined by the co-ordinating conjunctions *og, eller, men, for*: Dei kom, og vi gjekk. Han spurde om dei ville gå, eller om dei ville ta bil.
   Note: We always put a comma before the word *men*, even when it is not followed by a clause: Ikkje berre ho, men han også.
   b) Always after a subordinate clause if it comes first in a sentence: Då dei kom, gjekk vi. Dersom du les, vil det gå bra.

200

c) Always *after* an inserted clause, but not before it unless it is non-restrictive: Han som går der, er onkelen min. But: Roy Eisel, som no bur i Wisconsin, er flink i norsk.

d) When writing decimal numbers: 0,5 l (liter), 3,8 l (not decimal points).

Two cases should be commented on in particular:

a) We do not use a comma in front of the conjunctions *og* and *eller*, or abbreviations like *etc., osv.* in an enumeration: Alle var der: mannen, alle barna, kona og tenestejenta. Du kan få brød, ost, smør, poteter eller frukt. Dei les norsk, engelsk, tysk osv.

b) We do not put a comma after an adverbial phrase, even though it comes first in a sentence: *Etter å ha arbeidt ein heil månad reiste han bort. Etter mi meining bør han slutta. I det store og heile har han gjort ein god jobb.*

3. Quotation marks

In writing, the first set of the quotation marks is placed at the bottom of the line (,, . . ."); in print the English system is normally used (". . ."). Quotation marks are usually used when giving the titles of books, paintings, the names of ships, etc.: «Bondestudentar», «Fuglane», «Haust», «Ut mot havet», «Nordfjord». In fiction, quotation marks are often replaced by a dash (–) to introduce direct discourse as in *Nokre stubbar* (5D). Notice that a colon is always put in front of direct speech: Ho sa: «Kva ønskjer du deg til jul?»

21D Hesten

Dagen var heit og lang – no skal han gå.
No er det kveld, og alle ljod er få.
Ei småjente labbar inn døra naken: God natt til far!
Ho smeller ein kyss, og går til sitt svale putevar.

Han går ikkje sjølv. Stilnar til. Ved eit rotet bord.
Papir og bøker. Skrivne og prenta ord.
Jentekyssen på kinnet var varm og rund,
men gløymest likevel bort i same stund.

No er det arbeid. Og tida får gå som ho vil.
Omsider han ser mot ruta – og rykker til:
Ute er mørkt. Då kan ein arbeide best.
– Men no ligg det inn på ruta eit andlet: Ein hest!

Eit veldig hestandlet. Grått som leir.
Med svarte djupe auge. Ein ser ikkje meir.
Og ikkje ei rørsle i det. Men heile ruta dekt.
– Ein faren, underleg tidbolk blir opp att vekt.

Han stirer på synet. Ja! hesten er grå.
Mange slitsame dagar såg denna attende på
då han vart skoten bak gjerdet. Med krøkte kne
låg han velt der i kleggsurr. Far stod gripen attved.

Kring denna gråe hesten var allting arbeid og onn.
Vognrammel, solsteik, høylukt, regn, vassing i fonn.
Taumen fila den unge handa. Ho lære fekk
i alle årstider det å styre ein hest som gjekk og gjekk.

– Og no er han komen på ruta. Og kallar fram
alt som var rikt og enkelt, i trollande ham.
Å nei, det er ikkje for moro. Ikkje kjem han med fred.
Spørsmålet står inn strengt og stumt: Kva driv du med?

Kva gjer du ved detta bordet? Er du klar
til møte som barn som før, med alt du har?
Det skjer gjennom ord og papir. Det trenger inn
til det som gjeld om bakom: ،heilt sinn.

Kva kan han svara? Det er som allting lyer.
Han ser mot det mørke auga, og angest sigler som skyer.
Det er hans eiga store og dyre barneverd
som no har møtt opp med hesten og går han nær.

Då møter frå verda *no* det reinaste: Far, godnatt!
Og trykket av lepper på kinnet synest å vera der att.
Velsigna den som strålar ut kraft frå si pute.
Hesten får stå der han står med spørsmål ute.

Av Tarjei Vesaas

Tarjei Vesaas (1897–1970) var frå Vinje i Vest-Telemark, same
bygda som Vinje var frå. I 1934 gifte han seg med Halldis Moren og
slo seg ned på garden Midtbø i Vinje. Vesaas var ofte på reiser i
utlandet, og fekk då mange inntrykk som sette djupe spor i diktinga
hans. Han skreiv over tretti bøker – romanar, noveller, skodespel og
dikt.

heit – hot
eit ljod /jo:/ – sound
å labba (labbar, labba, labba) –
   to plod, to jog

å smella (smeller, smelte,
   smelt/ – to smack
ein kyss /kjyss/ – kiss
sval – cool

eit putevar – pillowcase
å stilna til (stilnar, stilna, stilna) – to become calm
å prenta (prentar, prenta, prenta) – to print
å gløymast (gløymest, gløym-
dest, gløymst) – to be forgotten
i same stund – at once
omsider /om'si:der/ – at last, at
length
ei rute – window pane
å rykkja til (rykkjer or rykker
(optional form), rykte, rykt) –
to give a start
ei leire – clay
å dekkja (dekkjer, dekte, dekt) –
to cover
faren /"fa:ren/ – gone
ein tidbolk /"ti:bålk/ – period of
time
underleg /"underleg/ – strange
å stira (stirer, stirte, stirt) – to
stare
eit syn – sight
slitsam – hard, toilsome
denna, detta – dialect forms for
denne, dette
eit gjerde /"jæ:re/ – fence
å velta (velter, velte, velt) – to
tip over, to knock over
ein klegg – horsefly
eit surr – buzz, hum
gripen – moved
attved – by, beside
ei onn – seasonal work
ein rammel /'rammel/ – rattle,
clatter
ein vognrammel – rattle from a
wagon
ein solsteik – broiling heat of
the sun

ei høylukt – smell of hay
ei vassing – wading
ei fonn /fånn/ – snowdrift
ein taum – rein
å fila (filer, filte, filt) – to file
ei årstid /'å:rsti:/ – season
trollande – bewitched, transformed
ein ham – figure, form
streng – strict, precise
stum – silent
å driva med noko (driv, dreiv,
drive) – to be doing smth.
klar – ready
å skjera (skjer, skar, skore) – to
cut
bakom – behind
eit sinn – mind
å lya = å lyda (lyder, lydde,
lydt) – to listen
ein angest – anxiety
å sigla (sigler, siglde, siglt) – to
sail
ei sky /sjy:/ – cloud
ei barneverd /"ba:rnevæ:r/ –
childhood world
å møta opp – to show up, to
appear
eit trykk – impression; pressure
ei leppe – lip
å vera att – to remain
velsigna /vel'signa/ – blessed
å stråla ut – to radiate
ei kraft – power
å gifta seg med nokon – to
marry smb.
å slå seg ned (slår, slo, slege) –
to settle
eit spor – mark, sign
å setja spor i – to influence
ei novelle /no"velle/ – short
story

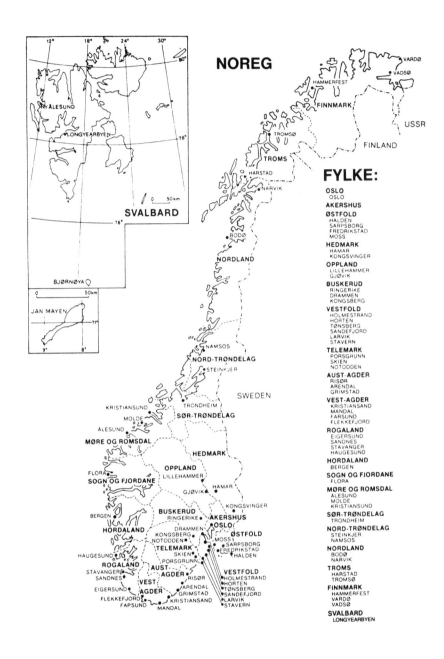

Fig. 21.2 Noreg er delt inn i 19 fylke, og kvart fylke med unntak av Oslo er delt inn i kommunar.

Alphabetical Wordlist

The present wordlist covers the dialogues and reading texts of lessons 1–21. Students are referred to Theodore Slette's Norsk-engelsk ordbok for more extensive definitions and examples of usage.

The letters æ, ø, å are listed at the end of the alphabet in that order.

The gender of nouns is indicated by the appropriate indefinite article (ein, ei, eit), and in the case of irregular nouns all forms are given. This is also true of irregular adjectives and irregular verbs. Verbs are listed with four forms: the infinitive, the present tense, the past tense, and the past participle.

The system used for showing the pronunciation is the same as that used in previous parts of the book. For an explanation see Sounds and Letters, p. 19. Pronunciations are omitted, however, whenever the word is identical with the regular spelling. For all words which are left unmarked it is assumed that:
1. The stress is on the first syllable.
2. The stressed vowel is long if it is final or followed by one consonant, short if followed by more than one consonant.
3. The stressed syllable has Toneme 1 in monosyllables, Toneme 2 in polysyllables if nothing else is indicated.

The stress and toneme mark is always placed in front of the stressed syllable.

A

ein administrasjon /administra-'sjo:n/ – administration
ei adresse /a'dresse/ – address
eit akademisk /aka'de:misk/ borgarbrev – certificate of matriculation
aktiv /'akti:v/ adj. – active
ein alboge – elbow
ein alderdom /'alderdom/ – old age
ein alderspensjon /'alderspen-sjo:n/ – old age pension
aldri – never
alle saman – all of them

alltid /'allti:/ – always
alt adv. – already
alt pron. – everything
altfor /'altfår/ adv. – too
altså /'altså:/ adv. – that is .
alvorleg /al'vå:rleg/ adj. – serious
eit amatørteater /ama'tø:rtea:-ter/ – amateur theater
eit andlet – face
andre pron., num. – other, second
annleis adj. – different
ein angest – anxiety

205

å arbeida (arbeider, arbeidde, arbeidt) – to work
å arbeida hardt – to work hard
Arbeidarpartiet – the Labor Party
arbeidsfolk n.pl. – working people
ein arbeidsgjevar – employer
ei arbeidsgrein – branch of work
ei arbeidsløyse – unemployment
arbeidslaus adj. – unemployed
eit arbeidsområde – field of activity
ei arbeidsoppgåve – task
ein arbeidsplass – job
ein arkitekt /arki'tekt/ – architect
ein arm – arm
ein artikkel (artikkelen, pl. artiklar, artiklane) /ar'tikkel/ – article
arveleg adj. – hereditary
at /att/ conj. – that
att adv. – back; again
attmed prep. – close by, near
attved prep. – by, beside, near
eit auga (auga, pl. augo, augo) – eye
å auka (aukar, auka, auka) – to increase
å ausa opp (auser, auste, aust) – to scoop
Austlandet – Eastern Norway
ei austlandsbygd – ei bygd in Austlandet
av prep. – of
av og til – now and then
ei avdeling /av'de:ling/ – section, department

ei avgift /''a:vjift/ – fee
ei avis /a'vi:s/ – newspaper
avliden, pl. avlidne /'a:vli:den/ adj. – dead, deceased

B

eit bad – bath; bathroom
bad – see å be
ei badstove – room for hot steam baths, sauna
ein bagasje /ba'ga:sje/ – luggage, baggage
bak prep. – behind, in back of
å baka (bakar, baka, baka) – to bake
ei bakeplate – baking sheet
ein bakke – hill
bakom prep., adv. – behind
eit bakstebord – baking table
å banka (bankar, banka, banka) – to beat; to knock
eit barn (barnet, pl. barn or born, barna or borna) – child
eit barnekinn – child's cheek, face
ein barneskule – elementary school
ei barneverd – childhood world
ein bauta /'bæuta/ – monolith
å be(da) (bed, bad, bede) – to ask, to pray
å be til – to worship
ei bedrift /be'drift/ – company
eit bein – leg; bone
beisk adj. – bitter
ein beisk strid – a bitter struggle
å bera (ber, bar, bore) – to carry
eit berg – rock
berre /''bærre/ adv. – only, just
berre bra – just fine

best – see god
å bestemma (bestemmer, be-
    stemte, bestemt) – to decide,
    to determine
    å bestemma seg for – to make
    up one's mind to
ein bestefar (-faren, pl. -fedrar,
    -fedrane) – grandfather
ei bestemor (-mora, pl. -mødrer,
    -mødrene) – grandmother
å betala (betaler, betalte, betalt)
    /be'ta:la/ – to pay
    å betala attende – to pay back
betre – see god
å bia `(biar, bia, bia) – to wait
ein bil – car; cab
eit bilete – picture
ein billett /bi'lett/ – ticket
billeg adj. – cheap
eit bispesete – episcopal resi-
    dence, cathedral city
bjart adj. – bright
ei bjølle – bell
ei bjørk – birch tree
eit blad – newspaper
blank adj. – bright, shining
bleik adj. – pale
å blenkja (blenkjer, blenkte,
    blenkt) – to shine
blind adj. – blind
ei blodprøve – blood test
eit blodtrykk – blood pressure
ei blokk /blåkk/ – writing pad;
    apartment house
ein blom – flower
ein blyant /'bly:ant/ – pencil
å bløma (blømer, blømde,
    blømt) – to flourish, to
    blossom
blå (n. blått) adj. – blue
ei bok (boka, pl. bøker, bøkene)
    – book

ein bolk /bålk/ – period
ein bonde (bonden, pl. bønder,
    bøndene) – farmer
cin bondchcim – farmers' inn,
    hotel
ein bondeklasse – the farmers
ein bondestudent – student
    from the country
eit bord – table
ein bork /bårk/ – bark
bra adj. – good, nice
ei bragd – deed, achievement
    ei lysande bragd – a brilliant
    exploit
å braka (brakar, braka, braka) –
    to bang, to crack
brei adj. – broad, wide
eit brev – letter
eit brevkort – postcard
ein brisk – bunk
ein bror (broren, pl. brør, brør-
    ne) – brother
å bruka (bruker, brukte, brukt) –
    to use
    folk bruker å seia – people
    usually say
ei bru – bridge
brun adj. – brown
ei brur – bride
eit bryst – chest
ei brødskive /''brø:sji:ve/ – slice
    of bread
å bu (bur, budde, butt) – to live
ein bukk – billy-goat, he-goat
ein bunad /''bu:na/ – national
    (regional) costume
ein buskap – cattle, livestock
ei bustadblokk = ei bustad-
    plattform
ei bustadplattform – platform
    containing living quarters,
    cabins

ein butikk /bu'tikk/ – store
ein by – city
ein byborgar /'by:bårgar/ – city-dweller
ein bydialekt /'by:dialekt/ – urban dialect
byfolk /'by:fålk/ n.pl. – townspeople
ei bygd – rural district, community
på bygdene – in the countryside
ein bygdekultur – rural (peasant) culture
eit bygdesamfunn – rural community
ein bygdeungdom – young person from a rural district
å byggja (byggjer, bygde, bygt) – to build
ein byggjekostnad – construction cost
ein bystudent /'by:student/ – student from a city
ein bygning – building
å byrja (byrjar, byrja, byrja) – to begin
å byrja på – to begin at
ein bærbusk – berry bush
å bøya (bøyer, bøygde, bøygt) – to bend; to inflect
ei bøyingsform – grammatical form
både ... og conj. – both ... and (can be used with any number of objects, not just two!)
bårut adj. – wavy, billowy
ein båt – boat
ein båtmotor – boat engine
ein båttype – type of boat

D

ein dag – day
dag ut og dag inn – day after day
god dag – hello; how do you do
midt på dagen – in the middle of the day
til dagleg – ordinarily, every day
eit dagtog – morning (day) train
ein dal – valley
ein dans – dance
å dansa (dansar, dansa, dansa) – to dance
dansk adj. – Danish
på dansk – in Danish
dansketida f. – the Danish period (1400–1814)
daud /dæu/ adj. – dead
dauv /dæu/ adj. – deaf
dauvvoren adj. – indifferent
de pron. pl. – you
De – you (polite form)
deg pron. sing. – you
dei pron. – they
deim pron. – them (old form)
deira pron. – their, theirs
eit dekar /'de:kar/ – decare, ca. ¼ acre
eit dekk – deck
å dekkja (dekkjer, dekte, dekt) – to cover
å dekkja til – to cover up
ein del – part
demokratisk /demo'kra:tisk/ adj. – democratic
den (det, dei) /denn, de:, dæi/ art. – the (when followed by an adj.)

den (det, dei) pron. – it, that, those
denne (dette, desse) pron. – this, these
der adv. – where; there
der borte – over there
deretter /'dæ:retter/ adv. – then, after that
derfor /'dærfår/ adv. – therefore
derifrå /'dæ:rifrå/ adv. – from there
dersom /'dæ:rsåm/ conj. – if
desse – see denne
ein dessert /de'sæ:r/ – dessert
dessutan /'dessu:tan/ adv. – in addition, besides
dessverre /des'værre/ adv. – unfortunately
det – see den
ein detaljhandel /de'talj-/ – retail trade
dette – see denne
di – see din
di ... di adv. conj. – the ... the
ein dialekt /dia'lekt/ – dialect
diger /'di:ger/ adj. – big
eit dikt – poem
ein diktar – author, poet
ei dikting – fiction, poetry
din (di, ditt, dine) pron. –|your, yours
dine – see din
ein direktør /direk'tø:r/ – director
ein distriktshøgskule /di'strikts-/ – regional state college
ein djervskap – daring, boldness
djup /ju:p/ adj. – deep
å dominera (dominerer, domi-

nerte, dominert) /domi'ne:ra/ – to dominate
ei domkyrkje /'dommkjyrkje/ – cathedral
ei dotter (dottera, pl. døtrer, døtrene) – daughter
eit drag – trait, characteristic
å dra(ga) (dreg, drog, drege) – to go; to pull
å dra av stad – to leave
å dra på seg – to put on
å dra sin veg – to leave
å dra til – to go to
å dra ut på – to go on
ein draum – dream
dreg – see å dra
å drikka (drikk, drakk, drukke) – to drink
å driva (driv, dreiv, drive) – to run; to move
å driva idrett – to engage in athletic activities
å driva lagsarbeid – to carry out lagsarbeid
å driva med noko – to be doing smth., to be into smth.
å driva stort – to do big business
ein drosje – taxi
du pron. – you
ein dusj – shower
ein dusk – tassel
ei duskeluve – tasseled cap, esp. a black cap worn by those who have passed the matriculation examination
eit dyr – animal
dyr adj. – expensive
å dyrka (dyrkar, dyrka, dyrka) – to cultivate; to grow; to adore; to worship
eit dødsfall /'døtsfall/ – death

209

å døy (døyr, døydde, døytt) – to die

då adv. – then

då conj. – when (single past event, cf. når)

ein dåd – deed; achievement

dårleg adj. – bad, poor

E

ein edruskap – promotion of temperance

effektiv /'effekti:v/ adj. – effective, efficient

eg pron. – I

eit egg – egg

ei – see ein

å eiga (eig, åtte, ått) – to own

eige – see eigen

eigen (f. eiga, n. eige, pl. eigne) adj. – own

eigentleg adv. – actually, in reality

ein (ei, eit) art. – a, an

ein (ei, eitt) num. – one
den einaste – the only one

ei eining – unit

einskild /''æinsjild/ adj. – individual

eit – see ein

eitt – see ein

å ekspedera (ekspederer, ekspederte, ekspedert) /ekspe'de:-ra/ – to send, to dispatch

ei ekspeditrise /ekspedi'tri:se/ – saleswoman

ein ekspeditør /ekspedi'tø:r/ – salesman, clerk, agent

ein ekspert /ek'spært/ – expert

å eksportera (eksporterer, eksporterte, eksportert) /ekspor-'te:ra/ – to export

ein eksportartikkel /ek'sportar-tikkel/ – export article

ekte adj. – real, genuine

ein eldstad – fireplace

ein elev /e'le:v/ – pupil, student

ein elite /e'li:te/ – elite

eller /''eller/ conj. – or

eit emne – subject; bit of material

eit emblem /em'ble:m/ – emblem

ei endring – change

endå adv. – still, yet
endå mindre – even smaller

ein engros-handel /an'gro:-/ – wholesale business

enkel /''enkel/ (n. enkelt, pl. enkle) adj. – simple

enn conj. – than

eit ensemble /an'sambel/ – cast

eit eple – apple

er /æ:r/ – see å vera

å eta (et, åt, ete) – to eat
for å eta – in order to eat

etter prep. – after
etter kvart – little by little, gradually
etter tur – respectively

ein ettermiddag – afternoon
om ettermiddagen – in the afternoon

eit etternamn – family name, surname

etterpå adv. – afterward

evangelisk-luthersk – evangelical Lutheran

eit eventyr – folktale

evig adj., adv. – everlasting; eternally

F

ein fabrikkeigar /fa'brikkæigar/
– factory owner
ein fabrikktrålar /fa'brikktrå:lar/
– big trawler, factory trawler
eit fag – subject
fager /'fa:ger/ adj. – beautiful
å falla (fell, fall, falle) – to fall
falsk adj. – false
ein familie /fa'mi:lie/ – family
frå familie til familie – from
one family to another
fann – see å finna
ein fantasi /fanta'si:/ – imagination
ein far (faren, pl. fedrar, fedra-
ne) – father
å fara (fer, fór, fare) – to go; to
leave
å fara frå plassen – to leave
the farm
ein fare – danger
faren past part. – gone
ein farge – color
eit farge-TV – color TV
eit farsnamn /'fa:rsnamn/ – father's name
eit farvatn – waters
ein fasong /fa'sång/ – fashion,
cut, style
fast adj. – regular
å fastsetja (fastset, fastsette,
fastsett) /'fastsekjkja/ – to determine
fattig adj. – poor
ein fattigdom – poverty
eit fedreland – mother country
å feira (feirar, feira, feira) – to
celebrate
feit adj. – fat
eit feitt – fat; lard
fell – see å falla

felles /'felles/ adj. – common
femti /'femti/ num. – fifty
fenge past part. of å få, old form
– got
ein ferie /'fe:rie/ – vacation
ein feriestad /'fe:riesta:/ – vacation place
ei ferje – ferryboat
fersk adj. – fresh
ein fest – party; celebration
fest i ungdomslaget – entertainment and dance in the
Young People's Society
på fest – at a party
ein festdag /'festda:g/ – holiday
festleg adj. – festive
å fila (filer, filte, filt) – to file
fin adj. – nice, pretty
å vera fin i målet – to have a
nice voice
det ville vera fint – that
would be nice
ein finger /'finger/ – finger
å finna (finn, fann, funne) – to
find
å finna fram – to find one's way
å finnast (finst, fanst, funnest) –
to be, to exist
ein firedel num. – one fourth
ein fisk – fish
å fiska (fiskar, fiska, fiska) – to
fish, to catch fish
ein fiskar – fisherman
eit fiskaryrke – fisherman's
trade
eit fiske – fishing
ein fiskebåt – fishing boat
eit fiskefelt – fishing ground(s)
ei fiskemengd – quantity of fish
ein fiskereiskap – fishing tackle
ein fiskeressurs – fishing resource

ei fiskerinæring – fishing industry

eit fiskeskjer – fishing ground near a skerry

eit fjell – rocky upland; mountain

ein fjellregel – guideline for hiking in the mountains

fjong /fjång/ adj. – elegant, smart

ein fjord /fjo:r/ – fjord

ein fjordarm – arm of larger fjord

eit fjøs – cow barn, cow-shed

flat adj. – flat

eit flatbrød /'flattbrø:/ – flatbread

flaug – see å *flyga*

dei fleste – most people

flott /flått/ adj. – elegant, smart

eit fly – (air)plane, aircraft

å flyga (flyg, flaug, floge) – to fly

å flytta (flyttar, flytta, flytta) – to move

ei flytting – moving, change of residence

ein flåte – raft, float

folk n.pl. – people
folk flest – the broad majority of the people, people in general

ein folkedans – folk dancing

ein folkehøgskule – folk high school

ein folkemusikk – folk music

eit folketal – population
etter folketalet – in proportion to the population

ei folketrygd – national insurance

ei folkevise – folk song, popular ballad

ein folkeviseleik – dancing accompanying singing of folk songs

ei fonn /fånn/ – snowdrift

for /fårr/ conj. – for, because

for prep. – for
for det meste – for the most part
for å – in order to
for lenge – too long

for . . . sidan adv. – ago

forboden /får'bå:den/ adj. – illegal, forbidden

å fordela (fordeler, fordelte, fordelt) /får'de:la/ – to distribute

foreldre /får'eldre/ n.pl. – parents

ein forfattar /får'fattar/ – author

forholdsvis adv. – relatively

å forklara (forklarer, forklarte, forklart) /får'kla:ra/ – to explain

forkledd /får'kledd/ adj. – disguised

ei form /fårm/ – form
eg er i god form – I'm in good shape

å fornorska (fornorskar, fornorska, fornorska) /får'nårska/ – to Norwegianize

ei fornorsking /får'nårsking/ – Norwegianization

forresten /få'resten/ adv. – by the way

ei forretning /få'retning/ – store, shop; business

å forsterka (forsterkar, forsterka, forsterka) /får'stærka/ – to strengthen

forstod – see å *forstå*

å forstå (forstår, forstod, forstått) /får'stå:/ – to understand
eg forstår – I see

forståeleg /får'stå:eleg/ adj. – understandable

å forsyna seg (forsyner, forsyn-te, forsynt) /får'sy:na/ – to help oneself
å forsyna seg med – to help oneself to
no må du berre forsyna deg – please help yourself

forsynt /får'sy:nt/ adj. – full

å fortelja (fortel, fortalde, fortalt) /får'telja/ – to tell

ein forteljekunst – art of telling a story

ein foss /fåss/ – waterfall

ein fot (foten, pl. føter, føtene) – foot

ein frakk – overcoat

fram /framm/ adv. – ahead, forward
fram til – until

framand adj. – strange

framfor prep. – in front of

ein framgrunn – foreground

framleis adv. – still

ei framstelling /'frammstelling/ – presentation

ei framsyning – performance

ei framtid – future
for framtida – for the future

ein fred – calm; peace

fredeleg adj. – calm, peaceful

å freista (freistar, freista, freista) – to try

fri adj. – free; gratis

ein fridom – freedom

frilyndt adj. – liberal
den frilyndte ungdomsrørsla – the Liberal Association of Youth

eit frimerke /'fri:mærke/ – stamp

frisk adj. – healthy, sound

ein fritidskjole /'fri:ti:skjo:le/ – casual dress

ei fruktdyrking /'fruktdyrking/ – growing fruit

eit frukttre /'fruktre:/ – fruit tree

frå prep. – from

ein fugl – bird

full adj. – complete; full

eit fylke – county

eit fylkeslag – county organization

eit fylkesting – county council

å fylla (fyller, fylte, fylt) – to fill
å fylla sju år – to turn seven

å fyra (fyrer, fyrte, fyrt) – to fire

fæl adj. – terrible

fødd past part. – born

ei føde – nourishment

ein fødsel /'føtsel/ – birth

å følgja (følgjer, følgde, følgt) – to follow
å følgja med – to keep up

ei følgje – consequence

å føra (fører, førte, ført) – to lead
å føra fram – to put on, to present
å føra med seg – to lead to
å føra til – to lead to

ein førelaupar – forerunner, precursor

ei førelesning (førelesninga, pl. førelesningar, førelesninga-ne) – lecture
førelesning om – lecture on

eit føremål – purpose

eit førenamn – given name

først adj. – first
først og fremst – above all
først ikring – not until about

første num. – first

få (comp. færre – fewer, sup. færrast – fewest) adj. – few

å få (får, fekk, fått) – to get
eg får vel – I guess I may as
well
å få bort – to get rid of
å få fatt i – to get hold of
å få fyr i omnen – to light the
fire
å få hug til – to get a mind to,
to like
å få lov til – to be permitted
to
å få å seia for – to become
important for
fått – see å få

G

gammal (n. gammalt, pl. gamle)
adj. – old
ein gammaldans – old-
fashioned dancing
gammalnorsk adj. – Old Norwegian
ein gang – hallway, corridor
på gangen – in the hallway
ein gard /ga:r/ – farm
eit gardsarbeid /'ga:rsarbæi/ –
work on a farm
eit gardsbruk /'ga:rsbru:k/ –
farm
eit gardsnamn /'ga:rsnamn/ –
farm name
å gapa (gaper, gapte, gapt) – to
open one's mouth wide
eit garn – net
ei gate – street
gav – see å gje
ei geit /jæit/ – goat
ein generaldirektør /gener'a:l-/
– managing director

å gifta seg med nokon (gifter,
gifte, gift) /'jifta/ – to marry
smb.
gild /jild/ adj. – kind
ver gild og betal i kassen –
please pay at the cash register
det var gildt – it was much
fun
gje (gjev, gav, gjeve) /je:/ – to
give
å gje ut – to publish
å gje rom for – to give room
for
gjev eg var – I wish I were
gjekk – see å gå
å gjelda (gjeld, galdt, golde)
/'jelda/ – to be valid; to be a
question of
det gjeld følgjande – they are
the following
når det gjeld – as far as . . . is
concerned
gjennom /'jennom/ prep. –
through
å gjennomføra (gjennomfører,
gjennomførte, gjennomført) –
to carry out, to accomplish
å gjennomgå – to go through
å gjera (gjer, gjorde, gjort)
/'je:ra/ – to do
å gjera noko for nokon – to do
smth. for smb.
å gjera seg feit – to get fat
eit gjerde /'jæ:re/ – fence
gjerne /'jærne/ adv. – gladly;
possibly
eg vil gjerne koma – I would
like to come
gjerrig /'jærri/ adj. – stingy
gjort – see å gjera
glad /gla:/ adj. – happy
glad i – fond of

gladeleg adv. – gladly
eit glas – glass
eit glas vatn – a glass of water
ei glede joy
med glede – gladly
å glo (glor, glodde, glott) – to
stare
å gløyma (gløymer, gløymde,
gløymt) – to forget
å gløymast (gløymest, gløym-
dest, gløymst) – to be forgotten
god (comp. betre – better, sup.
best – best) adj. – good
ver så god – please; here you
are; you're welcome
god dag – hello
god tur – have a nice trip
i dei gode gamle dagane – in
the good old days
godsleg adj. – friendly, pleasant
godt /gått/ n. sing. of god –
good, well
dette var godt – this is good
godt unna – far away
ein gong /gång/ – once; time,
occurrence
eit golv /gålv/ – floor
ei golvflate – floor area
ei gran – spruce
granbar n. – spruce twigs with
needles
ei granne – neighbor
å grava (grev, grov, grave) – to
dig
å grava seg ned – to dig
oneself a hole in the snow to
stay in
å greia (greier, greidde, greitt) –
to manage
å greia seg – to get along, to
manage

ei grend – group of farms in
close vicinity to one another
gripen adj. – moved
grov – see å grava
grov adj. – coarse
å vera grov i målet – to have a
coarse voice
grublande adj. – brooding
ein grunn – reason
på grunn av – on account of
eit grunnlag – basis, foundation
grunnlagd – see å grunnleggja
å grunnleggja (grunnlegg,
grunnla, grunnlagt) – to
establish, to found
ei grunnlov – constitution
ein grunnskule – basic school
ei gruppe – group, class
gruv adj. – bent forward,
stooping
grøn adj. – green
å grønka (grønkar, grønka, grønka) – to grow (or become)
green
grønsaker pl. – vegetables
ei grønsakdyrking – truck-
gardening; vegetable gardening
ein grønsakhage – (vegetable)
garden
ein gråstein – gray rock
Gudbrandsdalen – valley in
Eastern Norway
gul adj. – yellow
ei gulrot (gulrota, pl. gulrøter,
gulrøtene) – carrot
ein gut – boy
ein gymnastikksal /gymna-
'stikksa:l/ – gymnasium
å gå (går, gjekk, gått) – to go; to
walk; to leave
å gå att – to recur

215

å gå føre seg – to take place
å gå i – to wear
å gå inn på – to enter, to go into
å gå ned – to decrease
å gå omkring – to walk around
å gå over til – to go over to, to change into
å gå på ein skule – to attend a school
å gå på ski – to go skiing
å gå saman – to merge
å gå til sengs – to go to bed
det gjekk ikkje så bra – it didn't turn out so well
gått – see å gå

H

å ha (har, hadde, hatt) – to have
ha det – bye-bye
ha det bra så lenge – so long
å ha det triveleg – to enjoy oneself
å ha det vondt – to be miserable
å ha god kondisjon – to be in good shape
å ha lov til – to be allowed to
å ha med seg – to bring
å ha å seia – to be important
hadde – see å ha
ein hage – garden
eit hagearbeid – gardening
ei hake – chin
å halda (held, heldt, halde) – to hold
å halda eit kurs – to give a course
å halda fram – to continue

å halda på med – to be doing smth.
hallo /ha'lo:/ interj. – hello
ein hals – throat
eg har vondt i halsen – I've a sore throat
halv adj. – half
ein ham – figure, form
ei hamn – port
eit hamskifte – changing of the outer appearance; transfiguration
han pron. – he
ei hand (handa, pl. hender, hendene) – hand
ein handel /'handel/ – trade, commerce
ein handelsfridom – freedom of trade
ein handelsmann – merchant
ein handelsstad – trading center, store
å handla (handlar, handla, handla) – to buy; to shop; to trade
ein handled – wrist
ei handling – action
å hanga (heng, hang, hange) – to hang
det heng saman med – it is related to
hans pron. – his
eit hav – ocean
havgåande adj. – seafaring
ein havtorsk = skrei – spawning cod that gather on the banks offshore in winter
hei /hæi/ interj. – hi
ein heidenskap – paganism
heil adj. – whole
i det heile – on the whole
heilnorsk adj. – wholly Norwegian

216

heilt adv. – quite
ein heim – home
heim adv. – home
heimanfrå adv. – (away) from home
heime adv. – at home
heimleg adj. – home, homelike
heit adj. – hot
å heita (heiter, heitte, heitt) – to be called
eg heiter – my name is
kva heiter du – what's your name
heldigvis adv. – fortunately
eit helikopterdekk – helicopter pad
heller /'heller/ adv. – either; rather
heller ikkje – nor
ei helse – health
ein helt – hero
ein helteglorie – heroic halo
her /hæ:r/ adv. – here
heve – has (old form)
å hindra (hindrar, hindra, hindra) – to prevent
historie /hi'sto:rie/ f. – history
hit adv. – here
eit hjarta (hjarta, pl. hjarto, hjarto) – heart
å hjelpa (hjelper, hjelpte, hjelpt) /'jelpa/ – to help
det hjelper godt – it helps a lot
ho pron. – she
eit hol /hå:l/ – cavity; hole
ei hofte /'håfte/ – hip
eit hopprenn /'håpprenn/ – jumping competition
ei hoppski /'håppsji:/ – jumping ski
eit hovud /'hå:vu/ – head

hovud – main
ein hovudinstruktør – producer
ein hovudstad – capital
ein hovudtanke – basic idea
å hugsa (hugsar, hugsa, hugsa) – to remember, to recall
humørfylt /hu'mø:rfylt/ adj. – humorous
hundre num. – hundred
ein hunger /'honger/ – hunger
«hurtigruta» – the costal express
ei husleige – rent
ein huslyd – family
ein husmann – cottager, tenant farmer
ein husmannsplass – cotter's farm
ein husmannsskipnad – system of tenant farmers
ein husmannsson – son of a husmann
høfleg adj. – polite
ei høgd – story; floor; height
Høgre – the Conservative Party
høgre adj. – right
til høgre – to the right
på høgre sida – on the right-hand side
ein høgskule – college
høgtidsam adj. – solemn
å høva (høver, høvde, høvt) – to suit, to fit
eit høy – hay
ei høylukt – smell of hay
å høyra (høyrer, høyrde, høyrt) – to hear
å høyra med til – to belong to
å høyra på – to listen to
eit hår – hair

I

i prep. – in
i fjor – last year
i går – yesterday
i staden for – instead of
i utkanten av – on the outskirts of
iallfall adv. – at any rate
ein idé /i'de:/ – idea
ein idrett – athletics, sports
ein idrettsplass – athletic fields
igjen /i'jenn/ adv. – again
ikkje adv. – not
  ikkje enno – not yet
  ikkje på lenge – not for a long time
ein ikkje-røykjar – non-smoker
i orden – all right
ikring /i'kring/ adv. – about
ein immatrikuleringsdag – day of university matriculation
imot /i'mo:t/ prep. – against
eit industriland /indu'stri:land/ – industrial country
ei industrialisering /industriali-'se:ring/ – industrialization
ingen pron. – nobody
ingenstad adv. – nowhere
ingenting pron. – nothing
innanfor adv. – within
ein innbyggjar – inhabitant
å innebera (inneber, innebar, innebore) – to imply
å innehalda (inneheld, inneheldt, innehalde) – to contain
å innføra (innfører, innførte, innført) /'innfø:ra/ – to introduce
ei innmark – cultivated land
ei inntekt – income

eit innslag – element
eit inntrykk – impression
å inspirera (inspirerer, inspirerte, inspirert) /inspi're:ra/ – to inspire
ein institusjon /institu'sjo:n/ – institution
ein instruksjon /instruk'sjo:n/ – instruction
eit instrument /instru'ment/ – instrument
interessant /intre'sant/ adj. – interesting
ei interesse /inter'esse/ – interest
interessert /intre'se:rt/ adj. – interested
å invitera (inviterer, inviterte, invitert) /invi'te:ra/ – to invite

J

ja adv., interj. – yes
  ja, det er det – yes, it is
  ja, det har eg – yes, I have
  ja, det gjer eg – yes, I do
  ja vel – okay
jamvel om conj. – even though
januar /janu'a:r/ – January
ein jarnbanefunksjonær – railroad official
ei jarnbaneline – railway line
ein jarnvegsstasjon – railway station
jau adv., interj. – yes (in answer to a question which contains a doubt or a negation)
ei jente – girl
ein jobb /jåbb/ – job
  på jobben – at work

ei jord /joːr/ – earth; soil
på jorda – on earth
eit jordbruk – agriculture,
farming
eit jordbruksområde – farming
district
eit jordgolv – dirt floor
ei jordlov /ˮjoːrlå:v/ – law relating to land problems
jul f. – Christmas
til jul – before Christmas

K

ein kafeteria /kafeˈteːria/ – cafeteria
kaffi m. – coffee
ei kaffistove – coffee house
ein kai – pier, quay
å kalla (kallar, kalla, kalla) – to
call
å kalla opp – to name after
å kallast (kallast, kallast, kallast) – to be called
kald adj. – cold
ein kalv – calf
ein kamerat /kameˈraːt/ – friend
kan – see å kunna
kanskje adv. – perhaps
ei kantine /kanˮtiːne/ – canteen,
snack bar
eit kapell /kaˈpell/ – chapel
eit kart – map
ein kasse – cash register, cashier's window; box
å kasta (kastar, kasta, kasta) – to
throw
å kasta av – to take off
eit kav – deep, the depths of the
sea

eit kinn /kjinn/ – cheek
ein kinosal /ˈkjiːnosaːl/ – movie
theater
ein kiosk /kjåsk/ – kiosk, newsstand
ei kiste /ˮkjiste/ – trunk, chest
ein kjake – jaw
ei kjedeforretning – chain store
kjem – see å koma
kjend adj. – well-known; acquainted
eg er ikkje kjend der – I'm not
acquainted there
å kjenna (kjenner, kjende,
kjent) – to know; to feel
å kjenna seg framand – to feel
a stranger
kjenslevar adj. – sensitive
ei kjerring – woman, wife
å kjevla ut (kjevlar, kjevla, kjevla) – to roll out with a rolling
pin
ein kjole – dress
kjær adj. – dear
kjære vene – (pretty) please
kjærleg adj. – loving
ein kjærleik – love
ein kjærleikssong – love song
eit kjøken /ˈkjøːken/ – kitchen
ein kjøkenbenk – kitchen
counter
eit kjøleskap – refrigerator
å kjøpa (kjøper, kjøpte, kjøpt) –
to buy
eit kjøt – meat
ei kjøtkake – meat patty
eit kjøtpålegg – meat topping
for bread
klar adj. – ready
klartenkt adj. – clear thinking
ein klasse – grade; class
ei klauv /klæu/ – hoof

å kle (kler, kledde, kledt) – to suit, to fit
dei kler meg ikkje – they don't suit me
klede /"kle:e/ n.pl. – clothes
ein klegg – horsefly
å klippa (klipper, klipte, klipt) – to cut
ei klokke – watch
klokka ni – at 9 o'clock
å kløyva ved (kløyver, kløyvde, kløyvt) – to cut up firewood
å knaka (knakar, knaka, knaka) – to creak, to crack
knapt adv. – scarcely, hardly
knapt nok – just barely, hardly enough
å knasa (knasar, knasa, knasa) – to smash
eit kne – knee
eit knippe – bunch
ein kniv – knife
å knyta (knyter, knytte, knytt) – to tie
å knyta seg til – to be attached to
ein kokk /kåkk/ – cook
å kolna (kolnar, kolna, kolna) – to run cold, to shudder
å koma (kjem, kom, kome) /"kå:ma/ – to come
å koma innom – to drop by
å koma til orde – to appear, to be expressed
ein komfyr /kom'fy:r/ – stove, range
ein kommune /ko'mu:ne/ – municipality (city, town, or village)
eit kommunestyre – local council
ein kompass /kom'pass/ – compass

ei kone /"kå:ne/ – wife; woman
eit konferanserom /konfe'ranseromm/ – conference room
ein konge /"kånge/ – king
eit kongedøme – monarchy
kontant /kon'tant/ adj. – cash
eit kontor /kon'to:r/ – office
ein kontrakt /kon'trakt/ – contract
ein kontraktpris – contract price
å kontrollera (kontrollerer, kontrollerte, kontrollert) /kontro-'le:ra/ – to check, to control
konstitusjonell /konstitusjo-'nell/ adj. – constitutional
ein kopi /ko'pi:/ – copy
ein kopp /kåpp/ – cup
ein kopp kaffi – a cup of coffee
ei korndyrking – grain cultivation
korleis adv. – how
korleis har du det – how are you
korleis står det til – how are you
å kosa seg (kosar, kosa, kosa) – to enjoy oneself
koseleg adj. – nice
ein kost /kåst/ – food
å kosta (kostar, kosta, kosta) /"kåsta/ – to cost
kva kostar denne kjolen – how much is this dress
ein kove /"kå:ve/ – alcove, small room
ei kraft – power
ein kraftblokkbåt /'kraftblåkbå:t/ – fishing boat equipped with a purse net, seine
kraftig adj. – substantial; strong

ei krambu – general store

eit krambuliv – *krambu* culture

kringom adv. – round, about

Kristeleg Folkeparti – the Christian Democratic Party

kristendomen – Christianity

ei krone – the monetary unit of Norway

å krympa i hop (krympar, krympa, krympa) – to shrink

å kryssa (kryssar, kryssa, kryssa) – to cross

krøkt adj. – bent, stooped

ei ku (kua, pl. kyr, kyrne) – cow

kulturell /kultu'rell/ adj. – cultural

ein kulturfaktor /kul'tu:rfaktor/ – cultural factor

å kunna (kan, kunne, kunna) – can, to be able to
du kan nok ikkje – I'm afraid you can't

kunstnarleg adj. – artistic

ein kupé /ku'pe:/ – compartment

kva pron. – what

ein kvadratmeter /kva'dra:tme:ter/ – square meter

ein kvalitet /kvali'te:t/ – quality

kvar adv. – where

kvar pron. – everybody

ein kvardag – weekday, workday

ein kvardagshelt – everyday hero

ein kveld – evening
god kveld – good evening
i kveld – tonight
om kvelden – in the evening

ein kveldsmat – supper

kven pron. – who

kvifor /'kvi:får/ – why

ei kvinne – woman

kvit adj. – white

ein kvote – quota

ei kyrkje /"kjyrkje/ – church

kyrkjeleg adj. – religious, biblical

ein kyss /kjyss/ – kiss

ein kyst /kjyst/ – coast
utanfor kysten – off the coast

å køyra (køyrer, køyrde, køyrt) /"kjøyra/ – to drive
køyr varsamt – drive carefully
å køyra slalåm – to do slalom skiing

ein køyrebane – roadbed; traffic lane

ein kål – cabbage

L

å labba (labbar, labba, labba) – to plod, to jog

eit lag – team; company; organization

å laga (lagar, laga, laga) – to make
det lagar seg vel – things will be all right, I guess

eit lagsarbeid /'la:gsarbæi/ – work carried out by the (ung-doms)laget

ein lampe – lamp

ein lampett /lam'pett/ – bracket lamp, sconce

eit land – country

ei landlege – time ashore because of bad weather

ein landhandel – general store
ein landsdel /'lansde:l/ – region
eit landsnamn /'lansnamn/ – name of a country
ein landssamskipnad /'lans-samsji:pna/ – national organization
lang adj. – long
eit langrenn – cross-country race
langs prep. – along
ein langtur – long trip
langvarig adj. – long-lasting
å lata (lèt, lét, late) – to let
lat oss byrja med – let us start with
latinsk /la'ti:nsk/ adj. – Latin
å lava (laver, lavde, lavt) – to hang down in rich clusters
ledig adj. – vacant
ei lefse – kind of soft flatbread buttered and served folded or rolled
ein legg – lower leg (between the knee and the foot)
å leggja (legg, la, lagt) to lay
å leggja ned – to desert
å leggja om – to change, to reorganize
å leggja til grunn – to use as a basis
å leggja utpå – to set out on
å leggja vekt (vinn) på – to emphasize
lei adj. – sorry, unhappy
eg er lei for at – I'm sorry that
leiande adj. – leading
ein leiar – leader
å leiga (leiger, leigde, leigt) – to rent, to lease
å leiga ut – to let, to rent out
ei leige – rent

ein leik – play, playing
å leika (leikar, leika, leika) – to play
å leika seg – to play together
ein leikeplass – playground
ei leire – clay
å leita (leitar, leita, leita) – to look for, to search
å leita etter – to look for
på leiting etter – in search of
ei lekse – homework, assignment; lesson
ein lenestol – easy chair
lenge adv. – a long time, long
å lengta etter (lengtar, lengta, lengta) – to long for
ei leppe (or lippe) – lip
å lesa (les, las, lese) – to read
å lesa lekser – to do one's homework
å lesa om – to read about
eit leserom – reading room
eit lesestoff – reading material
lett adj. – easy; light (in weight)
lettdriven adj. – easily operated or run
å leva (lever, levde, levt) – to live
å leva av – to live off
å leva for – to live for
levande adj. – living, vital
ein levestandard – standard of living
ein leveveg – way to make a living, employment
ei li – hillside
å liggja (ligg, låg, lege) – to lie, to be located
å lika (liker, likte, likt) – to like
å lika seg – to like it
likevel /like've:l/ adv. – all the same

liksom /'liksåm/ adv., conj. – like, as; as if
ein linjal – ruler
liten (comp. mindre – smaller, sup. minst – smallest) adj. – small, little
litt pron. – some, a little
litt etter litt – little by little
ein livbåt – lifeboat
eit ljod /jo:/ – sound; voice
ljos /jo:s/ adj. – light
ein ljå /jå:/ – scythe
loden /"lå:den/ adj. – hairy
Lofothavet /"Loffo:tha:ve/ – the Lofoten Sea
lokal /lo'ka:l/ adj. – local
eit lokallag – local organization
ei lokalavis – local newspaper
ei lov /lå:v/ – law, regulation
eit lovord – word of praise
ei lue – cap
ei luft – air
ein lugar /lu'ga:r/ – cabin
å lyda (lyder, lydde, lytt) – to listen; to obey
eit lynne – character, temperament
lys adj. – light, bright
å lysa (lyser, lyste, lyst) – to shine
ei lysing – advertisement
ei lyspære – light bulb
ei lyst – desire
  eg har lyst på kaffi – I would like coffee
  eg har lyst til å kjøpa bilen – I would like to buy the car
ei lækjarhjelp – medical treatment
å læra (lærer, lærte, lært) – to learn; to teach
  å læra opp – to train, to instruct

eit lærarrom – teachers' common room, lounge
ein lærarskule – teachers training college, college of education
ei lære – doctrine
ein læremeister – teacher
lærerik adj. – informative, instructive
å løna (løner, lønte, lønt) – to pay (wages, salary)
  å løna seg – to pay, to be profitable
  det løner seg – it pays
å løysa (løyser, løyste, løyst) – to solve
  å løysa inn – to buy
  å løysa opp – to dissolve
låg – see å liggja
eit lån – loan
å låna (låner, lånte, lånt) – to borrow; to lend
  å låna hjå – to borrow from
  å låna nokon – to lend smb.
eit lånord – loanword
eit lår – thigh
ein låve – barn

M

ein mage – stomach
mager /'ma:ger/ adj. – thin
  mager jord – lean (or poor) soil
ein makrell /ma'krell/ – mackerel
ei makt – power
å makta (maktar, makta, makta) – to manage
mang (n. mangt, pl. mange, comp. fleire, sup. flest) adj. – many

mange adj. pl. – many. See *mang*

mangt adj. n. – see *mang*

ein mann, pl. menn – man

ein mannsbunad /'mannsbu:na/ – man's national costume

mat m. – food

å mata (matar, mata, mata) – to feed

å mata seg – to feed oneself

ein matskikk /"ma:tsjikk/ – eating custom

med /me:/ prep. – with

medan /"me:an/ conj. – while

ein medlem, pl. medlemer – member

ei medlemsavgift – membership fee

meg pron. – me

å meina (meiner, meinte, meint) – to think, to be of the opinion that

meir – see *mykje*

å mekra (mekrar, mekra, mekra) – to bleat

å melda frå om (melder, melde, meldt) – to report, to tell

ei melding – notice, message

mellom prep. – between

mellomalderen m. – the Middle Ages

eit mellomrom – interval

med jamne mellomrom – at regular intervals

den mellomste – the middle one

men /menn/ conj. – but

ei mengd – a lot of

eit menneske – human being, person

ein menneskerett – human right

ein merg – marrow

mest – see *mykje*

mi – see *min*

ein middag /'middag/ – dinner

eit miljø /mil'jø:/ – surroundings; setting

ein million /milli'o:n/ – million

min (mi, mitt, mine) /minn/ pron. – my, mine

mindre /'mindre/ – see *liten*

mindreverdig /'mindreværdi/ adj. – inferior

mine – see *min*

eit minne – memory

til minne om – in memory of

å minna om (minner, minte, mint) – to remind of

å missa (misser, miste, mist) – to lose

mitt – see *min*

eit mjøl – flour

ei mjølk – milk

ein modell /mo'dell/ – fashion, style; model

moderne /mo'dærne/ adj. – modern

modfallen adj. – discouraged, downcast

å modnast (modnast, modnast, modnast) – to ripen

ei mold /måld/ – soil, earth

eit monarki /monar'ki:/ – monarchy

ei mor (mora, pl. mødrer, mødrene) – mother

ein morgon /"mårgon/ – morning

i morgon – tomorrow

om morgonen – in the morning

ei moro – fun

ei morshand /'mo:rshand/ – mother's hand

224

eit mosjonsrom /mo'sjo:ns-romm/ – room for physical exercise

mot prep. – against

ein mote – fashion, style

ikkje på moten – not in style

eit motiv /mo'ti:v/ – subject

eit musikkrom /mu'sikkromm/ – music room

mykje (comp. meir – more, sup. mest – most) adj. – much

meir enn nokon annan – more than anybody else

ei myrsnipe – sandpiper

møblar n.pl. – furniture

eit mønster /'mønster/ – model, pattern

mørk adj. – dark

å møta (møter, møtte, møtt) – to meet

å møta opp – to show up, to appear

på eit møte – at a meeting

eit møtehus – assembly hall

møtte – see å møta

må – see å måtta

eit mål – goal; language; one thousand square meters

eit målblad – nynorsk newspaper

målfolk n.pl. – adherents of nynorsk

eit målføre – dialect

eit mållag – nynorsk linguistic society

ei målreising – language movement

ei målrørsle – linguistic movement

ei målsak – language movement

eit måltid – meal

ein månad (månaden, månader, månadene) – month

ein måte – way

på ein måte – in a way

på ingen måte – not at all

på mange måtar – in many ways

på same måten som – in the same way as

å måtta (må, måtte, måtta) – must, to have to

N

naken (n. nake, pl. nakne) adj. – bare, naked

ein nakke – (back of) neck

ein nase – nose

nasjonal /nasjo'na:l/ adj. – national

ei nasjonalforsamling – national assembly, parliament

ein nasjonalromantikk – national romanticism, national feeling

ei natt (natta, pl. netter, nettene) – night

god natt – good night

eit nattog – night train

ein natur /na'tu:r/ – nature, scenery

naturleg /na'tu:rleg/ adj. – natural, logical

ei naud /næu/ – difficulty, peril

naudsynt adj. – necessary

nedanfor adv., prep. – further down, below

ned adv. – down

nedi adv. – down in

nedlagd /'ne:lagd/ adj. – deserted

ein nedlagd gard – a deserted farm

225

nedtyngd /'ne:tyngd/ adj. – weighed down

nemleg adv. – namely, that is, you see

å nemna (nemner, nemnde, nemnt) – to mention

no adv. – now

nok /nåkk/ adv. – enough

noko – see nokon

nokolunde adv. – somewhat, to a certain degree

nokon (f.noka, n. noko, pl. nokre) /"nå:kon/ pron. – some-(one), something, any, anything

nokre få – a few

nordisk /'nordisk/ adj. – Nordic, Scandinavian

Nordisk Råd – the Nordic Council

ein Nordlands-båt – special type of boat from the county of Nordland

ein nordmann /"no:rmann/ – Norwegian

nordpå /'no:rpå/ adv. – in the north

Nordsjøen – the North Sea

å normera (normerer, normerte, normert) /når'me:ra/ – to standardize, to normalize

norsk /nårsk/ adj. – Norwegian

Den norske kyrkja – the Norwegian Church

Det Norske Teatret – theater in Oslo that gives all performances in nynorsk

Norskekysten – the Norwegian coast

ei not (nota, pl. nøter, nøtene) – seine, trawl net

eit notbruk – the use of seine

ei novelle /no"velle/ – short story

eit nummer /'nommer/ – number

ny (n. nytt, pl. nye) adj. – new

ein nynorsk /"ny:nårsk/ – New Norwegian

ei nynorskavis – newspaper in nynorsk

å nytta (nyttar, nytta, nytta) – to use

det nyttar ikkje – it's useless

nær adv. – close

ei næringsgrein – branch of industry

eit næringsliv – economic life of a nation, esp. commercial and industrial life, trade, industry

ein næringsveg – (branch of) trade (or industry)

å nærma seg (nærmar, nærma, nærma) – to get close to, to approach

nørdst /nørst/ adj. – northernmost

å nå (når, nådde, nått) – to reach

når conj. – when (referring to what usually happens or happened or what will happen in the future)

O

obligatorisk /obliga'to:risk/ adj. – compulsory

ein odelsbonde /'o:delsbonde/ – allodial owner

ein odelsrett /'o:delsrett/ – allodial rights

offisiell /åfisi'ell/ adj. – official

ofte (comp. oftare, oftast) /''åfte/ adv. – often

og /å:g/ conj. – and

også /''åkså/ adv. – also

oktober /ok'to:ber/ – October

oliven /o'li:ven/ adj. – olive

eit oljeavfall – oil residue

ei oljeboring – drilling for oil

eit oljeeventyr – oil adventure

eit oljefelt – oil field

ei oljeleiting – oil exploration

eit oljesøl – oil slick

om conj. – if, whether

om lag /om 'la:g/ – approximately

omkring /om'kring/ adv. – about

ein omn /åmn/ – stove; furnace

ei omlegging /'omlegging/ – change, rearrangement

eit område – area, region

å omsetja (omset, omsette, omsett) – to translate

omsider /om'si:der/ adv. – at length, at last

eit omskifte /''omsjifte/ – change

eit omsyn – consideration

ein onkel /'onkel/ – uncle

ei onn /ånn/ – seasonal work

å opna (opnar, opna, opna) – to open

ei opningsframsyning – opening performance

opp /opp/ adv. – up

å oppdaga (oppdagar, oppdaga, oppdaga) – to discover

oppe /''oppe/ adv. – upstairs

å oppfatta (oppfattar, oppfatta, oppfatta) – to conceive, to understand

ei oppgåve – task; purpose; exercise

eit opphav – origin

ein oppkjøpar – buyer

å oppleva (opplever, opplevde, opplevt) – to experience

ei opplysning /opp'ly:sning/ – piece of information

eit opprør – protest, rebellion

oppteken (n. oppteke, pl. opptekne) /'oppte:ken/ – occupied, taken

oppå prep., adv. – upon

eit ord /o:r/ – word

eit ordtak /''o:rta:k/ – proverb, saying

ein organisasjon /årganisa'sjo:n/ – organization

eit orgel /'årgel/ – organ

å orka (orkar, orka, orka) – to manage

orsak /''å:rsa:k/ – excuse me

osv. = og så vidare – and so forth

ein ost – cheese

eit overhovud – head

å overtaka (overtek, overtok, overteke) – to take over

P

å pakka inn (pakkar, pakka, pakka) – to wrap up

ein pakke – parcel

ei panne – forehead

eit par – couple

ein parkeringsplass – parking lot

å peika ut (peikar, peika, peika) – to point out, to distinguish

ein peis – fireplace

pengar /''pengar/ m.pl. – money

ei pensjonsordning /pen'sjo:ns-
årdning/ – pension system
ein periode /peri'o:de/ – period
ein person /per'so:n/ – person
ei pipe – chimney; pipe
ein pipekonsert – jeering
å pla (plar, pla, pla) – to be
accustomed to, to be used to
vi plar ha – we usually have
å plaga (plagar, plaga, plaga) –
to bother
ei plante – plant
ein plass – place; room, space
god plass – plenty of room
ei plattform /'plattfårm/ – platform
ein plen – lawn
ein plenklippar – lawn mower
ei plikt – duty
ei plomme – plum
ein politikk /poli'tikk/ – policy;
politics
politisk /po'li:tisk/ adj. – political
populær /popu'læ:r/ adj. – popular
ein portier /porti'e:/ – doorman
ein porto /'porto/ – postage
ein post /påst/ – mail
eit postkontor /'påstkonto:r/ –
post office
ei potet /po'te:t/ – potato
ein prat – talk, chat
å prata (pratar, prata, prata) – to
talk, to chat
å prega (pregar, prega, prega) –
to mark
å prenta (prentar, prenta, prenta) – to print
ein prest – minister, clergyman
ei primærnæring /pri'mæ:r-
næ:ring/ – primary industry

ein pris – price; prize
privat /pri'va:t/ adj. – private
ein produksjon /produk'sjo:n/ –
production
produktiv /'proddukti:v/ – productive
ein prosent /pro'sent/ – percent
å prøva (prøver, prøvde, prøvt)
– to try
ei prøve – test; sample
eit prøverom – fitting room
ein puls – pulse
eit putevar – pillowcase
på prep. – on, in, at
eit pålegg /''på:legg/ – anything
laid or spread on buttered
bread to make a smørbrød
å påleggja nokon (pålegg, påla,
pålagt) /'på:legjgja/ – to impose on smb., to tell smb. to
ei påske – Easter
ei påskehelg – Easter holidays

R

ein rabatt /ra'batt/ – discount
ein rammel /'rammel/ – rattle,
clatter
rask adj. – quick, fast
raud /ræu/ adj. – red
ei reform /re'fårm/ – reform
reformasjonen /refårma'sjo:nen/
– the Reformation
ein regel /'re:gel/ – rule; guideline
som regel – as a rule
ei regjering /re'je:ring/ – government; Cabinet
ein regjeringsmedlem – member of the Cabinet
ein regjeringssjef – head of government

å regna (regnar, regna, regna) – to rain

rein adj. – clean

å reisa (reiser, reiste, reist) – to travel; to erect, to build
  å reisa attende – to go back
  å reisa med båt – to travel by boat
  å reisa seg opp – to get up, to rise

ei reise – journey

eit reisebyrå – travel agency

eit reisegods – baggage, luggage

ei reisetid – traveling time

eit reisingsarbeid – restoration of the essentially Norwegian in language and culture

ei rekkje – row
  i fremste rekkja – at the front of the line

å rekna med (reknar, rekna, rekna) – to count on
  å verta rekna som – to be considered as

rekommandert /rekoman'de:rt/ adj. – registered

ein religion /religi'o:n/ – religion

eit repertoar /repærto'a:r/ – repertoire

ein representant /represen'tant/ – representative

ein rest – rest, remainder

ein restriksjon /restrik'sjo:n/ – restriction

rett adj. – right, correct; upright
  du har rett – you're right
  rett fram – straight ahead
  rett overfor – right across from
  rett som det var – in a little while, then all at once

ein rett – dish, course

å retta seg opp (rettar, retta, retta) – to straighten one's back

rettkomen adj. – just, legitimate

ei retning – direction

ein revolusjon /revolu'sjo:n/ – revolution

ein rikdom – wealth

eit riksvåpen /'riksvå:pen/ – national coat of arms

rimeleg adj. – reasonable

ein ring – circle, ring

å ringja (ringjer, ringde, ringt) – to call

eit riveskaft – rake handle

å ro (ror, rodde, rott) – to row

ein roman /ro'ma:n/ – novel

romantisk /ro'mantisk/ adj. – romantic

romsleg adj. – spacious

ei rorbu – fisherman's shanty

ein ros – praise

ei rose – rose

rotut adj. – disorderly, messy

ein rudning – clearing, piece of land

ruskut adj. – rough, stormy

å rusla (ruslar, rusla, rusla) – to walk slowly

ei rute – window pane

å røda (røder, rødde, rødt) – to talk, to discuss

ein rømmegraut – cream porridge

ei rørsle – movement

å røykja (røykjer, røykte, røykt) – to smoke

ein røykjekupé – smoking compartment

røynd adj. – experienced

røynde fjellfolk – experienced mountain people

å røysta (røystar, røysta, røysta) – to vote

å rydda ut (ryddar, rydda, rydda) – to kill off, to exterminate

ryddig adj. – tidy

å rydja (ryd, rudde, rudt) – to clear (land of trees, bushes, and stones)

ein rygg – back
rett rygg – straight back
med rett rygg – upright
eg har vondt i ryggen – I have a sore back

å ryka på (ryk, rauk, roke) – to attack

å rykkja til (rykkjer, rykte, rykt) – to give a start

eit råsegl – square sail

S

sa – see å seia

ei saft – juice

å sakna (saknar, sakna, sakna) – to miss

ein salat /sa'la:t/ – salad (lettuce)

ein salong /sa'lång/ – lounge

eit salongbord /sa'långbo:r/ – coffee table

saman /'sa:man/ adv. – together

ein samanheng – connection

å samanlikna (samanliknar, samanlikna, samanlikna) – to compare

å samarbeida med (samarbeider, samarbeidde, samarbeidt) – to cooperate with, to collaborate with

eit samband – contact, communication
i samband med – in connection with

same adj. – same
med det same – immediately

eit samfunn – society; community

ei samkome – meeting, gathering

å samla inn (samlar, samla, samla) – to gather, collect

ein samlingsfaktor – uniting factor

ei sanning – truth

sams adj. – common

samstundes adv. – simultaneously, at the same time

eit samsvar – accordance
i samsvar med – in accordance with

å samsvara med (samsvarar, samsvara, samsvara) – to correspond to

sat – see å sitja

ein scene /''se:ne/ – stage

ei segn – legend

å seia (seier, sa, sagt) – to say

seig adj. – slow, tough

sein adj. – late

eit sekretariat /sekretari'a:t/ – secretariat

eit sel – living-house of a mountain outfarm

å senda (sender, sende, sendt) – to send

ei seng – bed

ei sengeeining – bed unit

ein sengeplass – bed

eit senter (senteret, pl. senter, sentra) /'senter/ – center

Senterpartiet – the Center Party

230

ei sentralisering /sentrali'se:r-ing/ – centralization
eit sentrum /'sentrum/ – center
ser – see å sjå
ein serie /'se:rie/ – series
eit sesongfiskeri /se'sångfiskeri/ – seasonal fishing
ei seter (setra, pl. setrar, setrane) /'se:ter/ – summer dairy (usually in the mountains)
å setja (set, sette, sett) /''sekjkja/ – to set, to put
å setja spor i – to influence
si – see sin
ei side – page; side
ved sida av – in addition to; next door
å sigla (sigler, siglde, siglt) – to sail
å sigra (sigrar, sigra, sigra) – to win, to prevail
ei sild – herring
eit sildemjøl – herring meal
sin (si, sitt, pl. sine) /sinn/ pron. – his, her, its, their (own)
sine – see sin
eit sinn – mind
sinna adj. – angry
sist adj. – last
å sitja (sit, sat, sete) – to sit
å sitja oppe – to sit up
å sitja rett – to sit straight; to fit well
sitt – see sin
ein sjekk – check
sjeldan adv. – seldom
sjuk adj. – sick, ill
ein sjukdom – disease
ei sjukestove – nurse's office, infirmary
sjølveigande adj. – freeholding
ein sjølveigande bonde – freeholding farmer
sjølvsagt adv. – of course, obviously
å sjå (ser, såg, sett) – to see
dette ser bra ut – this looks good
det ser ut til – it looks as if
å sjå ned på – to look down on
å sjå på – to think of; to look at
å sjå seg nøydd til – to feel forced to
å sjå seg om – to look around
å sjå ut på – to look out at
å sjå ut som – to look like
å skaffa (skaffar, skaffa, skaffa) – to provide
å skaffa seg – to get hold of
skakk adj. – out of plumb, not perpendicular
på skakke – on one side
ei skam – shame
skal – see å skulla
å skapa (skaper, skapte, skapt) – to create
ei skapingsevne – creative ability
ein skatt – tax, income tax
skaut – see å skyta
ei skei /sjæi/ – spoon
skeiv /skjæiv/ adj. – crooked
skeiv rygg – curvature of the spine, crooked back
ei ski /sji:/ – ski
ein skikk /sjikk/ – custom
å skildra (skildrar, skildra, skildra) /''sjildra/ – to describe, to depict
ei skildring (skildringa, pl. skildringar, skildringane) – description

å skilja (skil, skilde, skilt) /''sji-lja/ – to distinguish
ein skilling /'sjilling/ – obsolete coin
ein skilnad /''sjilna/ – difference
eit skilt /sjilt/ – sign
ei skiløype /'sji:løype/ – ski track, ski trail
ein skismurning /'sji:smurning/ – ski wax
ein skitype /'sji:ty:pe/ – type of ski
eit skip /sji:p/ – ship
å skipa (skipar, skipa, skipa/ /''sji:pa/ – to establish
ein skipsfart /'sjipsfa:rt/ – shipping industry
ei skive /''sji:ve/ – slice of bread`
eit skjer /sje:r/ – skerry, rock
å skjera (skjer, skar, skore) /''sje:ra/ – to cut
å skjøna (skjønar, skjøna, skjøna) /''sjø:na/ – to understand, to realize
eit skodespel – play
ein skodespelar – actor
ein skog – woods, forest
eit skogbruk – forestry, lumbering
ei skogsak – protection and preservation of forest
ein skolt /skålt/ – head
skral adj. – poor
eit skriftmål /'skriftmå:l/ – written language
å skrika (skrik, skreik, skrike) – to shout
skrinn adj. – barren, poor
  skrinn jord – barren soil
å skriva (skriv, skreiv, skrive) – to write

å skriva noko – to charge smth.
eit skrivepapir – writing paper
skrivesaker f.pl. – writing material
ei skulder /'skulder/ – shoulder
ein skule – school
  på skulen – at school
eit skulehus – school building
  sjølve skulehuset – the school building itself
ein skulelækjar – school doctor
skulepengar m.pl. – tuition
ei skuleplikt – compulsory school attendance
eit skulesystem – educational system
å skulla (skal, skulle, skulla) – to be going to
  det skal vera visst – to be sure, decidedly so
  eg skulle ha – I would like to have
ei sky /sjy:/ – cloud
skyldfolk /''sjyldfålk/ n.pl. – relatives, kinsmen
å skyta (skyt, skaut, skote) /''sjy:ta/ – to shoot
ein skyttar /''sjyttar/ – hunter
eit slag – kind, sort
  kva slags – what kind
ei slalåmski /'sla:låmsji:/ – slalom ski
ei slekt – family
  i slekt med – related to
slik pron., adj., adv. – such; thus, so
  slik som i – as in
slik at conj. – so that
eit slit – hard work, toil
slitsam adj. – toilsome, hard
eit slott /slått/ – palace

ein slutt – end
 i slutten av – at the end of
 til slutt – finally
å slå (slår, slo, slått) – to strike;
 to cut
 å slå gras – to cut grass
 å slå saman – to combine
 å slå seg ned – to settle
ein slått – mowing
å smaka (smakar, smaka, smaka) – to taste
 å smaka på noko – to taste
 smth.
å smella (smeller, smelte,
 smelt) – to smash
eit smør – butter
eit smørbrød – sandwich (open-
 faced)
ei småkake – cooky
småved m. – kindling
eit snakk – talk
å snakka (snakkar, snakka,
 snakka) – to speak, to talk
ein snarkjøpsbutikk – self-
 service store
snart adv. – soon
 så snart eg kan – as soon as I
 can
snill adj. – kind
 ver så snill – please
 det var veldig snilt av deg –
 that's very kind of you
å snu (snur, snudde, snutt) – to
 turn
 å snu i tide – to turn in time
 å snu seg – to turn around
ei snurpenot – purse net, purse
 seine
ein snø – snow
ein snøggbåt – fast ship
ei snøyde – desolate region
so adv. – so, then (old form)

ein sofa /'so:fa/ – sofa
ei soge /''så:ge/ – story, yarn
ein solsteik – broiling heat of
 the sun
som /såmm/ pron. – who, which,
 that
som om /såmm/ conj. – as if
ein sommar (sommaren, pl.
 somrar, somrane) – summer
 om sommaren – in the
 summer
somme pron. – some (people)
ein son (sonen, pl. søner, sønene) – son
eit songspel – musical
sosial /sosi'a:l/ adj. – social
Sosialistisk Venstreparti – the Socialist Left Party
å sova (søv, sov, sove) – to sleep
eit soverom – bedroom
spanande adj. – exciting
å spara (sparer, sparte, spart) –
 to save
ein spegel – mirror
ein spekemat – salt-cured meat
å spela (speler, spelte, spelt) –
 to play
 å spela orgel – to play the
 organ
eit spelerom – game room
ei spelferd – tour
ei spelform – style, form
eit spelstykke – play
spesialisert /spesiali'se:rt/ adj. –
 specialized
eit spor – mark, sign
spreidd adj. – spread
ei spreiing – spread, diffusion
sprek adj. – active, vigorous
å springa (spring, sprang,
 sprunge) – to run
eit språk – language

ein språkpolitikar – politician involved in the language conflict

ein språkstrid – language conflict

spurde – see å spørja

å spørja (spør, spurde, spurt) – to ask

å spørja etter – to ask for

St. /sankt/ – Saint (St.)

ein stad (staden, pl. stader, stadene) – place

eit stadnamn – place name

ein standard /'standar/ – standard, quality

å stanga (stangar, stanga, stanga) – to butt, to push with horns

ein stat – state

Statens Lånekasse – the State Loan Office

ei statskyrkje /'sta:tskjyrkje/ – state church

ein statsminister – prime minister

ein statsråd – Cabinet minister, member of the Cabinet

eit statsråd – Cabinet meeting

ei steinrøys – heap of stones, cairn

å stella (steller, stelte, stelt) – to work

å stella med – to take care of

ei stemning – mood

å stengja (stengjer, stengde, stengt) – to close

sterk adj. – strong

å stikka ut (stikk, stakk, stukke) – to poke out

ei stille – silence

stilistisk /sti'listisk/ adj. – stylistic

å stilna til (stilnar, stilna, stilna) – to become calm

å stira (stirer, stirte, stirt) – to stare

stod – see å stå

ei stode /''stå:e/ – situation

å stogga (stoggar, stogga, stogga) /''stågga/ – to stop

ein stol – chair

stor (comp. større, sup. størst) adj. – big, great

for stor – too big

ein storleik – size

ein storm /stårm/ – storm

storparten av – the greater part of, the majority of

Stortinget n. – the Parliament

stortingsbygningen m. – the Parliament building

ei stove /''stå:ve/ – living room

straks adv. – immediately

ei strand – beach

streng adj. – strict, precise

ein strid – conflict, controversy

eit strok /strå:k/ – area

eit grisgrendt strok – sparsely populated area

eit strå – stem or stalk of tall grass

å stråla ut (strålar, stråla, stråla) – to radiate

ein stubb – yarn, short tale

ein studentheim /stu'denthæim/ – residence hall, dorm

å studera (studerer, studerte, studert) /stu'de:ra/ – to study

å studera vidare – to continue with one's study

eit studiearbeid /'stu:diearbæi/ – studying activity

eit studium (studiet, pl. studium, studia) /'stu:dium/ – study

234

stum adj. – silent
ei stund – while, time, moment
  frå første stund – right from
  the start
  i same stund – at once
  om ei lita stund – in a little
  while
stundom adv. – now and then
stur adj. – solemn
stutt adj. – short
stygg adj. – ugly
eit styggevêr – nasty weather
eit stykke – piece; copy
  eit stykke herifrå – some distance from here
  eit stykke sør for – a little
  ways south of
å styra (styrer, styrte, styrt) – to
  govern; to steer
ei styreform – form of government
ein styreformann – chairman of
  the board
styremaktene f.pl. – the authorities
styven adj. – stupid
å stø (stør, stødde, støtt) – to
  support
ein stønad – support, relief
større – see stor
å støypa (støyper, støypte,
  støypt) – to cast
å stå (står, stod, stått) – to stand
ein sundag /'sunda:g/ – Sunday
  på sundagar – on Sundays
sundsprengd /'sundsprængd/
  adj. – put at variance
Sunnmørs-bunad – bunad from
  Sunnmøre
ei suppe – soup
eit surr – buzz, hum
sval adj. – cool
eit svar – answer

å svara (svarar, svara, svara) –
  to answer
å svara på – to answer
svart-kvitt adj. – black and
  white
å svida (svid, sveid, svide) – to
  hurt, to burn
svolten (n. svolte, pl. svoltne)
  /''svålten/ adj. – hungry
svært adv. – very
ein symjehall – swimming pool
eit syn – opinion; sight
  etter mitt syn – in my opinion
eit syltety – jam
å syna (syner, synte, synt) – to
  show
å synast (synest, syntest, synst)
  – to think, to be of the opinion that
  å synast om – to like
  eg synest at – I think that
  det synest å gå i retning av –
  it seems to go in the direction
  of
å syngja (syng, song, sunge) – to
  sing
sysken /''sysjen/ pl. – brothers
  and sisters
å sysselsetja (sysselset, sysselsette, sysselsett) – to employ
ei syster – sister
å syta for (syter, sytte, sytt) – to
  provide
særleg adv. – particularly
særmerkt adj. – distinctive
særprega adj. – distinctive
ei særstode – exceptional position
så adv. – then; besides
eit såkorn – seed
såleis adv. – thus

235

T

eit tak – ceiling; roof
å ta(ka) (tek, tok, teke) – to take
  å ta båt – to go by boat
  å ta ein skitur – to go on a ski trip
  å ta fly – to go by air
  å ta fram – to take out
  å ta i bruk – to take into use
  å ta med – to bring
  å ta omsyn til andre – to have consideration for others
  ta plass – sit down, take your seats
  å ta til – to begin
  å ta til å gjelda – to become effective
takk – thanks, thank you
  takk for i kveld – thank you for this evening
  takk for maten – thank you for the food
  takk for sist – 'thanks for last time'
  takk skal du ha – thank you
  mange takk – many thanks
  tusen takk – thanks a lot
  sjølv takk – the same to you
ei taklampe – ceiling light
eit tal – number
  på 1700-talet – in the 18th century
å tala (talar, tala, tala) – to speak, to talk
eit talemål – spoken language, speech
ei tann (tanna, pl. tenner, tennene) – tooth
ei tante – aunt
eit tap – loss
ein teatersjef /te'a:tersje:f/ – theater manager

å teikna (teiknar, teikna, teikna) – to design; to draw
ei teikning – design; drawing
tek – see å taka
ein tekst – text
ein telefon /tele'fo:n/ – telephone
eit telefonnummer – telephone number
å tena (tener, tente, tent) – to serve
  å tena til – to help to, to serve to
ein tendens /ten'dens/ – tendency, trend
eit tenesteyrke – service industry
å tenkja (tenkjer, tenkte, tenkt) – to think
  å tenkja på – to think of
ein tettstad – densely populated area, town
ei tjørn /kjø:rn/ – pond, small lake
ti num. – ten
ei tid – time
  ho hadde ikkje tid til – she didn't have the time to
  før i tida – formerly, in the old days
  i denne tida – in this period
  i eldre tid – in former times
  i 7-tida – about 7 o'clock
  etter ei tid – after some time
  på den tida – at that time
  på rett tid – at the right time
ein tidbolk – period of time
tidleg adv. – early
  frå tidleg til seint – early and late
ei tidløyse – state of being busy
tidt /titt/ adv. – often

ein tikroning – ten crown bill

til /till/ prep. – for, to

  til og med – even

  til saman – all together

  til slutt – finally

eit tilhøve – relationship

å tilhøyra (tilhøyrer, tilhøyrde, tilhøyrt) /'tillhøyra/ – to belong to

eit tillegg – addition

  i tillegg til – in addition to

å tilseia (tilseier, tilsa, tilsagt) /'tillsæia/ – to indicate

eit tilskot /"tillskå:t/ – support

ei tilslutning /'tillslutning/ – approval, support

tilsvarande /'tillsva:rande/ adv. – proportionally

eit tilvære – life

ein time – hour

ein ting (pl. ting, tinga) – thing, object

å tinga (tingar, tinga, tinga) – to book, to make reservations

ein tinntallerk – pewter plate

to num. – two

eit toalett /toa'lett/ – toilet

eit tog /to:g/ – train

tok – see å taka

tolv /tåll/ num. – twelve

ein tomannslugar – cabin for two

ein tomat /to'ma:t/ – tomato

ei tomt – building lot

ein torsk /tårsk/ – cod

ein trafikkregel /tra'fikkre:gel/ – traffic law, regulation

å trampa (trampar, trampa, trampa) – to tramp

travel /'tra:vel/ – busy

ein trass – defiance, obstinacy

å trekkja (trekkjer, trekte, trekt) – to pull

å trekkja lodd om – to cast, draw lots for

å trena (trenar, trena, trena) – to exercise.

å trengja ut (trengjer, trengde, trengt) – to push, force out

å trenga (treng, trong, trunge) – to need

ei trening – training

å trippa (trippar, trippa, trippa) – to trip

eit troll /tråll/ – troll, monster

trollande adj. – bewitched, transformed

å tru (trur, trudde, trutt) – to think

  eg trur ikkje at – I don't think that

  eg skulle tru – I should think

eit trugsmål /'tru:gsmå:l/ – threat

ei trygd – insurance

trygg adj. – safe

eit tryggingstiltak – security measure

eit trykk – impression; pressure

ei trøyst – comfort

ein trål – trawl net

ei tuft – (building) site

eit tun – yard (courtyard, farm yard)

tung (comp. tyngre, sup. tyngst) adj. – heavy

ein tur – trip

  på tur – on a trip

ein turist /tu'rist/ – tourist

ei turski /'tu:rsji/ – cross country ski

eit tusen /'tu:sen/ num. – thousand

tyngre – see tung

typisk /'ty:pisk/ adj. – typical

tysk adj. – German

ei tønne – barrel, cask

tørr adj. – dry

å tøya (tøyar, tøya, tøya) – to thaw

ei tå (tåa, pl. tær, tærne) – toe

U

ubrukt adj. – unused

ufør adj. – disabled

ein uførleik – disability

eit ulende – rugged ground

ulik adj. – different

under prep. – under

underleg prep. – strange

å undersøkja (undersøkjer, undersøkte, undersøkt) – to examine

eit underverk /'underværk/ – miracle

ei undervisning /under'vi:s-ning/ – education

ung (comp. yngre, sup. yngst) adj. – young

ein ungdom – youth

eit ungdomslag – youth association

eit ungdomsliv – life of a youth

ein ungdomsskule – junior high school

ein union /uni'o:n/ – union

universell /univær'sell/ – universal, general

eit universitet /univærsi'te:t/ – university

eit unntak – exception

urettferdig adj. – unfair

ei urinprøve /u'ri:nprø:ve/ – specimen of urine

uråd f. – impossibility

det er uråd å – it is impossible to

utan prep. – without

utan å . . . – without . . .ing

eit utdrag – extract, excerpt

ute adv. – out

ei utgift /'u:tjift/ – expense

å utgjera (utgjer, utgjorde, utgjort) /'u:tje:ra/ – to constitute

utlandet /'u:tlande/ – the outside world, foreign countries

ein utlending – foreigner

ei utmark – uncultivated land, pasture

utmed prep. – along, near

ei utnytting /'u:tnytting/ – exploitation

eit utsal – sale

på utsal – on sale

ei utvandring /'u:tvandring/ – emigration

å utvida (utvidar, utvida, utvida) – to expand

å utvikla (utviklar, utvikla, utvikla) /'u:tvikla/ – to develop

ei utvikling /'u:tvikling/ – development

uvanleg /'u'va:nleg/ adj. – unusual

eit uvêr – storm

V

vakker (n. vakkert, pl. vakre) adj. – pretty, beautiful

vaksen (n. vakse, pl. vaksne) adj. – grown-up

eit val – election; choice

valfri /'va:lfri:/ adj. – optional
eit valfritt fag – elective
ein valperiode /'va:lperio:de/ –
electoral period
å vandra (vandrar, vandra,
vandra) – to walk, to stroll
vanleg adj. – ordinary, regular
til vanleg – usually
ein vanske – difficulty
var – see å vera
å vara (varer, varte, vart) – to
last
ei vare – article
eit varehus – department store
ein variant /vari'ant/ – variant
varm adj. – hot, warm
å varma opp (varmar, varma,
varma) – to warm up
varsam adj. – careful
vart – see å verta
ein vask – sink, washbasin
ei vassing – wading
ei vasskraft – water power
eit vatn – lake; water
eit vederlag – compensation
veit – see å vita
ein veg – road; way
kan De seia meg vegen til –
can you tell me the way to
det har aldri vore noko i
vegen med – there has never
been anything wrong with
ei veke – week
midt i veka – in the middle of
the week
eit vekeblad – weekly magazine
å vekkja (vekkjer, vekte, vekt) –
to wake, to awaken
å vekkja opp att – to call
forth, to revive
å vekkja til nytt liv – to
revive, to start again

å veksa (veks, voks, vakse) – to
increase, to grow
å veksa fram – to develop
å veksla (vekslar, veksla, veksla) – to change
vel /vell/ adv. – probably, well,
I suppose
veldig adv. – very, terribly
å velja (vel, valde, valt) – to
choose
velkomen /vel'kå:men/ adj. –
welcome
velsigna /vel'signa/ adj. –
blessed
å velta (velter, velte, velt) – to
tip over, to knock over
ein ven (venen, pl. vener, venene) – friend
ven adj. – pretty, beautiful
venstre adj. – left
på venstre sida – on the left-
hand side
Venstre – the Liberal Party
å venta (ventar, venta, venta) –
to expect; to wait
å venta på – to wait for
eit vêr – weather
å vera (er, var, vore) – to be
å vera att – to remain
å vera forkjølt – to have a
cold
å vera redd for – to fear
å vera med på – to take part
in, to join in
å vera usamd – to disagree
å vera utrusta – to be
equipped, fitted out
ei verd /væ:r/ – world
eit verde /"væ:re/ – value
verdsdramatikken – the world's
dramatic literature
verkeleg adv. – really

ei verksemd – activity

ei vêrmelding – weather fore-cast

vesentleg /'ve:sentleg/ adj. – es-sential

å verta (vert, vart, vorte) – to become, to get

å verta borte – to disappear

vi pron. – we

å via livet sitt til (vier, vigde, vigt) – to dedicate one's life to

vid /vi:/ adj. – broad

ein vidaregåande skule – senior high school, upper second-ary school

ei vik (vika, pl. vikar, vikane) – bay

eit vikingskip – viking ship

vikingtida f. – the viking period

viktig adj. – important

vil – see å vilja

å vilja (vil, ville, vilja) – to want to, to wish

eg vil gjerne – I would like to

eg ville berre – I only wanted to

eg ville no helst ha – I would rather prefer

vil du ha meir – would you like to have more

ein vilje – will

å vinna (vinn, vann, vunne) – to win

å vinna seg ein trygg plass – to acquire a solid position

ein vinter (vinteren, pl. vintrar, vintrane) /'vinter/ – winter

i vinter – this winter

vinterstid /'vintersti:/ adv. – in winter

å visa respekt for (viser, viste, vist) – to show respect for

eit viskelêr – eraser

ei vis – way

viss adj. – certain

å vita (veit, visste, visst) – to know

så vidt eg veit – as far as I know

å vitja (vitjar, vitja, vitja) /"vikj-kja/ – to visit

å vitna om (vitnar, vitna, vitna) – to tell about

ein voggesong /"våggesång/ – lullaby

ei vogn /vågn/ – coach, car; wagon

eit vognrammel – rattle from a wagon

ein voksterstad /'våkstersta:/ – place of growth

ei von – hope

å vona (vonar, vona, vona) – to hope

Vosse-bunad m. – bunad from Voss

eit vær – place where men gather to form fishing expe-ditions, fishing station

ein væreigar – owner of a vær

vår (n. vårt, pl. våre) pron. – our, ours

Vårherre – Our Lord

ei vårsol – spring sun

vårt – see vår

Y

yngre – see ung

ypparleg adj. – excellent

Æ

ei ætt – family
eit ættarland – land of forefathers
ein ættled (ættleden, pl. ættleder, ættledene) – generation
ættestolt adj. – proud of one's family

Ø

ein økonomi /økono'mi:/ – economy
økonomisk /øko'no:misk/ adj. – economic, financial
eit øl – beer
eit ønske – wish
å ønskja (ønskjer, ønskte, ønskt) – to wish
eit øre – the smallest monetary unit

å øva inn (øver, øvde, øvt) – to rehearse
øvst adv. – at the top of
øvst oppe – at the top
ei øy (øya, pl. øyar, øyane) – island
å øydeleggja (øydelegg, øydela, øydelagt) – to ruin, to destroy
eit øyra (øyra, pl. øyro, øyro) – ear

Å

åleine /å"læine/ adv. – alone
eit år – year
  i år – this year
  neste år – next year
-årig adj. – year(s), year old
ei årstid /'å:rsti:/ – season
åt prep. – to
åtti /'åtti/ num. – eighty

241

Index of Topics

The numerals and capital letters after the entries refer to the section in which the topic is discussed.

242

Tonemes (word tone)

Intonation (speech melody)

Spelling

B. **Grammar**

Nouns

Verbs

Basic Books

Aasen, Ivar	Norsk Grammatik. Christiania, P. T. Malling, 1864.
Beito, Olav T.	Nynorsk grammatikk. Lyd- og ordlære. Oslo, Det Norske Samlaget, 1970.
Fossestøl – Lundeby – Torvik	Morsmålet. Norsklære for ungdomsskulen. 7.–9. år. Oslo, J. W. Cappelens Forlag, 1966.
Halland, Nils	Engelsk-nynorsk ordbok. Oslo, Gyldendal Norsk Forlag, 1955.
Heggstad, Leiv	Fornorskingsordliste. Oslo, Olaf Norlis Forlag, 1958.
Hellevik, Alf	Norsk på ny. Nynorsk. Oslo, Det Norske Samlaget, 1968.
Hellevik, Alf	Nynorsk ordliste. Større utgåve. Oslo, Det Norske Samlaget, 1980.
Slette, Theodore	Norsk-engelsk ordbok. Oslo, Det Norske Samlaget, 1977.
Vikør, Lars S.	The New Norse Language Movement. Oslo, Novus, 1975.

Credits

Figs. 3, 7.1, 7.2, 8.1, 9.1, 10.1, 13, 14.2, 15, 16, 17, 18.3, 19.2, 21.1, 21.2	Courtesy Norwegian Information Service
Figs. 18.1, 18.2	Petter Torvholm
Fig. 1	Aslaug Mundal
Fig. 2	Ivar Torvanger
Fig. 11	Bjarne Rabben
Fig. 12.1	Lasse Kornberg
Fig. 6	Per Nesje-Nilsen
Fig. 8.2	Peter Hallaråker